CLINICAL HANDBOOK
FOR
PEDIATRIC

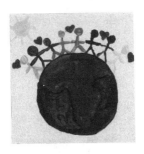

Jane W. Ball, RN, CPNP, DrPH
Executive Director
Emergency Medical Services for Children
National Resource Center, Children's National Medical Center
Washington, District of Columbia

Ruth C. Bindler, RNC, PhD
Associate Professor
Washington State University
Intercollegiate College of Nursing
Spokane, Washington

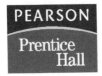

PEARSON
Prentice
Hall

Upper Saddle River, New Jersey 07458

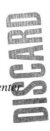

Library of Congress Cataloging-in-Publication Data

Ball, Jane

    Clinical handbook for pediatric nursing / Jane W. Ball, Ruth C. Bindler.
       p. ; cm.
    Includes bibliographical references and index.
    ISBN 0-13-113316-0
    1. Pediatric nursing–Handbooks, manuals, etc.   I. Bindler, Ruth McGillis.
II. Title.
    [DNLM: 1. Pediatric nursing–methods–Handbooks. 2. Child Develop-
ment–Handbooks. 3. Nursing Assessment–Handbooks.   WY 49 B187c
2006]
    RJ245.B345 2006
    618.92'00231–dc22

                                        2005032298

Notice: Care has been taken to confirm the accuracy of the information presented in this book. The authors, editors, and the publisher, however, cannot accept any responsibility for errors or omissions or for consequences from application of the information in this book and make no warranty, express or implied, with respect to its contents.

    The authors and the publisher have exerted every effort to ensure that drug selections and dosages set forth in this text are in accord with current recommendations and practice at time of publication. However, in view of ongoing research, changes in government regulations, and the constant flow of information relating to drug therapy and drug reactions, the reader is urged to check the package inserts of all drugs for any change in indications of dosage and for added warnings and precautions. This is particularly important when the recommended agent is a new and/or infrequently employed drug.

    The authors and the publisher disclaim all responsibility for any liability, loss, injury, or damage incurred as a consequence, directly or indirectly, of the use and application of any of the contents of this volume.

    All photographs/illustrations not credited on page, under or adjacent to the piece, were photographed/rendered on assignment and are the property of Pearson Education/Prentice Hall Health.

Pearson Education Ltd.
Pearson Education Singapore, Pte. Ltd.
Pearson Education Canada, Ltd.
Pearson Education—Japan
Pearson Education Australia PTY, Limited
Pearson Education North Asia Ltd.
Pearson Education de Mexico, S.A. de C.V.
Pearson Education Malaysia, Pte. Ltd.
Pearson Education, Upper Saddle River, New Jersey

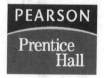

CONTENTS

PREFACE

As a nursing student and practicing nurse, you will face challenging client situations that test your knowledge base, your ability to prioritize, and your familiarity with certain clinical skills. The *Clinical Handbook for Pediatric Nursing* has been created to help you in situations like these. The handbook provides general information on growth and development, vital signs, assessment, and more, with information specific to the care of children in the community or hospital. Included are principles of pediatric medications, pain management, immunization schedules, and an overview of clinical and nursing management for conditions organized by body systems. Each content area includes key information about clinical therapy as well as how to use the nursing process to plan appropriate nursing management. Critical nursing assessments and interventions are identified, and specific examples are given regarding documentation of care.

As a valuable resource, the *Clinical Skills Manual for Pediatric Nursing, Third Edition,* can be consulted for detailed instructions on how to perform the techniques and procedures referred to in this book.

Although the handbook provides condensed information about each subject area, critical aspects of nursing practice have been included. It is our hope that this book will enhance pediatric nursing practice, provide a quick overview in the clinical setting, and help nurses provide safe, competent care to all children.

We'd also like to acknowledge and thank the following contributors and reviewers for their helpful feedback and participation:

Missy Ofe Fleck, RN, MSN
Assistant Professor
University of Nebraska
  Medical Center
Lincoln, Nebraska

Wendee Johnson, RNC, MSN
Clinical Associate Professor
Arizona State University
Phoenix, Arizona

Andrea Kline, RN, MS, PCCNP, PNP, CCRN
Pediatric Critical Care Nurse
  Practitioner
Children's
  Memorial Hospital
Chicago, Illinois

Sara Mitchell, RN, PhD, CPNP
Assistant Professor
Mercer University
Atlanta, Georgia

Deborah Persell, MSN, RN, CPNP
Assistant Professor
Arkansas State University
Jonesboro, Arkansas

Deborah Roberts, RN, EdD
Assistant Professor
Humboldt University
Arcata, California

Diane Van Os, MS, RN
Professor
Westminster College
Salt Lake City, Utah

Jane W. Ball
Ruth C. Bindler

1. Growth and Development

GENERAL CONCEPTS

Growth refers to an increase in physical size; growth represents quantitative changes such as height, weight, blood pressure, and number of words in the child's vocabulary.

Development refers to an increase in capability or function; developmental skills unfold in a complex manner as a relationship between the child's innate, unfolding capabilities with the stimuli and support provided in the environment.

Growth and development, or quantitative and qualitative, changes in body organ functioning, ability to communicate, and performance of motor skills unfold over time and are key components in the process of planning pediatric healthcare.

Each child displays a unique maturational pattern during the process of development; although the exact age at which skills emerge differs, the sequence, or order, of skill performance is uniform among children.

Development that proceeds from the head downward through the body and toward the feet is called *cephalocaudal* development

Development that proceeds from the center of the body outward to the extremities is called *proximodistal* development.

Major theoretical frameworks used to understand and analyze the development of children include the following:

- Psychoanalytic theory of Sigmund Freud
- Psychosocial theory of Erik Erikson
- Cognitive theory of Jean Piaget
- Moral development theory of Lawrence Kohlberg
- Social learning theory of Albert Bandura
- Ecologic theory of Urie Bronfenbrenner
- Temperament theory of Stella Chase and Alexander Thomas
- Resilience theory

See Table 1–1 for a description of nursing applications to the theories of Freud, Erikson, and Piaget.

The nurse is instrumental in performing developmental assessments throughout childhood and adolescence to identify

Table 1–1 Nursing Applications of Theories of Freud, Erikson, and Piaget

Age Group	Developmental Stages	Nursing Applications
Infant (birth to 1 year)	Oral stage (Freud): The baby obtains pleasure and comfort through the mouth.	When a baby is to have nothing by mouth, offer a pacifier if not contraindicated. After painful procedures, offer a baby a bottle or pacifier, or have the mother breastfeed.
	Trust versus mistrust stage (Erikson): The baby establishes a sense of trust when basic needs are met.	Hold the hospitalized baby often. Offer comfort after painful procedures. Meet the baby's needs for food and hygiene. Encourage parents to room in. Manage pain effectively with use of pain medications and other measures.
	Sensorimotor stage (Piaget): The baby learns from movement and sensory input.	Use crib mobiles, manipulative toys, wall murals, and bright colors to provide interesting stimuli and comfort. Use toys to distract the baby during procedures and assessments.
Toddler (1–3 years)	Anal stage (Freud): The child derives gratification from control over bodily excretions.	Ask about toilet training and the child's rituals and words for elimination during admission history. Continue child's normal patterns of elimination in the hospital. Do not begin toilet training during illness or hospitalization. Accept regression in toileting during illness or hospitalization. Have potty chairs available in hospital and childcare centers.
	Autonomy versus shame and doubt stage (Erikson): The child is increasingly independent in many spheres of life.	Allow self-feeding opportunities. Encourage child to remove and put on own clothes, brush teeth, or assist with hygiene. If restraint for a procedure is necessary, proceed quickly, providing explanations and comfort.
	Sensorimotor stage (end); preoperational stage (beginning) (Piaget): The child shows increasing curiosity and explorative behavior. Language skills improve.	Ensure safe surroundings to allow opportunities to manipulate objects. Name objects and give simple explanations.

(continued)

Table 1–1 Nursing Applications of Theories of Freud, Erikson, and Piaget (Continued)

Age Group	Developmental Stages	Nursing Applications
Pre-schooler (3–6 years)	Phallic stage (Freud): The child initially identifies with the parent of the opposite sex but by the end of this stage has identified with the same-sex parent.	Be alert for children who appear more comfortable with male or female nurses, and attempt to accommodate them. Encourage parental involvement in care. Plan for playtime and offer a variety of materials from which to choose.
	Initiative versus guilt stage (Erikson): The child likes to initiate play activities.	Offer medical equipment for play to lessen anxiety about strange objects. Assess children's concerns as expressed through their drawings. Accept the child's choices and expressions of feelings.
	Preoperational stage (Piaget): The child is increasingly verbal but has some limitations in thought processes. Causality is often confused, so the child may feel responsible for causing an illness.	Offer explanations about all procedures and treatments. Clearly explain that the child is not responsible for causing the illness.
School age (6–12 years)	Latency stage (Freud): The child places importance on privacy and understanding the body.	Provide gowns, covers, and underwear. Knock on door before entering. Explain treatments and procedures.
	Industry versus inferiority stage (Erikson): The child gains a sense of self-worth from involvement in activities.	Encourage the child to continue school work while hospitalized. Encourage child to bring favorite pastimes to the hospital. Help child adjust to limitations on favorite activities.
	Concrete operational stage (Piaget): The child is capable of mature thought when allowed to manipulate and see objects.	Give clear instructions about details of treatment. Show the child equipment that will be used in treatment.

(continued)

Table 1-1   Nursing Applications of Theories of Freud, Erikson, and Piaget (Continued)

Age Group	Developmental Stages	Nursing Applications
Adolescent (12–18 years)	Genital stage (Freud): The adolescent's focus is on genital function and relationships.	Ensure access to gynecologic care for adolescent girls. Provide information on sexuality. Ensure privacy during healthcare. Have brochures and videos available for teaching about sexuality.
	Identity versus role confusion stage (Erikson): The adolescent's search for self-identity leads to independence from parents and reliance on peers.	Provide a separate recreation room for teens who are hospitalized. Take health history and perform examinations without parents present. Introduce adolescent to other teens with same health problem.
	Formal operational stage (Piaget): The adolescent is capable of mature, abstract thought.	Give clear and complete information about healthcare and treatments. Offer both written and verbal instructions. Continue to provide education about the disease to the adolescent with a chronic illness, as mature thought now leads to greater understanding.

children at risk of delays, to plan appropriate interventions, and to offer interventions that encourage the child's continued development.

See Tables 1–2 through 1–11 for descriptions of the physical and psychosocial growth parameters of children and adolescents.

Table 1–2 Physical Growth and Development during Infancy

Age	Physical Growth	Fine Motor Ability	Gross Motor Ability	Sensory Ability
Birth to 1 month	Gains 5–7 oz (140–200 g)/week Grows 1.5 cm (0.5 in.) in first month Head circumference increases 1.5 cm (0.5 in.)/month	Holds hand in fist Draws arms and legs to body when crying	Inborn reflexes such as startle and rooting are predominant activity May lift head briefly if prone Alerts to high-pitched voices Comforts with touch	Prefers to look at faces and black and white geometric designs Follows objects in line of vision
2–4 months	Gains 5–7 oz (140–200 g)/week Grows 1.5 cm (0.5 in.)/month Head circumference increases 1.5 cm (0.5 in.)/month Posterior fontanel closes Eats 120 mL/kg/24 hr (2 oz/lb/24 hr)	Holds rattle when placed in hand Looks at and plays with own fingers Readily brings objects from hand to mouth	Moro reflex fading in strength Can turn from side to back and then return Decrease in head lag when pulled to sitting; sits with head held in midline with some bobbing When prone, holds head and supports weight on forearms	Follows objects 180 degrees Turns head to look for voices and sounds
4–6 months	Gains 5–7 oz (140–200 g)/week Doubles birth weight 5–6 months Grows 1.5 cm (0.5 in.)/month Head circumference increases 1.5 cm (0.5 in.)/month	Grasps rattles and other objects at will; drops them to pick up another offered object Mouths objects Holds feet and pulls to mouth Holds bottle	Head held steady when sitting No head lag when pulled to sitting Turns from abdomen to back by 4 months and then back to abdomen by 6 months	Examines complex visual images Watches the course of a falling object Responds readily to sounds

(continued)

Table 1–2   Physical Growth and Development during Infancy (Continued)

Age	Physical Growth	Fine Motor Ability	Gross Motor Ability	Sensory Ability
4–6 months (continued)	Teeth may begin erupting by 6 months Eats 100 mL/kg/24 hr (1.5 oz/lb/24 hr)	Grasps with whole hand (palmar grasp) Manipulates objects	When held standing supports much of own weight	
6–8 months	Gains 3–5 oz (85–140 g)/week Grows 1 cm (0.375 in.)/month Growth rate slower than first 6 months	Bangs objects held in hands Transfers objects from one hand to the other Beginning pincer grasp at times	Most inborn reflexes extinguished Sits alone steadily without support by 8 months Likes to bounce on legs when held in standing position	Recognizes own name and responds by looking and smiling Enjoys small and complex objects at play
8–10 months	Gains 3–5 oz (85–140 g)/week Grows 1 cm (0.375 in.)/month	Picks up small objects Uses pincer grasp well	Crawls or pulls whole body along floor by arms Creeps by using hands and knees to keep trunk off floor Pulls self to standing and sitting by 10 months Recovers balance when sitting	Understands words such as "no" and "cracker" May say one word in addition to "mama" and "dada" Recognizes sound without difficulty
10–12 months	Gains 3–5 oz (85–140 g)/week Grows 1 cm (0.375 in.)/month Head circumference equals chest circumference Triples birth weight by 1 year	May hold crayon or pencil and make mark on paper Places objects into containers through holes	Stands alone Walks holding onto furniture Sits down from standing	Plays peek-a-boo and patty cake

Table 1–3 Psychosocial Development during Infancy

Age	Play and Toys	Communication
Birth to 3 months	Prefers visual stimuli of mobiles, black-and-white patterns, mirrors Auditory stimuli are music boxes, tape players, soft voices Responds to rocking and cuddling Moves legs and arms while adult sings and talks Likes varying stimuli—different rooms, sounds, visual images	Coos Babbles Cries
3–6 months	Prefers noise-making objects that are easily grasped—e.g., rattles Enjoys stuffed animals and soft toys with contrasting colors	Vocalizes during play and with familiar people Laughs Cries less Squeals and makes pleasure sounds Babbles multisyllabically ("mamamamama")
6–9 months	Likes teething toys Increasingly desires social interaction with adults and other children Soft toys that can be manipulated and mouthed are favorites	Increases vowel and consonant sounds Links syllables together Uses speechlike rhythm when vocalizing with others
9–12 months	Enjoys large blocks, toys that pop apart and go back together, nesting cups and other objects Laughs at surprise toys such as jack-in-the-box Plays interactive games such as peek-a-boo Uses push-and-pull toys	Understands "no" and other simple commands Says "dada" and "mama" to identify parents Learns one or two other words Receptive speech surpasses expressive speech

Table 1–4 Physical Growth and Development during Toddlerhood

Age	Physical Growth	Fine Motor Ability	Gross Motor Ability	Sensory Ability
1–2 years	Gains 8 oz (227 g) or more/month Grows 3.5–5.0 in. (9–12 cm) during this year Anterior fontanel closes	By end of second year, builds a tower of four blocks Scribbles on paper Can undress self Throws a ball	Runs Walks up and down stairs Likes push and pull toys	Visual acuity 20/50

(continued)

Table 1–4 Physical Growth and Development during Toddlerhood (Continued)

Age	Physical Growth	Fine Motor Ability	Gross Motor Ability	Sensory Ability
2–3 years	Gains 1.4–2.3 kg (3–5 lb)/year Grows 5.0–6.5 cm (2–2.5 in.)/year	Draws a circle and other rudimentary forms Learns to pour Learning to dress self	Jumps Kicks ball Throws ball overhand	

Table 1–5 Psychosocial Development during Toddlerhood (Age 1–3 Years)

Play and Toys	Communication
Refines fine motor skills by use of cloth books, large pencil and paper, wooden puzzles	Increasingly enjoys talking
Facilitates imitative behavior by playing kitchen, grocery shopping, toy telephone	Exponential growth of vocabulary, especially when spoken and read to
Learns gross motor activities by riding Big Wheel tricycle, playing with soft ball and bat, molding water and sand, tossing ball or bean bag	Needs to release stress by use of pounding board toy, frequent gross motor activities, and occasional temper tantrums
Cognitive skills develop by educational television shows, music, stories, and books	Likes contact with other children and learns interpersonal skills

Table 1–6 Physical Growth and Development during Preschool

Physical Growth	Fine Motor Ability	Gross Motor Ability	Sensory Ability
Gains 1.5–2.5 kg (3–5 lb)/year Grows 4–6 cm (1.5–2.5 in.)/year	Uses scissors Draws circle, square, cross Draws at least a six-part person Enjoys art projects such as pasting, stringing beads, using clay Learns to tie shoes at end of preschool years Buttons Brushes teeth	Throws a ball overhand Climbs well Rides tricycle	Visual acuity continues to improve Can focus on and learn letters and numbers

Table 1-7 Psychosocial Development during Preschool (Age 3–6 Years)

Play and Toys	Communication
Associative play is facilitated by simple games, puzzles, nursery rhymes, songs	All parts of speech are developed and used, occasionally incorrectly
Dramatic play is fostered by dolls and doll clothes, play houses and hospitals, dress-up clothes, puppets	Communicates with a widening array of people
Stress is relieved by pens, paper, glue, scissors	Play with other children is a favorite activity
Cognitive growth is fostered by educational television shows, music, stories, and books	Health professionals can
	▶ Verbalize and explain procedures to children
	▶ Use drawings and stories to explain care
	▶ Use accurate names for bodily functions
	▶ Allow the child to talk, ask questions, and make choices

Table 1-8 Physical Growth and Development during School Age

Physical Growth	Fine Motor Ability	Gross Motor Ability	Sensory Ability
Gains 1.4–2.2 kg (3–5 lb)/year	Enjoys craft projects	Rides two-wheeler	Can read
Grows 4–6 cm (1.5–2.5 in.)/year	Plays card and board games	Jumps rope	Able to concentrate for longer periods on activities by filtering out surrounding sound
		Roller skates or ice skates	

Table 1-9 Psychosocial Development during School Age (Age 6–12 Years)

Activities	Communication
Gross motor development is fostered by ball sports, skating, dance lessons, water and snow skiing/boarding, biking	Mature use of language
A sense of industry is fostered by playing a musical instrument, gathering collections, starting hobbies, playing board and video games	Ability to converse and discuss topics for increasing lengths of time
Cognitive growth is facilitated by reading, crafts, word puzzles, school work	Spends many hours at school and with friends in sports or other activities
	Health professionals can
	▶ Assess child's knowledge before teaching
	▶ Allow the child to select rewards following procedures
	▶ Teach techniques such as counting or visualization to manage difficult situations
	▶ Include both parent and child in health-care decisions

Table 1–10   Physical Growth and Development during Adolescence

Physical Growth	Fine Motor Ability	Gross Motor Ability	Sensory Ability
Variation in age of growth spurt During growth spurt, girls gain 7–25 kg (15–55 lb) and grow 2.5–20.0 cm (2–8 in.); boys gain approximately 7.0–29.5 kg (15–65 lb) and grow 11–30 cm (4.5–12.0 in.)	Skills are well developed	New sports activities attempted and muscle development continues Some lack of coordination common during growth spurt	Fully developed

Table 1–11   Psychosocial Development during Adolescence (Age 12–18 Years)

Activities	Communication
Sports—ball games, gymnastics, water and snow skiing/boarding, swimming, school sports School activities—drama, yearbook, class office, club participation Quiet activities—reading, school work, television, computer, video games, music	Increasing communication and time with peer group—movies, dances, driving, eating out, attending sports events Applying abstract thought and analysis in conversations at home and school

2. Normal Vital Signs

Table 2–1 Normal Respiratory Rate Ranges for Each Age Group

Age	Respiratory Rate Per Min
Newborn	30–60
1 year	20–40
3 years	20–30
6 years	16–22
10 years	16–20
17 years	12–20

Table 2–2 Heart Rate Ranges and Average Heart Rates for Each Age Group

Age	Heart Rate Range (Beats/Min)	Average Heart Rate (Beats/Min)
Preterm	100–180	110–160 when stabilized
Newborns	100–180	120–160 when stabilized
Infants to 2 years	80–130	110
2–6 years	70–120	100
6–10 years	70–110	90
10–16 years	60–100	85

Table 2–3 Blood Pressure Levels for Boys by Age and Height Percentile*

Age (Year)	BP Percentile	Systolic BP (mm Hg)							Diastolic BP (mm Hg)						
		Percentile of Height							Percentile of Height						
		5th	10th	25th	50th	75th	90th	95th	5th	10th	25th	50th	75th	90th	95th
1	50th	80	81	83	85	87	88	89	34	35	36	37	38	39	39
	90th	94	95	97	99	100	102	103	49	50	51	52	53	53	54
	95th	98	99	101	103	104	106	106	54	54	55	56	57	58	58
	99th	105	106	108	110	112	113	114	61	62	63	64	65	66	66
2	50th	84	85	87	88	90	92	92	39	40	41	42	43	44	44
	90th	97	99	100	102	104	105	106	54	55	56	57	58	58	59
	95th	101	102	104	106	108	109	110	59	59	60	61	62	63	63
	99th	109	110	111	113	115	117	117	66	67	68	69	70	71	71
3	50th	86	87	89	91	93	94	95	44	44	45	46	47	48	48
	90th	100	101	103	105	107	108	109	59	59	60	61	62	63	63
	95th	104	105	107	109	110	112	113	63	63	64	65	66	67	67
	99th	111	112	114	116	118	119	120	71	71	72	73	74	75	75
4	50th	88	89	91	93	95	96	97	47	48	49	50	51	51	52
	90th	102	103	105	107	109	110	111	62	63	64	65	66	66	67
	95th	106	107	109	111	112	114	115	66	67	68	69	70	71	71
	99th	113	114	116	118	120	121	122	74	75	76	77	78	78	79
5	50th	90	91	93	95	96	98	98	50	51	52	53	54	55	55
	90th	104	105	106	108	110	111	112	65	66	67	68	69	69	70
	95th	108	109	110	112	114	115	116	69	70	71	72	73	74	74
	99th	115	116	118	120	121	123	123	77	78	79	80	81	81	82
6	50th	91	92	94	96	98	99	100	53	53	54	55	56	57	57
	90th	105	106	108	110	111	113	113	68	68	69	70	71	72	72
	95th	109	110	112	114	115	117	117	72	72	73	74	75	76	76
	99th	116	117	119	121	123	124	125	80	80	81	82	83	84	84
7	50th	92	94	95	97	99	100	101	55	55	56	57	58	59	59
	90th	106	107	109	111	113	114	115	70	70	71	72	73	74	74
	95th	110	111	113	115	117	118	119	74	74	75	76	77	78	78
	99th	117	118	120	122	124	125	126	82	82	83	84	85	86	86
8	50th	94	95	97	99	100	102	102	56	57	58	59	60	60	61
	90th	107	109	110	112	114	115	116	71	72	72	73	74	75	76
	95th	111	112	114	116	118	119	120	75	76	77	78	79	79	80
	99th	119	120	122	123	125	127	127	83	84	85	86	87	87	88
9	50th	95	96	98	100	102	103	104	57	58	59	60	61	61	62
	90th	109	110	112	114	115	117	118	72	73	74	75	76	76	77
	95th	113	114	116	118	119	121	121	76	77	78	79	80	81	81
	99th	120	121	123	125	127	128	129	84	85	86	87	88	88	89
10	50th	97	98	100	102	103	105	106	58	59	60	61	61	62	63
	90th	111	112	114	115	117	119	119	73	73	74	75	76	77	78
	95th	115	116	117	119	121	122	123	77	78	79	80	81	81	82
	99th	122	123	125	127	128	130	130	85	86	86	88	88	89	90

(continued)

Table 2–3 Blood Pressure Levels for Boys by Age and Height Percentile* (Continued)

Age (Year)	BP Percentile	Systolic BP (mm Hg) Percentile of Height							Diastolic BP (mm Hg) Percentile of Height						
		5th	10th	25th	50th	75th	90th	95th	5th	10th	25th	50th	75th	90th	95th
11	50th	99	100	102	104	105	107	107	59	59	60	61	62	63	63
	90th	113	114	115	117	119	120	121	74	74	75	76	77	78	78
	95th	117	118	119	121	123	124	125	78	78	79	80	81	82	82
	99th	124	125	127	129	130	132	132	86	86	87	88	89	90	90
12	50th	101	102	104	106	108	109	110	59	60	61	62	63	63	64
	90th	115	116	118	120	121	123	123	74	75	75	76	77	78	79
	95th	119	120	122	123	125	127	127	78	79	80	81	82	82	83
	99th	126	127	129	131	133	134	135	86	87	88	89	90	90	91
13	50th	104	105	106	108	110	111	112	60	60	61	62	63	64	64
	90th	117	118	120	122	124	125	126	75	75	76	77	78	79	79
	95th	121	122	124	126	128	129	130	79	79	80	81	82	83	83
	99th	128	130	131	133	135	136	137	87	87	88	89	90	91	91
14	50th	106	107	109	111	113	114	115	60	61	62	63	64	65	65
	90th	120	121	123	125	126	128	128	75	76	77	78	79	79	80
	95th	124	125	127	128	130	132	132	80	80	81	82	83	84	84
	99th	131	132	134	136	138	139	140	87	88	89	90	91	92	92
15	50th	109	110	112	113	115	117	117	61	62	63	64	65	66	66
	90th	122	124	125	127	129	130	131	76	77	78	79	80	80	81
	95th	126	127	129	131	133	134	135	81	81	82	83	84	85	85
	99th	134	135	136	138	140	142	142	88	89	90	91	92	93	93
16	50th	111	112	114	116	118	119	120	63	63	64	65	66	67	67
	90th	125	126	128	130	131	133	134	78	78	79	80	81	82	82
	95th	129	130	132	134	135	137	137	82	83	83	84	85	86	87
	99th	136	137	139	141	143	144	145	90	90	91	92	93	94	94
17	50th	114	115	116	118	120	121	122	65	66	66	67	68	69	70
	90th	127	128	130	132	134	135	136	80	80	81	82	83	84	84
	95th	131	132	134	136	138	139	140	84	85	86	87	87	88	89
	99th	139	140	141	143	145	146	147	92	93	93	94	95	96	97

BP, blood pressure.

Note: Use the child's height percentile for the age and sex from the standard growth charts found in Chapter 4. A blood pressure value at 50th percentile for the child's age, sex, and height percentile is considered the midpoint of the normal range. A reading above the 95th percentile indicates hypertension.

*The 90th percentile is 1.28 SD, the 95th percentile is 1.645 SD, and the 99th percentile is 2.326 SD over the mean.

Note: From National Heart, Lung, and Blood Institute. (2004). Blood pressure tables for children and adolescents from the fourth report on the diagnosis, evaluation, and treatment of high blood pressure in children and adolescents. http://www.nhlbi.nih.gov/guidelines/hypertension/child_tbl.htm, accessed 6/11/2004, with permission.

Table 2–4 Blood Pressure Levels for Girls by Age and Height Percentile*

Age (Year)	BP Percentile	Systolic BP (mm Hg) Percentile of Height							Diastolic BP (mm Hg) Percentile of Height						
		5th	10th	25th	50th	75th	90th	95th	5th	10th	25th	50th	75th	90th	95th
1	50th	83	84	85	86	88	89	90	38	39	39	40	41	41	42
	90th	97	97	98	100	101	102	103	52	53	53	54	55	55	56
	95th	100	101	102	104	105	106	107	56	57	57	58	59	59	60
	99th	108	108	109	111	112	113	114	64	64	65	65	66	67	67
2	50th	85	85	87	88	89	91	91	43	44	44	45	46	46	47
	90th	98	99	100	101	103	104	105	57	58	58	59	60	61	61
	95th	102	103	104	105	107	108	109	61	62	62	63	64	65	65
	99th	109	110	111	112	114	115	117	69	69	70	70	71	72	72
3	50th	86	87	88	89	91	92	93	47	48	48	49	50	50	51
	90th	100	100	102	103	104	106	106	61	62	62	63	64	64	65
	95th	104	104	105	107	108	109	110	65	66	66	67	68	68	69
	99th	111	111	113	114	115	116	117	73	73	74	74	75	76	76
4	50th	88	88	90	91	92	94	94	50	50	51	52	52	53	54
	90th	101	102	103	104	106	107	108	64	64	65	66	67	67	68
	95th	105	106	107	108	110	111	112	68	68	69	70	71	71	72
	99th	112	113	114	115	117	118	119	76	76	76	77	78	79	79
5	50th	89	90	91	93	94	95	96	52	53	53	54	55	55	56
	90th	103	103	105	106	107	109	109	66	67	67	68	69	69	70
	95th	107	107	108	110	111	112	113	70	71	71	72	73	73	74
	99th	114	114	116	117	118	120	120	78	78	79	79	80	81	81
6	50th	91	92	93	94	96	97	98	54	54	55	56	56	57	58
	90th	104	105	106	108	109	110	111	68	68	69	70	70	71	72
	95th	108	109	110	111	113	114	115	72	72	73	74	74	75	76
	99th	115	116	117	119	120	121	122	80	80	80	81	82	83	83
7	50th	93	93	95	96	97	99	99	55	56	56	57	58	58	59
	90th	106	107	108	109	111	112	113	69	70	70	71	72	72	73
	95th	110	111	112	113	115	116	116	73	74	74	75	76	76	77
	99th	117	118	119	120	122	123	124	81	81	82	82	83	84	84
8	50th	95	95	96	98	99	100	101	57	57	57	58	59	60	60
	90th	108	109	110	111	113	114	114	71	71	71	72	73	74	74
	95th	112	112	114	115	116	118	118	75	75	75	76	77	78	78
	99th	119	120	121	122	123	125	125	82	82	83	83	84	85	86
9	50th	96	97	98	100	101	102	103	58	58	58	59	60	61	61
	90th	110	110	112	113	114	116	116	72	72	72	73	74	75	75
	95th	114	114	115	117	118	119	120	76	76	76	77	78	79	79
	99th	121	121	123	124	125	127	127	83	83	84	84	85	86	87
10	50th	98	99	100	102	103	104	105	59	59	59	60	61	62	62
	90th	112	112	114	115	116	118	118	73	73	73	74	75	76	76
	95th	116	116	117	119	120	121	122	77	77	77	78	79	80	80
	99th	123	123	125	126	127	129	129	84	84	85	86	86	87	88

(continued)

Table 2–4 Blood Pressure Levels for Girls by Age and Height Percentile* (Continued)

Age (Year)	BP Percentile	Systolic BP (mm Hg) Percentile of Height							Diastolic BP (mm Hg) Percentile of Height						
		5th	10th	25th	50th	75th	90th	95th	5th	10th	25th	50th	75th	90th	95th
11	50th	100	101	102	103	105	106	107	60	60	60	61	62	63	63
	90th	114	114	116	117	118	119	120	74	74	74	75	76	77	77
	95th	118	118	119	121	122	123	124	78	78	78	79	80	81	81
	99th	125	125	126	128	129	130	131	85	85	86	87	87	88	89
12	50th	102	103	104	105	107	108	109	61	61	61	62	63	64	64
	90th	116	116	117	119	120	121	122	75	75	75	76	77	78	78
	95th	119	120	121	123	124	125	126	79	79	79	80	81	82	82
	99th	127	127	128	130	131	132	133	86	86	87	88	88	89	90
13	50th	104	105	106	107	109	110	110	62	62	62	63	64	65	65
	90th	117	118	119	121	122	123	124	76	76	76	77	78	79	79
	95th	121	122	123	124	126	127	128	80	80	80	81	82	83	83
	99th	128	129	130	132	133	134	135	87	87	88	89	89	90	91
14	50th	106	106	107	109	110	111	112	63	63	63	64	65	66	66
	90th	119	120	121	122	124	125	125	77	77	77	78	79	80	80
	95th	123	123	125	126	127	129	129	81	81	81	82	83	84	84
	99th	130	131	132	133	135	136	136	88	88	89	90	90	91	92
15	50th	107	108	109	110	111	113	113	64	64	64	65	66	67	67
	90th	120	121	122	123	125	126	127	78	78	78	79	80	81	81
	95th	124	125	126	127	129	130	131	82	82	82	83	84	85	85
	99th	131	132	133	134	136	137	138	89	89	90	91	91	92	93
16	50th	108	108	110	111	112	114	114	64	64	65	66	66	67	68
	90th	121	122	123	124	126	127	128	78	78	79	80	81	81	82
	95th	125	126	127	128	130	131	132	82	82	83	84	85	85	86
	99th	132	133	134	135	137	138	139	90	90	90	91	92	93	93
17	50th	108	109	110	111	113	114	115	64	65	65	66	67	67	68
	90th	122	122	123	125	126	127	128	78	79	79	80	81	81	82
	95th	125	126	127	129	130	131	132	82	83	83	84	85	85	86
	99th	133	133	134	136	137	138	139	90	90	91	91	92	93	93

BP, blood pressure.

Note: Use the child's height percentile for the age and sex from the standard growth charts found in Chapter 4. A blood pressure value at 50th percentile for the child's age, sex, and height percentile is considered the midpoint of the normal range. A reading above the 95th percentile indicates hypertension.

*The 90th percentile is 1.28 SD, the 95th percentile is 1.645 SD, and the 99th percentile is 2.326 SD over the mean.

Note: From National Heart, Lung, and Blood Institute. (2004). Blood pressure tables for children and adolescents from the fourth report on the diagnosis, evaluation, and treatment of high blood pressure in children and adolescents. http://www.nhlbi.nih.gov/guidelines/hypertension/child_tbl.htm, accessed 6/11/2004, with permission.

3. ASSESSMENT

ELEMENTS OF THE CHILD'S HISTORY

Patient identifying information: name, nickname, age, sex, ethnic origin, birth date, race, religion, contact information. Name of person providing information.

Chief complaint.

History of present illness or injury: detailed description of each current health problem, including onset, type of symptom, location, duration, severity, influencing factors, past evaluation of the problem, previous and current therapies.

Past history: detailed description of the child's prior health status.
- Birth history: prenatal history, description of delivery, condition of baby at birth, postnatal care and concerns.
- All major past illnesses and injuries: age at the time of each illness, injury, related surgery, or hospitalization; transfusions; treatment; outcome; complication or residual problem; and the child's reaction to the event.

Current health status: typical health status, allergies, current medications, immunization status, activities and exercise, sleep patterns, nutrition, safety measures used, and health maintenance care.

Family history: infectious diseases, allergies, disorders of the different body systems, cancer, problem pregnancies, learning problems. Identify the health status of each parent.

Review of systems: comprehensive overview of the child's health by body system (Table 3–1).

Psychosocial data: family composition, family members living in home, relationships, persons caring for child, financial resources, health insurance, description of housing and home environment, neighborhood, school or childcare arrangements, daily routines, spiritual life.

Developmental data: motor, cognitive, language, and social development; language, fine and gross motor milestones, and current skills; academic performance; interaction with other children, family members, and strangers.

Table 3–1   Review of Systems

Body Systems	Examples of Problems to Identify
General	General growth pattern, overall health status, active or tires easily, fever, sleep patterns; allergies, type of reaction (hives, rash, respiratory difficulty, swelling, nausea), seasonal or with each exposure; alertness of child
Skin and lymph	Rashes, dry skin, itching, changes in skin color or texture, tendency for bruising, swollen or tender lymph glands
Hair and nails	Hair loss, changes in color or texture, use of dye or chemicals on hair; abnormalities of nail growth or color, clubbing
Head	Headaches
Eyes	Vision problems, squinting, crossed eyes, "lazy eye," wears glasses; eye infections, redness, tearing, burning, rubbing, swelling eyelids
Ears	Ear infections, frequent discharge from ears, tubes in ears; hearing loss (hearing test ever done?); hearing aids or cochlear implants
Nose and sinuses	Nosebleeds, nasal congestion, runny nose, sinus pain or infections; nasal obstruction, difficulty breathing, snoring at night
Mouth and throat	Mouth breathing, difficulty swallowing, sore throats, strep infections; mouth odor; tooth eruption, cavities, braces; voice change, hoarseness, speech problems
Cardiac and hematologic	Heart murmur, anemia, hypertension, cyanosis, edema, rheumatic fever, chest pain
Chest and respiratory	Trouble breathing, choking episodes, cough, wheezing, cyanosis, exposure to tuberculosis, other infections
Gastrointestinal	Bowel movements, frequency, color, regularity, consistency, discomfort, constipation or diarrhea; abdominal pain, bleeding from rectum, flatulence; nausea or vomiting, appetite
Urinary	Frequency, urgency, dysuria, dribbling, enuresis, strength of urinary stream; age when day and night dryness attained

Reproductive
  Female
 	
  Male
 	
  Both
	For pubescent children
	    Menses onset, amount, duration, frequency, discomfort, problems; vaginal discharge, breast development
	    Puberty onset, emissions, erections, pain or discharge from penis, swelling or pain in testicles
	    Sexual activity, use of contraception, sexually transmitted diseases

(continued)

Assessment **17**

Table 3–1   Review of Systems (Continued)

Body Systems	Examples of Problems to Identify
Musculoskeletal	Weakness, clumsiness, poor coordination, balance, tremors, abnormal gait; painful muscles or joints, swelling or redness of joints, fractures
Neurologic	Seizures, fainting spells, dizziness, numbness, head injuries; cranial nerves functioning; learning problems, concentration, attention span, hyperactivity, memory problems

PHYSICAL EXAMINATION TECHNIQUES

Inspection is the purposeful observation of the child's physical features and behaviors and detection of odors with your nose.

Palpation is the use of touch to identify characteristics of the skin, internal organs, and masses (texture, moistness, tenderness, temperature, position, shape, consistency, and mobility of masses and organs).

Auscultation is listening to sounds produced by the airway, lungs, stomach, heart, and blood vessels to identify their characteristics.

Percussion is striking the surface of the body, either directly or indirectly, to set up vibrations that reveal the density of underlying tissues and borders of internal organs.

Standard precautions are used during the physical examination.

EQUIPMENT NEEDED

Stethoscope, sphygmomanometer, otoscope, ophthalmoscope, reflex hammer, cotton balls, penlight, and tongue blades.

GENERAL APPRAISAL

Procedure[1]	Findings[2]
Observe the child's general appearance and behavior.	Well-nourished and well-developed. Infants and young children may be fearful.
Measure the child's weight, length or height, and head circumference, and plot on appropriate growth curves. Calculate the body mass index.	Following a consistent growth channel for all measurements. Height and weight are proportional.

[1]Italics indicates caution to take with procedure.
[2]Italics indicates abnormal findings.

ASSESSING SKIN AND HAIR CHARACTERISTICS AND INTEGRITY

Procedure[1]	Findings[2]
Inspect the skin for color and the presence of imperfections, elevations, variations, or lesions. Identify lesion characteristics (location, size, type of lesion, pattern, and discharge). Inspect the buccal mucosa and tongue when a skin color abnormality such as jaundice or cyanosis is suspected.	Even color distribution; bruises are common on the knees, shins, and lower arms from falls. *See Chapter 27 for skin lesion descriptions. Suspect child abuse when bruises are on other parts of the body in various stages of healing. Pigmentation, pallor, mottling, bruises, erythema, cyanosis, or jaundice may indicate local or generalized conditions.*
Palpate skin for temperature, texture, moistness, and resilience, or turgor.	Feels cool, dry, soft, and smooth to the touch; taut, elastic, and mobile with good turgor. *Warm skin with fever or inflammation. Excessive sweating without exertion in an uncorrected congenital heart defect. Poor skin turgor with dehydration.*
Test capillary refill and small-vein filling times.	Capillary refill is less than 2 seconds and small-vein filling time is less than 4 seconds. *Prolonged times indicate poor circulation or hypovolemia.*

| Inspect the scalp hair for color, distribution, and cleanliness, presence of lice, and development of pubic and axillary hair. | Hair is evenly colored, shiny. Pubic and axillary hair at expected ages. *Hair loss due to tight braids. A low hairline on neck or forehead may indicate a congenital defect. Insects in scalp or eggs on hair shafts indicate head lice.* |
| Palpate the hair shafts for texture. | Soft or silky, with fine or thick shafts. |

ASSESSING THE HEAD FOR SKULL CHARACTERISTICS AND FACIAL FEATURES

Procedure[1]	Findings[2]
Inspect the head for shape.	The skull is rounded, with a prominent occipital area. *Abnormal skull shape with premature closure of the sutures. Flat, elongated skull in low-birth-weight infants.*
Inspect the face for symmetry when child rests, smiles, talks, and cries. Draw an imaginary line down the middle of the face to compare sides.	Symmetric facial features with expressions are expected. *Facial asymmetry with paralysis of cranial nerves V and VII. Coarse facial features, wide eye spacing, or disproportionate size may indicate a congenital anomaly. Tremors, tics, and twitching of facial muscles may indicate a seizure.*

| Palpate the sutures and fontanels of the skull. | No separation of sutures, fontanel is diamond-shaped. Posterior fontanel closes by 2–3 months. *Additional bone edges may indicate a skull fracture. Bulging fontanel indicates increased intracranial pressure. Sunken fontanel indicates dehydration.* |

ASSESSING THE EYE STRUCTURES, FUNCTION, AND VISION

Procedure[1]	Findings[2]
Inspect the external eye structures (eye size and spacing, eye color). Test the function of cranial nerves II, III, IV, and VI.	Eyes are equal and appropriately sized. Sclerae are white or ivory. *Bulging may indicate a tumor. A sunken appearance with dehydration. Hypertelorism may indicate mental retardation. Blue tinge to the sclerae indicates osteogenesis imperfecta.*
Inspect the eyelids for color, size, position, mobility, and condition of the eyelashes. Inspect palpebral slant. Inspect the conjunctivae.	Eyelids free of swelling or inflammation. Each lid covers part of the iris but none of the pupil. Conjunctivae are pink and glossy. No redness or excess tearing. An epicanthal fold in children of Asian descent. *Ptosis indicates injury of cranial nerve III. Sunset sign indicates hydrocephalus or retracted eyelids.*

Inspect the pupils for size and shape. Inspect the iris for the presence of Brushfield's spots. Test pupillary response to light and accommodation.	Pupils are round, clear, and equal in size and respond to light and accommodation. *Brushfield's spots with Down syndrome.*
Inspect eye muscles for extraocular movement and corneal light reflex, and perform cover-uncover test.	Both eyes move and track together. Symmetric light reflection on corneas. No obvious movement of either eye is seen with the cover-uncover test. *Asymmetric corneal light reflex after 6 months of age with strabismus.*
Assess visual acuity with standardized charts, and assess visual fields.	Infants fixate on and track an object. Expected visual acuity at 3 years is 20/40, at 4 years is 20/40, at 5 years is 20/30, and 6 years is 20/20 (American Academy of Pediatrics Committee on Practice and Ambulatory Medicine and Section of Ophthalmology, 2003).
Use an ophthalmoscope to inspect the internal eye structures.	A red reflex bilaterally. The retina is pink. The optic disc margin is sharply defined, round, and yellow to creamy pink. *A white reflex indicates a retinoblastoma.*

ASSESSING THE EAR STRUCTURES AND HEARING

Procedure[1]	Findings[2]
Inspect the position and characteristics of the pinna.	The pinna is appropriately formed and positioned, and the auditory canal is open. No discharge is apparent. *Low-set ears may indicate a congenital renal disorder.*
Inspect the tympanic membrane with the otoscope. Assess mobility of the tympanic membrane.	Tympanic membrane is pearly gray, translucent, and mobile. Light reflex and ossicles are visible. *A bulging, red tympanic membrane without movement indicates acute otitis media.*
Screen for hearing loss with noisemakers or whispering words.	Infants turn toward the noisemaker. Children repeat the whispered words accurately.
Weber test: place a vibrating tuning fork on the child's skull at midline, and ask if the sound is heard best in one ear or both ears. Rinne test: place the vibrating tuning fork on the mastoid process and when the sound is no longer heard, move and hold the tines next to the ear. Repeat for the other ear.	Sound is heard equally in both ears with the Weber test. The child hears the air-conducted sound twice as long as the bone-conducted sound.

ASSESSING THE NOSE AND SINUSES FOR AIRWAY PATENCY AND DISCHARGE

Procedure[1]	Findings[2]
Inspect the external nose for size, shape, symmetry, and midline placement on the face. Observe for nasal discharge.	The nose is proportional to other facial features and positioned midline. Symmetric nasolabial folds. No discharge. *A saddle-shaped nose with congenital defects such as cleft palate.*
Palpate the external nose for pain, break in contour, masses.	No tenderness, contour deviations, or masses.
Test for nasal patency by occluding one nostril at a time.	The child breathes through the open nostril with the mouth closed. *Nasal flaring is a sign of respiratory distress.*
Inspect the internal nose for color of the mucous membranes and the presence of any discharge, swelling, lesions, or other abnormalities. Do not touch the nasal septum with the speculum.	Mucous membranes and turbinates are dark pink and glistening; a film of clear discharge. Intact nasal septum. *Pale or bluish gray turbinates and polyps with allergies. A foul-smelling discharge in one nostril with a foreign body.*
Palpate the maxillary sinuses by pressing up under both zygomatic arches with the thumbs. Palpate the ethmoid sinuses by pressing up against the bone above both eyes with the thumbs.	No swelling or tenderness is expected. *Puffiness and swelling of the face around the sinuses and tenderness on palpation indicate sinusitis.*

ASSESSING THE MOUTH AND THROAT

Procedure[1]	Findings[2]
Inspect the lips for color, shape, symmetry, moisture, and lesions. *Avoid examining the mouth if there are signs of respiratory distress, high fever, drooling, and intense apprehension. These may be signs of epiglottitis. Inspecting the mouth may trigger a total airway obstruction.*	Lips symmetric with pink color in whites, more bluish in children of darker skin. *Pale, cyanotic, or cherry red lips are indicators of poor tissue perfusion.*
Inspect and count the child's teeth. Inspect the condition of the teeth; look for loose and missing teeth to assess tooth eruption.	Teeth are white, without a flattened, mottled, or pitted appearance. Discolored tooth crown may indicate a carie. *Discolored tooth surface with some medications and fluorosis.*
Inspect the gums for color and adherence to the teeth.	Gums are pink, with a stippled or dotted appearance. *Inflammation and tenderness with infection, poor nutrition.*
Inspect the mucous membranes for color and moisture. Inspect the tongue and floor of the mouth for color, moistness, size, tremors, and lesions.	Mucous membrane is pink. Patches of hyperpigmentation in children of darker skin. No redness, swelling, or ulcerative lesions. Tongue is pink and moist, without a coating. *A protuberant tongue with various genetic conditions, such as Down syndrome. A white, adherent coating may be thrush, a Candida infection.*

Inspect the hard and soft palate to detect any clefts, masses, or an unusually high arch.	Palate is pink, dome-shaped arch, no cleft. Uvula hangs freely.
Palpate the palate. Test the tongue's strength by asking the child to press the tongue against a finger on the cheek.	No clefts are palpated. Some pressure against the finger is normally felt.
Inspect the throat for color, swelling, lesions, and the condition of the tonsils. A tongue blade may be needed. Assess the gag reflex.	Throat is pink without lesions, drainage, or swelling. Tonsils are pink without exudate, but crypts (fissures) may be seen. The uvula rises symmetrically. *Swelling or bulging in the posterior pharynx with a peritonsillar abscess.*

ASSESSING THE NECK FOR CHARACTERISTICS, RANGE OF MOTION, AND LYMPH NODES

Procedure[1]	Findings[2]
Inspect the neck for size, symmetry, swelling, and any abnormalities, such as webbing.	Neck is symmetric, without swelling. Infants have short neck with skin folds. *Webbing may indicate Turner syndrome.*
Note the head control in infants.	Infants develop head control by 2 months. *Lack of head control can result from neurologic injury.*

Use the fingerpads to palpate both sides of the neck for lymph nodes. Use a gentle firm motion to define the characteristics of a palpated node.	Firm, clearly defined, nontender, movable lymph nodes up to 1 cm (0.5 in.) in diameter are common. *Enlarged, firm, warm, tender lymph nodes with infection. Enlarged, nontender, nonmovable lymph nodes with lymphomas.*
Palpate the trachea by placing the thumb and forefinger on each side of the trachea near the chin and slowly slide them down the trachea. In the lower neck, feel the isthmus of the thyroid, a band of glandular tissue crossing over the trachea.	The trachea is midline. Lobes of the thyroid are not usually palpable. *Any tracheal shift to the right or left of midline may indicate a tumor or a collapsed lung.*
Ask the child to touch the chin to each shoulder and to the chest and then to look at the ceiling. Move a light or toy in all four directions when assessing infants.	Freely moves the neck and head in all four directions, no pain. *Limited horizontal range of motion may be a sign of torticollis. Pain with neck flexion (Brudzinski sign) with meningitis.*

ASSESSING THE CHEST FOR SHAPE, MOVEMENT, RESPIRATORY EFFORT, AND LUNG FUNCTION

Procedure[1]	Findings[2]
Identify the topographic landmarks of the chest.	The intercostal spaces are the horizontal markers. The sternum and spine are the vertical landmarks.
Inspect the anterior and posterior chest for size and shape. Inspect the chest for any irregularities in shape.	The rib cage is prominent, thinner chest muscles and subcutaneous tissue. The rounded chest of infants becomes oval by 2 years.

	A rounded chest in a child may indicate a chronic obstructive lung condition. Scoliosis causes a lateral deviation of the chest.
Inspect for simultaneous chest expansion and abdominal rise. Count the respiratory rate when the child is quiet. See Chapter 2 for normal respiratory rate ranges by age.	Chest movement is symmetric bilaterally, and the abdomen rises simultaneously with the chest on inspiration. *Asymmetric chest rise with a collapsed lung. Retractions and a sustained respiratory rate of more than 60 breaths per minute indicate respiratory distress.*
Palpate the chest to confirm bilateral symmetry of chest motion. Palpate any depressions, bulges, or unusual chest wall shape.	Chest movement is symmetric. No tenderness, cysts, other growths, crepitus, or fractures.
Palpate the chest for tactile fremitus. Ask the child to repeat a series of words or numbers, such as Mickey Mouse or ice cream. Compare quality of vibrations side to side.	The vibration or tingling sensation is palpated over the entire chest. *Decreased sensations when air is trapped in the lungs. Increased sensations with lung consolidation.*

Auscultate the chest for the quality and characteristics of breath sounds. Compare sounds side to side. Listen to an entire inspiratory and expiratory phase at each location. See Figure 3–1.

To assess abnormal breath sounds, determine their location, the respiratory phase in which they are present, duration, intensity, and whether they change or disappear when the child coughs or shifts position.

Breath sounds have equal intensity, pitch, and rhythm bilaterally. Breath sounds usually heard on auscultation include the following:

- Vesicular breath sounds are low-pitched, swishing, soft, short expiratory sounds.

- Bronchovesicular breath sounds are medium-pitched, hollow, blowing sounds heard equally on inspiration and expiration in all age groups.

- Bronchial/tracheal breath sounds are hollow and higher pitched than vesicular breath sounds.

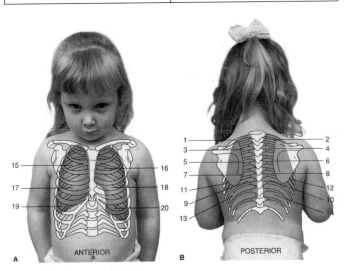

Figure 3–1 ■ Sequence for auscultating the chest.

	Absent or diminished breath sounds indicate a pneumothorax or obstruction. Abnormal breath sounds include crackles, rhonchi, and friction rubs.
Auscultate the chest while the child repeats a series of words to evaluate voice sound transmission.	Muffled, indistinct words and syllables heard throughout the chest. *Voice sounds absent or more muffled than usual with airway obstruction. Abnormal vocal resonance characteristics include the following:* • *Whispered pectoriloquy is present when syllables are heard distinctly in a whisper.* • *Bronchophony is increased intensity and clarity of sounds while the words remain indistinct.* • *Egophony is the transmission of the "eee" sound as a nasal "ay" sound.*
Note the quality of the voice and other audible sounds.	*Hoarseness with inflammation of the larynx. A cough is a reflexive clearing of the airway. Stridor is a high-pitched crowing sound from air moving through a narrowed airway. Wheezing results from passage of air through mucus or fluids in a narrowed lower airway.*

BREASTS

Procedure[1]	Findings[2]
Inspect the breasts. Inspect the anterior chest for supernumerary nipples (small, undeveloped nipples and areola that may be mistaken for moles).	The areola is normally round and more darkly pigmented than the surrounding skin. *Supernumerary nipples anywhere along the mammary line associated with congenital renal or cardiac anomalies.*
Inspect the breasts of sitting older children and adolescents for stage of development.	Breast development Stage I: preadolescent, only the nipple is raised above the level of the breast Stage II: budding stage; areola increased in diameter and surrounding area slightly elevated Stage III: breast and areola enlarged, no contour separation Stage IV: areola forms a secondary elevation above that of the breast in half of girls Stage V: areola is part of the general breast contour and strongly pigmented, nipple usually projects Breasts often develop at different rates and appear asymmetric. The mean age for breast development in black girls is 8.87 years and for white girls is 9.96 years (Herman-Giddens, Slora, Wasserman, et al., 1997).

	Breast development before 6 years of age in black girls and 7 years of age in white girls needs further evaluation (Kaplowitz & Oberfield, 1999).
Position the adolescent female on her back with one arm behind the neck at a time. Palpate the breast and axilla on that side in a concentric pattern covering all quadrants and the axilla, then around the nipple. Repeat on other side.	Breast tissue feels dense, firm, and elastic. *Abnormal masses or hard nodules need further investigation but are usually not malignancies.*
Palpate the breast tissue in adolescent boys to detect any masses.	Unilateral or bilateral breast enlargement during adolescence (gynecomastia).

ASSESSING THE HEART FOR HEART SOUNDS AND FUNCTION

Procedure[1]	Findings[2]
Place the child in a reclining or semi-Fowler's position. Observe the anterior chest for movement associated with the heart's contraction.	Symmetric rib cage. The apical impulse is where the left ventricle taps the chest wall during contraction. *Bulging of the left side of the chest wall or a heave may indicate an enlarged heart.*
Use the palmar surface of the fingers to palpate the precordium for pulsations, heaves, or vibrations. Use the topographic landmarks of the chest to describe their location.	Apical impulse felt as a slight tap against a fingertip. *A lift or thrill is usually abnormal. Estimate the diameter of the thrill.*

Use the bell of the stethoscope and position the child in both sitting and reclining positions to auscultate the heart. Note differences in heart sounds caused by a position change. Count the apical heart rate and compare to the radial or brachial pulse. See Chapter 2 for heart rate ranges by age. Assess the rhythm. If a rhythm irregularity is detected, ask the child to take a breath and hold it while you listen to the heart rate.

The brachial or radial pulse rate should be the same as the auscultated apical heart rate. Children often have a normal cycle of irregular rhythm associated with respiration called *sinus arrhythmia*; the rate is faster on inspiration and slower on expiration. The rhythm should become regular when the breath is held.

Other irregular rhythms are not expected.

Auscultate heart sounds at specific listening areas on the chest wall (see Figure 3–2). The heart sound heard simultaneously with the carotid pulsation is S_1. See Table 3–2 for best sites to auscultate S_1 and S_2. Auscultate heart sounds for quality (distinct versus muffled) and intensity (loud versus weak).

S_1 and S_2 heard in all listening areas. S_1, the first heart sound, is produced by closure of the tricuspid and mitral valves. S_2, produced by closure of the aortic and pulmonic valves, is sometimes heard as a single sound and at other times as a split sound, as the timing of the valve closure varies with respirations. The S_2 split sound is more apparent when the child takes a deep breath. Heart sounds are distinct and crisp in children with a thin chest wall.

Muffling, or indistinct sounds, with a heart defect or congestive heart failure. Fixed splitting that does not vary with respiration with an atrial septal defect.

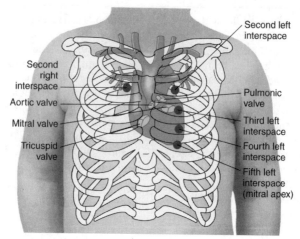

Figure 3–2 ■ Listening posts of the heart.

Table 3–2   Identification of the Sites for Auscultating the Quality and Intensity of Heart Sounds

Heart Sound	Locations Best Heard
S₁	Apex of the heart
	Tricuspid area
	Mitral area
S₂	Base of the heart
	Aortic area
	Pulmonic area
Physiologic splitting	Pulmonic area
S₃	Mitral area

Auscultate for other unexpected heart sounds and murmurs. Note characteristics of these heart sounds (intensity, presence of a thrill, location by listening post and topographical landmarks, change in character with position change, radiation, timing in relation to S_1 and S_2, and quality).	S_3 heard in diastole, louder in the mitral area than the pulmonic area, just after S_2, is found in some children. *Murmurs are abnormal sounds produced by blood passing through a defective valve, great vessel, or other heart structure. Intensity or loudness is described by grades:* *Grade 1: Barely heard in a quiet room* *Grade 2: Quiet, but clearly heard* *Grade 3: Moderately loud, no thrill palpated* *Grade 4: Loud, a thrill is usually palpated* *Grade 5: Very loud, a thrill is easily palpated* *Grade 6: Heard without the stethoscope in direct contact with the chest wall*
Auscultate for a venous hum over the supraclavicular fossa above the middle of the clavicle or over the upper anterior chest with the bell of the stethoscope.	A venous hum is a continuous low-pitched hum, may be loudest during diastole or when the child stands, does not change with respiration but may be quieted when the child turns the neck.

Assess the blood pressure; use correct cuff size for the extremity. Use the right arm. Take the blood pressure twice and average the two readings. The systolic and diastolic blood pressure reading should be compared to the values in Chapter 2. When any concern exists about a heart condition, obtain a blood pressure reading in both an arm and a leg, and then compare the readings.	The systolic reading is the onset of Korotkoff's sounds. The diastolic reading is the fifth Korotkoff's sound or the disappearance of Korotkoff's sounds in children and adolescents. The blood pressure in the leg should be the same or up to 10 mm Hg higher than the arm reading. *Confirm blood pressure values indicating hypertension with repeated readings on several visits. A lower blood pressure reading in the leg than the arm with coarctation of the aorta.*
Palpate the pulses in both extremities to assess the circulation. Assess rate, rhythm regularity, and strength. Compare findings bilaterally. Compare the strength of the femoral arteries with that of the brachial or radial pulse.	Detecting distal pulses in infants is often difficult. The femoral pulsations are stronger than or as strong as the brachial pulsations. *A weaker femoral pulse with coarctation of the aorta.*
Assess heart and tissue perfusion by observing color and capillary refill.	Mucous membranes pink. Capillary refill less than 2 seconds. *Cyanosis with a congenital heart defect in children. Prolonged capillary refill with poor tissue perfusion.*

ASSESSING THE ABDOMEN FOR SHAPE, BOWEL SOUNDS, AND UNDERLYING ORGANS

Procedure[1]	Findings[2]
Inspect the shape and contour, condition of the umbilicus and rectus muscle, and abdominal movement.	Abdomen is symmetric and rounded or flat when the child is supine. An umbilical hernia or a separation of the rectus muscle [depression may be up to 5 cm (2 in.) wide] may be seen. The abdomen rises with inspiration and falls with expiration in synchrony with the chest. *A scaphoid or sunken abdomen in dehydration or with a diaphragmatic hernia in a newborn. Peristaltic waves indicate an intestinal obstruction, such as pyloric stenosis.*
Auscultate the abdomen with the diaphragm of the stethoscope. Listen in each quadrant long enough to hear at least one bowel sound. Before determining that bowel sounds are absent, auscultate at least 5 minutes. Auscultate over the abdominal aorta and the renal arteries for a vascular hum or murmur.	High-pitched, tinkling, metallic bowel sounds every 10–30 seconds. No murmur. *Absence of bowel sounds with peritonitis or a paralytic ileus. Hyperactive bowel sounds with gastroenteritis or a bowel obstruction. A murmur may indicate a narrowed artery.*

While the child is supine, use indirect percussion to evaluate borders and sizes of abdominal organs and masses. Identify organ size, listening for a percussion tone change at the border of an organ.	Dullness over organs (liver, spleen, and a full bladder); tympany over the stomach or the intestines when an obstruction is present; resonance over other areas. The upper edge of the liver is near the fifth intercostal space at the right midclavicular line. The lower liver edge is 2–3 cm (approximately 1 in.) below the right costal margin in infants and toddlers, near the costal margin in older children.
To palpate the abdomen, position the child supine with knees flexed to relax the abdominal muscles. Use the edge of your fingers plus fingerpads, and palpate the entire abdomen. Watch the child's face for signs of pain (a grimace or constriction of the pupils).	
Use *light palpation* to evaluate the tenseness of the abdomen, the liver, the presence of any tenderness or masses, and any defects in the abdominal wall. Use a superficial, gentle touch that slightly depresses the abdomen. Palpate any bulging along the abdominal wall. Measure the diameter of the umbilical ring if open.	Abdomen is soft, no tenderness. An open umbilical muscle ring normally becomes smaller and closes by 4 years of age. The liver edge is palpated 2–3 cm (approximately 1 in.) below the right costal margin in infants and toddlers. It may not be palpable in older children.

To locate the lower liver edge, place the fingers in the right midclavicular line at the level of the umbilicus. Gently move the side of the index finger toward the costal margin during expiration. As the liver edge descends with inspiration, a flat, narrow ridge may be felt. Measure the distance of the liver edge from the right costal margin at the right midclavicular line.	*An enlarged liver, more than 3 cm (1.25 in.) below the right costal margin, with congestive heart failure or hepatic disease.*
Deep palpation is used to detect masses, define their shape and consistency, and identify tenderness in the abdomen. Press the fingers of one hand (for small children) or two hands (for older children) more deeply into the abdomen. Ask the child to take regular deep breaths when each area of the abdomen is palpated. Palpate for the spleen at the left costal margin in the midclavicular line. Palpate for the kidneys deep in the abdomen along each side of the spinal column. *If any abnormal mass is palpated, discontinue palpation. Continued palpation could potentially release cancer cells.*	The spleen tip may be felt when the child takes a deep breath. The kidneys are difficult to palpate in all children, except newborns. Feces feel like a tubular mass in the lower left or right quadrant. A distended bladder feels like a firm, central, dome-shaped mass above the symphysis pubis. *The spleen is enlarged when it is easily palpated below the left costal margin. If a kidney is palpated, an abnormal mass may be present. Any fixed mass that moves laterally, pulsates, or is located along the vertebral column may be a neoplasm.*

ASSESSING THE INGUINAL AREA

Procedure[1]	Findings[2]
Inspect the inguinal area for any change in contour, comparing sides.	*A small bulging over the femoral canal in girls may be a femoral hernia. A bulging in the inguinal area in boys may be an inguinal hernia.*
Palpate the inguinal area for lymph nodes and other masses.	Small lymph nodes, less than 1 cm (0.5 in.) in diameter, often present. *Tenderness, heat, or inflammation in lymph nodes with a local infection.*

ASSESSING THE GENITAL AND PERINEAL AREAS FOR EXTERNAL STRUCTURAL ABNORMALITIES

Procedure[1]	Findings[2]
Females Position young children on the parent's lap with their legs spread apart. Older children can be positioned on the examining table with their knees flexed and the legs spread apart like a frog. Gloves, lubricant, and a penlight are needed for the examination.	Pubic hair development Stage I: preadolescent, no growth of pubic hair Stage II: initial, scarcely pigmented straight hair, especially along medial border of the labia

Inspect the mons pubis for the presence of pubic hair and its characteristics. See Figure 3–3A for assessment of sexual maturity.	Stage III: sparse, dark, visibly pigmented curly pubic hair on labia Stage IV: hair coarse and curly, abundant but less than adults Stage V: lateral spreading in triangle shape to medial surface of thighs Stage VI: further extension laterally and upward
Inspect the external genitalia for color, size, and symmetry of the mons pubis, labia, urethra, and vaginal opening. Look for any swelling, inflammation, masses, lacerations, or discharge. Separate the labia minora for viewing structures in the vestibule. Inspect the vestibule for lesions or discharge.	In preadolescents Labia minora are thin and pale, hymen is a thin membrane with a crescent-shaped opening just inside the vaginal opening, no vaginal discharge.
An internal vaginal examination is performed by an experienced examiner when abnormal findings are noted.	After puberty The labia minora are dark pink and moist; vaginal opening is approximately 1 cm (0.5 in.) in adolescents when the hymen is intact; clear discharge without a foul odor; menses begin about 2 years after breast bud development at sexual maturity rating 4; no lesions or signs of inflammation around the urethral or vaginal opening.

	In young infants, the labia minora may be fused and cover the structures in the vestibule. A foul-smelling discharge may be a foreign body or vaginal infection.
Palpate the vaginal opening with a finger of your free hand.	*If the Bartholin's and Skene's glands are palpated in preadolescents, an infection such as gonorrhea may be present.*

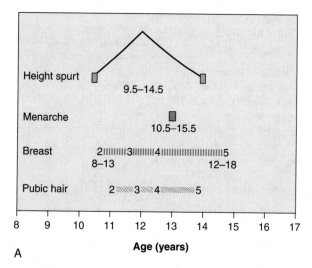

A

Figure 3–3 ■ Sexual maturity rating. Approximate timing of developmental changes. The numbers (2, 3, 4, 5) indicate stages of development. Range of ages during which some changes occur is indicated by the inclusive numbers below them. **A:** Females. **B:** Males. [A. Redrawn from Marshall, W. A. & Tanner, J. M. (1969). Variations in pattern of pubertal changes in girls. Archives of Disease in Childhood, 44, 291. B. Marshall, W. A. & Tanner, J. M. (1970). Variations in pattern of pubertal changes in boys. Archives of Diseases in Childhood, 45, 13, with permission.] (*continued*)

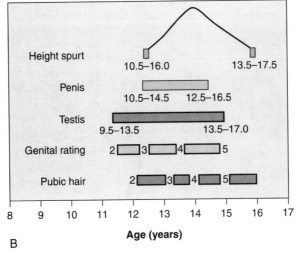

Height spurt
10.5–16.0   13.5–17.5

Penis
10.5–14.5   12.5–16.5

Testis
9.5–13.5   13.5–17.0

Genital rating   2 ⬜ 3 ⬜ 4 ⬜ 5

Pubic hair   2 ◼ 3 ◼ 4 ◼ 5 ◼

Age (years)

B

Figure 3–3 ◼ *(Continued)*

Males	
Seat boys in tailor position with legs crossed in front of them to push the testicles into the scrotum.	Pubic hair and external genital development
Inspect the pubertal development of the penis, scrotum, testicles, and pubic hair. See Figure 3–3B for assessment of sexual maturity.	Stage I: Preadolescent, hair present is same as that on abdomen; testes, scrotum, and penis are the same size and shape as young child.
	Stage II: Slightly pigmented, longer, straight pubic hair, often still downy, usually at base of penis, sometimes on scrotum; enlargement of scrotum and testes.

Stage III: Dark, definitely pigmented, curly pubic hair around base of penis; enlargement of penis, especially in length, further enlargement of testes, descent of scrotum.

Stage IV: Adult in type pubic hair, but spread no further than inguinal fold; continued enlargement of penis and sculpturing of glans, increased pigmentation of scrotum.

Stage V: Pubic hair spreads to medial surface of thighs in adult distribution; adult stage, scrotum ample, penis reaching nearly to bottom of scrotum.

Penile enlargement follows testicular enlargement. Pubic hair before 9 years of age is uncommon. Ejaculation at sexual maturity rating 3, with semen noted between sexual maturity ratings 3 and 4.

Delayed onset of testicular enlargement after 14 years of age needs evaluation.

Inspect the penis for size, foreskin, hygiene, and position of the urethral meatus. Inspect the urinary stream. Use gentle traction to evaluate the degree of foreskin retraction and the meatal location and size.

In the uncircumcised infant and child, avoid forcible retraction of the foreskin to prevent tearing of adhesions that could lead to fibrosis.

Inspect the scrotum for size, symmetry, presence of the testicles, and any abnormalities. To distinguish between a hydrocele and an incarcerated hernia, place a bright penlight under the scrotum and look for a red glow or transillumination.

The newborn penis length is 2–3 cm (1 in.). The penis is straight. Foreskin adhesions in infants and young boys, with opening large enough for a good urinary stream is normal, even when the meatus cannot be seen. The foreskin retracts easily by 5 years of age.

The glans penis is clean and smooth, no inflammation or ulceration. The urethral meatus is a slit-shaped opening near the tip of the glans. No discharge. Strong stream, no dribbling.

The scrotum is loose and pendulous, with rugae, or wrinkles. A hydrocele transilluminates; a hernia does not.

Erythema and edema of the glans (balanitis) from an infection or trauma. A round, pinpoint urethral meatus with meatal stenosis. Hypospadias or epispadias. A downward bowing of the penis (chordee) with hypospadias.

A small, undeveloped scrotum with undescended testicles. Enlargement of the scrotum may indicate an inguinal hernia, hydrocele, torsion of the spermatic cord, or testicular inflammation. A deep cleft in the scrotum may indicate ambiguous genitalia.

Palpate the shaft of the penis for nodules and masses.	No nodules or masses are present. The testicles are smooth and equal in size. They are approximately 1.0–1.5 cm (0.5 in.) in diameter until puberty, when they increase in size. The testicle is descendable when it can be moved into the scrotum. The spermatic cord feels solid and smooth without tenderness.
Palpate the scrotum for the presence of the testicles. Place your index finger and thumb over the inguinal canals on each side of the penis to keep the testicles from retracting. Gently palpate each testicle to identify the shape and size. If a testicle is not in the scrotum, palpate the inguinal canal for a soft mass. If found in the inguinal canal, try to move the testicle to the scrotum to palpate the size and shape.	
	An undescended testicle does not descend into the scrotum or cannot be palpated in the inguinal canal. A hard, enlarged, painless testicle may indicate a tumor. A scrotal mass that reduces may indicate an inguinal hernia; a hydrocele and an incarcerated hernia do not reduce.
When scrotal bulging or swelling is present, palpate the scrotum to identify the characteristics of the mass and attempt to reduce it. Determine if it is unilateral or bilateral.	
Palpate the length of the spermatic cord between the thumb and forefinger from the testicle to the inguinal canal.	
Anus and rectum	
Inspect the anus for sphincter control, inflammation, fissures, or lesions when the child is in supine or prone position.	The external sphincter is usually closed.
	Inflammation and scratch marks around the anus may indicate pinworms. A rectal wall prolapse or a hemorrhoid is seen as a protrusion from the rectum.

| Lightly touch the anal opening to stimulate an anal contraction or "wink." | *Absence of an anal contraction may indicate a lower spinal cord lesion.* |
| A rectal examination is performed by an experienced examiner. | |

ASSESSING THE MUSCULOSKELETAL SYSTEM FOR BONE AND JOINT STRUCTURE, MOVEMENT, AND MUSCLE STRENGTH

Procedure[1]	Findings[2]
Inspect and compare the arms for differences in alignment, contour, skin folds, length, and deformities. Count the fingers, and inspect the nails and creases on the palmar surface of each hand.	Extremities of equal length, circumference, and numbers of skin folds bilaterally. Arm alignment is straight, with a minimal angle at the elbows. All fingers and toes present; nails are convex and pink. Hand palms have multiple creases.
Assess the alignment of the lower extremities in infants and toddlers. Inspect the feet for in-toeing when the infant stands and walks. Inspect the feet for alignment, the presence of all toes, and any deformities. Inspect the feet for the presence of an arch when the child is standing.	Children up to 3 years of age appear to have flat feet due to a fat pad over the arch. Older children have a longitudinal foot arch. By 4 years, long bone alignment is straight. The infant's toes turn in due to tibial torsion.

If the toddler has bowlegs, stand the child on a firm surface with ankles together and measure the distance between the knees. To evaluate the child with knock-knees, stand the child on a firm surface with knees together and measure the distance between the ankles at the level of the medial malleoli.

Toddlers go through a skeletal alignment sequence of bowlegs (genu varum) and knock-knees (genu valgum) before the legs assume a straight alignment. No more than 3.5 cm (1.5 in.) between the knees and no more than 2 in. (5 cm) between the ankles is normal.

Inspect and compare the joints bilaterally for size, discoloration, and ease of voluntary movement.

Joints same color as surrounding skin; no swelling. Children flex and extend joints without pain.

Extra skin folds and a larger circumference may indicate a shorter extremity. Redness, swelling, and pain with movement may indicate injury or infection. Polydactyly or syndactyly is abnormal. A single crease that crosses the entire palm of the hand with Down syndrome. Clubbing of the nails with chronic respiratory and cardiac conditions.

Palpate the bones and muscles in each extremity for muscle tone, masses, or tenderness. Palpate each joint and surrounding muscles to detect any swelling, masses, heat, or tenderness.	Muscles feel firm, and bony masses are not present. *Doughy muscles indicate poor muscle tone. Rigid muscles or hypertonia with an active seizure or cerebral palsy. A mass over a long bone with a recent fracture or a bone tumor. Tenderness, heat, swelling, and redness around a joint with injury or inflammation.*
Inspect the standing posture from a front, side, and back view. Observe the height of the shoulders and hips. Ask the child to bend forward slowly at the waist, with arms extended toward the floor. Palpate each vertebra for a change in alignment.	Shoulders and hips are level; head is erect without a tilt, shoulder contour is symmetric. Thoracic convex and lumbar concave spinal curves after 6 years. No lateral curve. The lumbar concave curve flattens with forward flexion. *A lateral curve to the spine or a one-sided rib hump indicates scoliosis.*
Assess range of motion of all major joints during typical play activities (reaching for objects, climbing, and walking). Perform passive range of motion when a joint has limited active range of motion. Flex and extend, abduct and adduct, or rotate the affected joint cautiously to avoid causing extra pain.	Children spontaneously move joints through the full range of motion with play activities. No pain. *Limited active and passive range of motion indicates pain, malformation, injury, inflammation of a joint, or a muscle abnormality. Increased passive range of motion with muscle weakness.*

Assess the hips of young infants for dislocation or subluxation. Assess the skin folds on the upper legs. Check for a difference in knee height symmetry. Perform the Ortolani-Barlow maneuver. With the infant supine, flex the hips and knees at a 90-degree angle. Place a hand over each knee with the thumb over the inner thigh, and the first two fingers over the upper margin of the femur. Move the infant's knees together until they touch, and then put downward pressure on one femur at a time to see if the hips easily slip out of their joints or dislocate. Then, slowly abduct the hips, one at a time, moving each knee toward the examining table. Keep pressure on the hip joints with the fingers in a lever-type motion. Ask the child to stand on one leg and then the other.	Equal number of skin folds on each leg, knee height is even. The hips do not easily slip out of joint. The hips equally abduct, knees nearly touching the table. The iliac crests stay level when the child stands on each leg. *Uneven skin folds may indicate a hip dislocation or difference in leg length (Allis' sign). A hip that slips easily out of the joint, resistance to abduction, or a palpated clunk indicates a hip dislocation. If the iliac crest opposite the weight-bearing leg appears lower, the hip that is bearing weight may be dislocated.*
Assess muscle strength. Observe the child climbing onto an examining table, throwing a ball, clapping the hands, or moving around on the bed.	The child's ability to play indicates good muscle tone and strength. Good muscle strength bilaterally.

Assess the strength of specific muscles in the extremities. Ask the child to squeeze your fingers tightly with each hand, push against and pull your hands with the hands, lower legs and feet, and resist extension of a flexed elbow or knee. Compare muscle strength bilaterally. When generalized muscle weakness is suspected in a preschool- or school-age child, ask the child to stand up from the supine position.	*Unilateral muscle weakness may indicate a nerve injury.* *Bilateral muscle weakness from hypoxemia or a congenital disorder such as Down syndrome. Asymmetric weakness with cerebral palsy. Children who push their body upright from a supine position using the arms and hands have generalized muscle weakness, a sign of muscular dystrophy.*

ASSESSING THE NERVOUS SYSTEM FOR COGNITIVE FUNCTION, BALANCE, COORDINATION, CRANIAL NERVE FUNCTION, SENSATION, AND REFLEXES

Procedure[1]	Findings[2]
Observe level of consciousness and activity, including facial expressions, gestures, and interaction. Match the neurologic examination to the child's stage of development.	Alert and curious, easily aroused from sleep. Infants and toddlers seek the security of the parent. Older children are often anxious and watch all of the examiner's actions. Toddlers follow simple directions; by 3 years, speech can be understood.
Listen to speech articulation and words used. Compare the child's performance with standards of social development and speech articulation for the child's age.	*A lowered level of consciousness with brain injury, seizure, infection, or brain tumor. Lack of interest may indicate a serious illness. Excessive activity or an unusually short attention span with an attention deficit hyperactivity disorder. Delay in language and social skill development with mental retardation or hearing loss.*

Begin to evaluate recent memory at 4 years of age. Ask the child to remember a special name or object. Have the child recall the name or object 5–10 min later. Ask the child to repeat his or her address or birth date to assess remote memory.	By 5 or 6 years of age, children are able to recall this information without difficulty.
Observe the young child at play, walking, standing on one foot, and hopping to assess coordination and balance. Use the Romberg test to test balance in children older than 3 years. Have the child stand with eyes closed, and stand close to catch the child if needed.	Preschool-age children extend their arms to maintain balance; older children stand with their arms at their sides. Children do not stumble, fall, or limp. The iliac crests are level during walking. *Leaning or falling to one side with the Romberg test with poor balance, cerebellar dysfunction, or inner ear disturbance.*
Tests of coordination assess the smoothness and accuracy of movement. Assess fine motor skills in young children. After 6 years of age use the finger-to-nose, finger-to-finger, heel-to-shin, and alternating motion maneuvers.	*Jerky movements or inaccurate pointing (past pointing) indicates poor coordination.*
Inspect the child when walking from both a front and a rear view.	*A limp indicates injury or joint disease. Staggering or falling with cerebellar ataxia. Scissoring with cerebral palsy or other spastic conditions.*

Assess cranial nerves. See Table 3–3 for procedures and expected findings.	Abnormalities of cranial nerves with compression of an individual nerve, brain injury, or infections.
Assess sensory function and compare bilaterally the responses to stimulation. An infant's sensory function is not routinely assessed. Stroke the skin on the lower leg or arm with a cotton ball or a finger while the child's eyes are closed to test superficial tactile sensation. When the child's eyes are closed, touch the child on each arm and leg, alternating the sharp and dull ends of the tongue blade.	Equal responses bilaterally. Children older than 2 years can point to the location touched. Children older than 4 years can distinguish between a sharp and dull sensation each time. Withdrawal responses to painful procedures indicate normal sensory function in infants. *Loss of sensation with a brain or spinal cord lesion. Inability to identify superficial touch and pain sensation indicates sensory loss.*

Table 3–3   Cranial Nerve Assessment in Infants and Children

Cranial Nerve[a]	Assessment Procedure and Normal Findings[b]
I Olfactory	Infant: Not tested.
	Child: Not routinely tested. Give familiar odors to child to smell, one naris at a time. *Identifies odors such as orange, peanut butter, and chocolate.*
II Optic	Infant: Shine a bright light in eyes. *A quick blink reflex and dorsal head flexion indicate light perception.*
	Child: Test vision and visual fields if cooperative. *Visual acuity appropriate for age.*
III Oculomotor	Infant: Shine a penlight at the eyes and move it side to side. *Focuses on and tracks the light to each side.*
IV Trochlear	Child: Move an object through the six cardinal points of gaze. *Tracks objects through all fields of gaze.*
VI Abducens	All ages: Inspect eyelids for drooping. Inspect pupillary response to light. *Eyelids do not droop and pupils are equal sized and briskly respond to light.*
V Trigeminal	Infant: Stimulate the rooting and sucking reflex. *Turns head toward stimulation at side of mouth and sucking has good strength and pattern.*
	Child: Observe the child chewing a cracker. Touch forehead and cheeks with cotton ball when eyes are closed. *Bilateral jaw strength is good. Child pushes cotton ball away.*
VII Facial	All ages: Observe facial expressions when crying, smiling, frowning, and so forth. *Facial features stay symmetric bilaterally.*
VIII Acoustic	Infant: Produce a loud sound near the head. *Blinks in response to sound, moves head toward sound, or freezes position.*
	Child: Use a noisemaker near each ear or whisper words to be repeated. *Turns head toward sound and repeats words correctly.*
IX Glossopharyngeal	Infant: Observe swallowing during feeding. *Good swallowing pattern.*
X Vagus	All ages: Elicit gag reflex. *Gags with stimulation.*
XI Spinal accessory	Infant: Not tested.
	Child: Ask child to raise the shoulders and turn the head side to side against resistance. *Good strength in neck and shoulders.*
XII Hypoglossal	Infant: Observe feeding. *Sucking and swallowing are coordinated.*
	Child: Tell the child to stick out the tongue. Listen to speech. *Tongue is midline with no tremors. Words are clearly articulated.*

[a]Bracketed nerves are tested together.
[b]Italics indicate normal findings.

Primitive infant reflexes	Movements are equal bilaterally.
Moro reflex: Startle the infant with a sudden noise or change in position.	Moro reflex: The arms extend and the fingers form a C as they spread. The arms slowly move together as in a hug. The legs may make a similar movement. Present at birth and disappears by 6 months of age.
Palmar grasp: Place a finger across the infant's palm and avoid touching the thumb.	Palmar grasp: A strong grip of the finger occurs. Present at birth and disappears by 3 months of age.
Plantar grasp: Place finger across the foot at the base of the toes.	Plantar grasp: The toes curl as if gripping the finger. Present at birth and disappears at about 8 months of age.
Placing reflex: Hold the infant erect and touch the top of one foot with the edge of a table or chair.	Placing reflex: The infant lifts the foot as if to step up on the surface. Present within days of birth and disappears at various times.
Stepping reflex: Hold the infant erect and touch the bottom of the foot on the surface of a table or chair.	Stepping reflex: The feet lift in an alternating pattern as if to walk. Present at birth and disappears between 4 and 8 weeks of age.
Tonic neck reflex: When the supine infant is relaxed, turn the head to one side. Repeat by turning the head to the opposite side.	Tonic neck reflex: The arm and leg on the face side extend and the opposite arm and leg flex as if to assume a fencing position. Appears at about 2 months and disappears at no later than 6 months of age.
	An asymmetric response may indicate a serious neurologic problem.

Superficial reflexes	
The plantar reflex tests spine levels L4 through S2. Stroke the bottom of the foot from the heel, along the lateral side of the foot and curve over the ball of the foot. Watch the toes for plantar flexion or for fanning and dorsiflexion of the big toe (Babinski response).	The Babinski response in children younger than 2 years. Plantar flexion of the toes in older children. *A Babinski response in children older than 2 years indicates neurologic disease.*
Stroke the inner thigh of each leg to stimulate the cremasteric reflex.	The testicle and scrotum rise on the stroked side with intact T12, L1, and L2 function.
Deep tendon reflexes	
Tap a tendon near specific joints with a reflex hammer (or with the index finger for infants), and compare responses bilaterally. Inspect for movement in the associated joint and palpate the strength of the expected muscle contraction.	Bilaterally symmetric and active grade 2+ responses indicate intact spinal segments.
Biceps: Flex the child's arm at the elbow, and place your thumb over the biceps tendon in the antecubital fossa. Tap the thumb.	Biceps: Elbow flexion with biceps muscle contraction indicates intact C5 and C6 segments.

Triceps: Flex the child's arm at the elbow and tap the triceps tendon above the elbow.	Triceps: Elbow extension with triceps muscle contraction indicates intact C6, C7, and C8.
Brachioradialis: Lay the child's arm with the thumb upright over your arm. Tap the brachioradialis tendon 2.5 cm (1 in.) above the wrist.	Brachioradialis: Forearm pronation (palm facing downward) and elbow flexion indicate intact C5 and C6.
Patellar: Flex the child's knees, and tap the patellar tendon below the knee.	Patellar: Knee extension (knee jerk) with quadriceps muscle contraction indicates intact L2, L3, and L4.
Achilles: While the child's legs are flexed, support the foot and tap the Achilles tendon.	Achilles: Plantar flexion (ankle jerk) with gastrocnemius muscle contraction indicates intact S1 and S2.
	An absent response (grade 0) indicates decreased muscle tone and strength. Hyperactive responses (grade 4+) are associated with muscle spasticity.

4. Physical Growth Charts

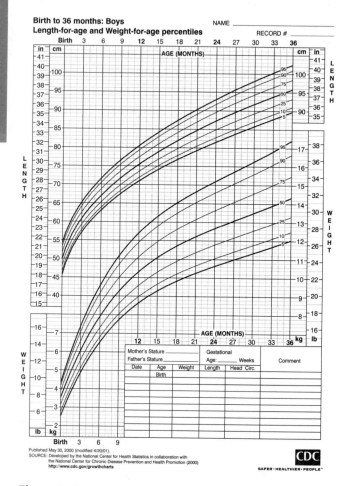

Figure 4–1 ■ Physical growth percentiles for length and weight—boys: birth to 36 months.
From CDC, 2001. http://www.cdc.gov/growthcharts.

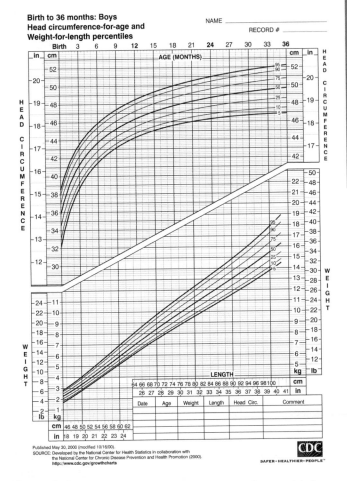

Figure 4–2 ■ Physical growth percentiles for head circumference, weight for length—boys: birth to 36 months.
From CDC, 2001. http://www.cdc.gov/growthcharts.

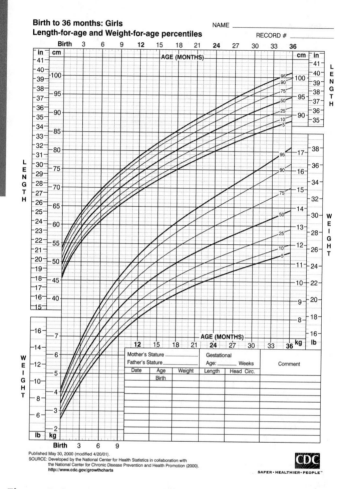

Figure 4–3 ■ Physical growth percentiles for length and weight—girls: birth to 36 months.

From CDC, 2001. http://www.cdc.gov/growthcharts.

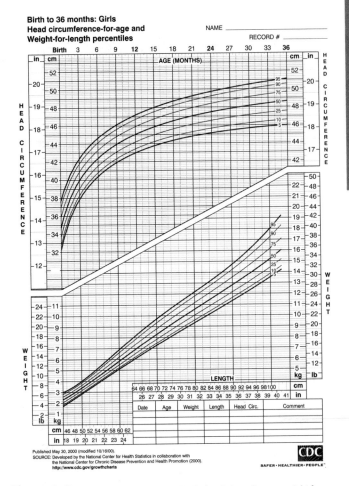

Figure 4–4 ■ Physical growth percentiles for head circumference, weight for length—girls: birth to 36 months.
From CDC, 2001. http://www.cdc.gov/growthcharts.

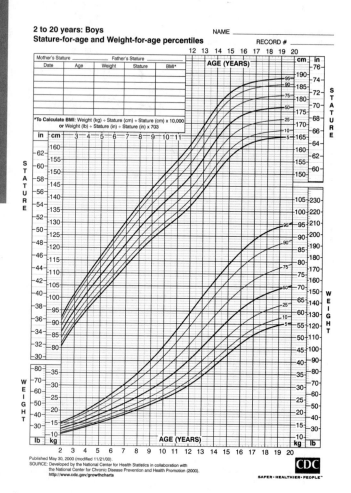

2 to 20 years: Boys
Stature-for-age and Weight-for-age percentiles

NAME _____

RECORD # _____

Published May 30, 2000 (modified 11/21/00).
SOURCE: Developed by the National Center for Health Statistics in collaboration with
the National Center for Chronic Disease Prevention and Health Promotion (2000).
http://www.cdc.gov/growthcharts

Figure 4–5 ▪ Physical growth percentiles for stature and weight according to age—boys: 2 to 20 years.
From CDC, 2001. http://www.cdc.gov/growthcharts.

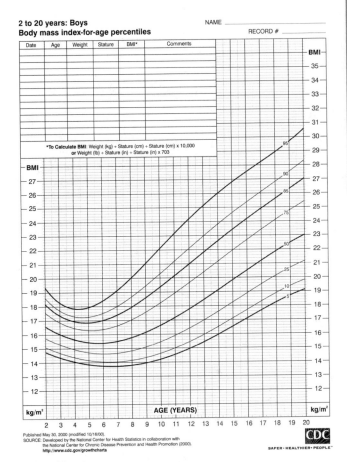

2 to 20 years: Boys
Body mass index-for-age percentiles

NAME _____

RECORD # _____

Figure 4–6 ■ Physical growth percentiles for body mass index (BMI) according to age—boys: 2 to 20 years.
From CDC, 2001. http://www.cdc.gov/growthcharts.

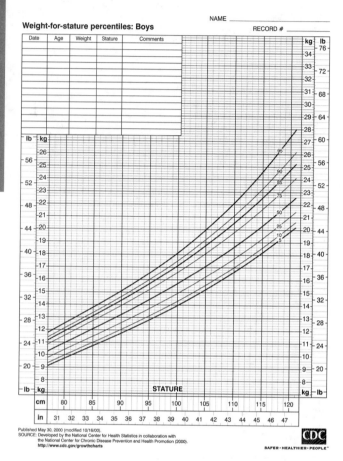

Figure 4–7 ■ Physical growth percentiles for weight for stature—boys: 2 to 20 years.
From CDC, 2001. http://www.cdc.gov/growthcharts.

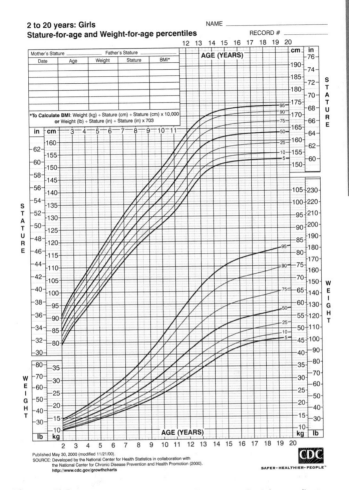

2 to 20 years: Girls
Stature-for-age and Weight-for-age percentiles

NAME _____

RECORD # _____

Published May 30, 2000 (modified 11/21/00).
SOURCE: Developed by the National Center for Health Statistics in collaboration with the National Center for Chronic Disease Prevention and Health Promotion (2000).
http://www.cdc.gov/growthcharts

Figure 4–8 ■ Physical growth percentiles for stature and weight according to age—girls: 2 to 20 years.
From CDC, 2001. http://www.cdc.gov/growthcharts.

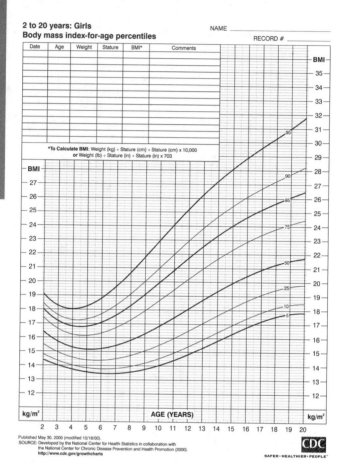

Figure 4–9 ■ Physical growth percentiles for body mass index (BMI) according to age—girls: 2 to 20 years.
From CDC, 2001. http://www.cdc.gov/growthcharts.

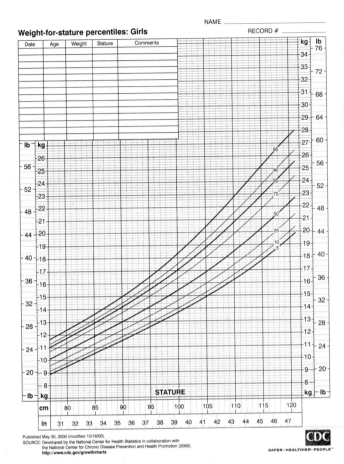

Weight-for-stature percentiles: Girls

Date	Age	Weight	Stature	Comments

STATURE

Published May 30, 2000 (modified 10/16/00).
SOURCE: Developed by the National Center for Health Statistics in collaboration with
the National Center for Chronic Disease Prevention and Health Promotion (2000).
http://www.cdc.gov/growthcharts

CDC
SAFER · HEALTHIER · PEOPLE™

Figure 4–10 ■ Physical growth percentiles for weight for stature—girls: 2 to 20 years.
From CDC, 2001. http://www.cdc.gov/growthcharts.

Section I: General Information

5. NUTRITION

RECOMMENDED DIETARY ALLOWANCES (RDAs)

	Age	Vitamin A (mcg/day)	Vitamin D (mcg/day)	Vitamin E (mcg/day) α-Tocopherol	Vitamin K (mcg/day)	Vitamin C (mg/day)	Thiamin (mg/day)	Riboflavin (mg/day)	Niacin (mg/day)	Vitamin B_6 (mg/day)
Infants	0–6 months	400*	5*	4*	2.0*	40*	0.2*	0.3*	~0.2*	0.1*
	7–12 months	500*	5*	5*	2.5*	50*	0.3*	0.4*	~0.4*	0.3*
Children	1–3 years	300	5*	6	30*	15	0.5	0.5	6	0.5
– –	4–8 years	400	5*	7	55*	25	0.6	0.6	8	0.6
Males	9–13 years	600	5*	11	60*	45	0.9	0.9	12	1.0
	14–18 years	900	5*	15	75*	75	1.2	1.3	16	1.3
Females	9–13 years	600	5*	11	60*	45	0.9	0.9	12	1.0
	14–18 years	700	5*	15	75*	65	1.0	1.0	14	1.2

*Values are adequate intakes rather than RDAs. All other values on chart are RDAs.
Note: All data from Institute of Medicine. (1997–2001). Dietary reference intakes. Washington DC: National Academy Press. Available also at http://www.iom.edu.

Folate (mg/ day)	Vita-min B_{12} (mg/ day)	Cal-cium (mg/ day)	Phos-pho-rus (mg/ day)	Magne-sium (mg/day)	Iron (mg/ day)	Zinc (mg/ day)	Iodine (mcg/ day)	Sele-nium (mcg/ day)
65*	0.4*	210*	100*	30*	0.27*	2.0*	110*	15*
80*	0.5*	270*	275*	75*	11	3	130*	20*
150	0.9	500*	460	80	7	3	90	20
200	1.2	800*	500	130	10	5	90	30
300	1.8	1,300*	1,250	240	8	8	120	40
400	2.4	1,300*	1,250	240	11	11	150	55
300	1.8	1,300*	1,250	410	8	8	120	40
400	2.4	1,300*	1,250	360	15	9	150	55

RDA FOR PROTEIN, CARBOHYDRATE, FAT

RDA

	Age	Protein	Carbohydrate	Polyunsaturated Fatty Acids n-6	Polyunsaturated Fatty Acids n-3	Total Fat	Fiber
Infants	0–6 months	9.1 g/day or 1.52 g/kg/day*	60 g/day	4.4 g/day	0.5 g/day	31 g/day	NE
	7–12 months	1.5 g/kg/day	95 g/day	4.6 g/day	0.5 g/day	30 g/day	NE
Children	1–3 years	13 g/day or 1.1 g/kg/day	130 g/day	7 g/day (linoleic)	0.7 g/day (α-linolenic)	NE	19 g/day
	4–8 years	0.95 g/kg/day or 19 g/day	130 g/day	10 g/day (linoleic)	0.9 g/day (α-linolenic)	NE	25 g/day
Males	9–13 years	0.95 g/kg/day or 34 g/day	130 g/day	12 g/day (linoleic)	1.2 g/day (α-linolenic)	NE	31 g/day
	14–18 years	0.85 g/kg/day or 52 g/day	130 g/day	16 g/day (linoleic)	1.6 g/day (α-linolenic)	NE	38 g/day
Females	9–13 years	0.95 g/kg/day or 34 g/day	130 g/day	10 g/day (linoleic)	1.0 g/day (α-linolenic)	NE	26 g/day
	14–18 years	0.85 g/kg/day or 46 g/day	130 g/day	11 g/day (linoleic)	1.1 g/day (α-linolenic)	NE	26 g/day

NE, not established.
*Values are adequate intakes rather than RDAs. All other values on charts are RDAs.
Note: All data from Institute of Medicine (2002). Dietary reference intakes. Washington DC: National Academy Press. Available also at http://www.iom.edu.

CLINICAL MANIFESTATIONS OF DIETARY DEFICIENCIES/EXCESSES

Nutrient	Deficiency Manifestation	Excess Manifestation
Vitamin A	Night blindness Skin dryness and scaling	Headache Drowsiness Hepatomegaly
Vitamin C	Abnormal hair (coiled shape) Skin abnormalities (dermatitis and lesions) Purpura Bleeding gums Joint tenderness Sudden heart failure	Usually none, excess is excreted in urine
Vitamin D	Rib abnormalities Bowed legs	Drowsiness
B vitamins	Weakness Decreased deep tendon reflexes Dermatitis	Usually none, excess is excreted in urine
Protein	Hepatomegaly Edema Scant, depigmented hair	Kidney failure
Carbohydrate	Emaciation Decreased energy Retarded growth and development	Overweight
Iron	Lethargy Slowed growth and developmental progression Pallor	Vomiting, diarrhea, abdominal pain Pallor Cyanosis Drowsiness Shock

FOOD GUIDE PYRAMID AND CANADIAN FOOD RAINBOW

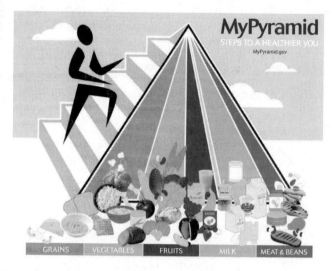

Figure 5–1 ■ The food guide pyramid and food rainbow are used to provide information about amounts of foods recommended for daily intake.
From U.S. Department of Agriculture and U.S. Department of Health and Human Services. (2005). http://www.mypyramid.gov/downloads/miniposter.pdf; Canada's Food Guide to Healthy Eating. (2003). http://www.hc-sc.gc.ca/fn-an/food-guide-aliment/fg_rainbow-arc_en_ciel_ga_e.html, accessed 10/26/2005. Reproduced with permission of the minister of Public Works and Government Services Canada, 2004. (*continued*)

GRAINS
Make half your grains whole

Eat at least 3 oz. of whole-grain cereals, breads, crackers, rice, or pasta every day

1 oz. is about 1 slice of bread, about 1 cup of breakfast cereal, or 1/2 cup of cooked rice, cereal, or pasta

VEGETABLES
Vary your veggies

Eat more dark-green veggies like broccoli, spinach, and other dark leafy greens

Eat more orange vegetables like carrots and sweet potatoes

Eat more dry beans and peas like pinto beans, kidney beans, and lentils

FRUITS
Focus on fruits

Eat a variety of fruit

Choose fresh, frozen, canned, or dried fruit

Go easy on fruit juices

MILK
Get your calcium-rich foods

Go low-fat or fat-free when you choose milk, yogurt, and other milk products

If you don't or can't consume milk, choose lactose-free products or other calcium sources such as fortified foods and beverages

MEAT & BEANS
Go lean with protein

Choose low-fat or lean meats and poultry

Bake it, broil it, or grill it

Vary your protein routine – choose more fish, beans, peas, nuts, and seeds

For a 2,000-calorie diet, you need the amounts below from each food group. To find the amounts that are right for you, go to MyPyramid.gov.

| Eat 6 oz. every day | Eat 2½ cups every day | Eat 2 cups every day | Get 3 cups every day; for kids aged 2 to 8, it's 2 | Eat 5½ oz. every day |

Find your balance between food and physical activity
- Be sure to stay within your daily calorie needs.
- Be physically active for at least 30 minutes most days of the week.
- About 60 minutes a day of physical activity may be needed to prevent weight gain.
- For sustaining weight loss, at least 60 to 90 minutes a day of physical activity may be required.
- Children and teenagers should be physically active for 60 minutes every day, or most days.

Know the limits on fats, sugars, and salt (sodium)
- Make most of your fat sources from fish, nuts, and vegetable oils.
- Limit solid fats like butter, margarine, shortening, and lard, as well as foods that contain these.
- Check the Nutrition Facts label to keep saturated fats, trans fats, and sodium low.
- Choose food and beverages low in added sugars. Added sugars contribute calories with few, if any, nutrients.

MyPyramid.gov
STEPS TO A HEALTHIER YOU

USDA
U.S. Department of Agriculture
Center for Nutrition Policy and Promotion
April 2005
CNPP-15

Figure 5–1 ■ (Continued)

Canada's Food Guide to Healthy Eating

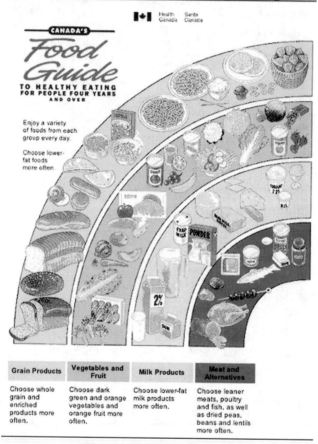

Grain Products	Vegetables and Fruit	Milk Products	Meat and Alternatives
Choose whole grain and enriched products more often.	Choose dark green and orange vegetables and orange fruit more often.	Choose lower-fat milk products more often.	Choose leaner meats, poultry and fish, as well as dried peas, beans and lentils more often.

Figure 5–1 ■ (Continued)

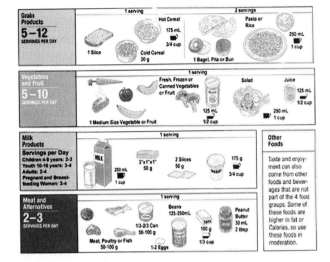

Different People Need Different Amounts of Food

The amount of food you need every day from the 4 food groups and other foods depends on your age, body size, activity level, whether you are male or female and if you are pregnant or breast-feeding. That's why the Food Guide gives a lower and higher number of servings for each food group. For example, young children can choose the lower number of servings, while male teenagers can go to the higher number. Most other people can choose servings somewhere in between.

Figure 5–1 ■ (Continued)

6. AVERAGE LABORATORY VALUES

All laboratory value ranges listed are approximate. Consult your local laboratory reference guide for normal values for the specific testing procedures used.

NORMAL VALUE RANGES: BLOOD*
Albumin (S)[1]
1 month–1 year: 2.8–4.8 g/dL
1–18 years: 3.2–4.7 g/dL

Alkaline Phosphatase (S)[1]

Age	Males Units/L	Females Units/L
1–30 days	75–316	48–406
1–3 years	104–345	108–317
4–6 years	93–309	96–297
7–9 years	86–315	69–325
10–12 years	42–362	51–332
13–15 years	74–390	50–162
16–18 years	52–171	47–119

Blood Chemistry
Chloride (S, P)[1]
Under 1 year: 96–111 mmol/L
1–17 years: 102–112 mmol/L

Glucose (S, P)[1]
54–117 mg/dL (3.0–6.49 mmol/L)

Magnesium (P, S)[1]
1.6–2.5 mg/dL (0.7–1.0 mmol/L)

Osmolality (S)[1]
280–300 mOsm/kg

Potassium (S, P)[1]
3.3–4.7 mmol/L

Sodium (P, S)[1]
132–141 mmol/L

---

*B, whole blood; P, plasma; S, serum.

Urea Nitrogen (S, P)[1]
1–13 years: 4–17 mg/dL (1.1–4.6 mmol/L)
14–19 years: 7–21 mg/dL (1.9–5.7 mmol/L)

Blood Gases
Carbon Dioxide, Partial Pressure (Pco2) (B)[1]
Infants: 27–41 mm Hg (3.6–5.5 kPa)
Children: 32–48 mm Hg (4.3–6.4 kPa)

Oxygen, Partial Pressure (Po2) (B)[1]
Over 1 day: 83–108 mm Hg (11.0–14.4 pKa)

Bicarbonate, Actual (P)[2]
Calculated from pH and $PaCO_2$
Newborns: 17.2–23.6 mmol/L
Children: 18–25 mmol/L

pH (B)[1]
0–6 months: 7.18–7.5
6–12 months: 7.27–7.49

Base Excess (B)[1]
Infants: –7 to –1 mmol/L
Children: –4 to +2 mmol/L
Thereafter: –3 to +3 mmol/L

Oxygen Saturation (B)[1]
Newborns: 85–90%
Thereafter: 95–99%

Cholesterol (S)[3]
Total Cholesterol
Borderline: greater than 170 mg/dL
Elevated: greater than 200 mg/dL

High-Density Lipoprotein
Less than 35 mg/dL

Low-Density Lipoprotein
Borderline: greater than 110 mg/dL
Elevated: greater than 130 mg/dL

Triglycerides
Less than 150 mg/dL

C-Reactive Protein (P, S)[1]
86–10,406 mcg/L

Hemoglobin A$_{1c}$ (B)[1]
Normal: 4–7%
Stable diabetic patients: 8–10%

Hemoglobin Electrophoresis (B)[2]
A$_1$ hemoglobin: 96.0–98.5% of total hemoglobin
A$_2$ hemoglobin: 1.5–4.0% of total hemoglobin

Hematology Values (B)
Values for children 2–12 years

Red Blood Cell[1]
$3.89–4.96 \times 10^{12}$/L

Hemoglobin[1]
10.2–13.4 g/dL

Hematocrit[1]
31.7–41%

Mean Corpuscular Volume[1]
72.7–86.5 micrometer^3

Mean Corpuscular Hemoglobin[1]
24.1–29.4 pg

Mean Corpuscular Hemoglobin Concentration[1]
32.4–35.3%

Reticulocyte Count[1]
0.8–2.2%

Sedimentation Rate (Micro)[2]
Under 2 years: 1–5 mm/hr
Over 2 years: 1–8 mm/hr

White Blood Cell[1]
$5.4–11.0 \times 10^9$/L

Differential[1]

Neutrophils	34.3–72.9%
Eosinophils	2.4–4.8%
Basophils	1%
Lymphocyte	13.5–52.8%
Atypical lymphocytes	2.6–5.6%
Monocytes	3.5–13.4%

Iron-Related Values
Ferritin (P, S)[1]
1–6 months: 47–449 ng/mL
Thereafter: 47–110 ng/mL

Iron (S, P)[1]
5–11 AM: 20–105 mcg/dL (3.6–18.8 micromole/L)

Iron-Binding Capacity (S, P)[1]
1–5 years: 268–441 mcg/dL (48–79 micromole/L)
6–9 years: 240–508 mcg/dL (43–91 micromole/L)
10–19 years: 290–575 mcg/dL (52–103 micromole/L)

Lead (B)[1]
0–15 years: less than 5 mcg/dL

Thyroid Hormones
Thyroid-Stimulating Hormone (P, S)[1]

Age	Males mUnit/mL	Females mUnit/mL
1–30 days	0.52–16	0.72–13.1
1 month–5 years	0.55–7.1	0.46–8.1
6–18 years	0.37–6	0.36–5.8

Thyroxine (T₄) (S, P)[1]

Age	Males mg/dL	Females mg/dL
1–30 days	5.9–21.5	6.3–21.5
1–6 years	6.1–13.1	7.1–14.1
7–12 years	6.7–13.4	6.1–12.1
13–15 years	4.8–11.5	5.8–11.2
16–18 years	5.9–11.5	5.2–13.2

Thyroxine, "Free" (Free T₄) (S, P)[1]
1–12 months: 0.76–2 ng/dL
1–5 years: 0.9–1.72 ng/dL
6–18 years: 0.81–1.68 ng/dL

Thyroxine-Binding Globulin (P)[1]
0–6 years: 16.2–33.8 mg/L
7–12 years: 15–29.2 mg/L
13–18 years: 13.4–28.7 mg/L

Triiodothyronine (T₃) (S)[1]

0–11 years: 90–260 ng/dL

12–18 years: 100–210 ng/dL

NORMAL VALUE RANGES: URINE

Addis Count[2]

Red cells (12-hr specimen): less than 1 million

White cells (12-hr specimen): less than 2 million

Casts (12-hr specimen): less than 10,000

Protein (12-hr specimen): less than 55 mg

Catecholamines (Norepinephrine, Epinephrine)[1]

Values in mmol/mol creatinine

Age	Norepinephrine	Epinephrine
Under 1 year	0.017–0.207	0–0.232
1–4 years	0.017–0.194	0–0.051
4–10 years	0.018–0.072	0.003–0.057
10–18 years	0.003–0.07	0.001–0.027

Chloride[2]

Infants: 1.7–8.5 mmol/24 hr

Children: 17–34 mmol/24 hr

Adults: 140–240 mmol/24 hr

Creatine[1]

18–58 mg/L (1.37–4.42 mmol/L)

Creatinine[1]

3–8 years: 0.11–0.68 g/24 hr

9–12 years: 0.17–1.41 g/24 hr

13–17 years: 0.29–1.87 g/24 hr

Adults: 0.63–2.5 g/24 hr

Osmolality[2]

Infants: 50–600 mOsm/L

Older children: 50–1,400 mOsm/L

Phosphorus, Tubular Reabsorption[2]

78–97%

Potassium[2]

26–123 mmol/L

Specific Gravity
1.010–1.030

NORMAL VALUE RANGES: SWEAT

Electrolytes[1]
Normal: less than 40 mmol/L for both sodium and chloride
Patients with cystic fibrosis: greater than 60 mmol/L for both sodium and chloride

NORMAL VALUE RANGES: CEREBROSPINAL FLUID

Protein[1]
Under 1 month: 15–153 mg/dL
Under 3 months: 15–93 mg/dL
Over 3 months: 15–45 mg/dL

Glucose[1]
All ages: 60–80% of blood glucose

Modified from:
[1]Soldin, S. J., Brugnara, C., & Wong, E. C. (2003). Pediatric reference ranges (4th ed.). Washington, DC: AACC Press.
[2]Hay, W. W., Hayward, A. R., Levin, M. J., Sondheimer, J.M. (2003). Current pediatric diagnosis and treatment (16th ed.). New York: Lange Medical Books/McGraw-Hill.
[3]Kavey, R. W., Daniels, S. R., Lauer, R. M., Atkins, D. L., Hayman, L. L., & Taubert, K. (2003). American Heart Association guidelines for primary prevention of atherosclerotic cardiovascular disease beginning in childhood. Journal of Pediatrics, 142(4), 368–372.

7. HEALTH PROMOTION AND HEALTH MAINTENANCE THROUGH CHILDHOOD

DEFINITIONS

Health is a state of complete physical, mental, and social well-being and not merely the absence of disease and infirmity (World Health Organization, 1996).

Health promotion refers to activities that increase well-being and enhance wellness or health (Pender, Murdaugh, & Parsons, 2002). These activities lead to actualization of positive health potential for all individuals, even those with chronic or acute conditions.

Health maintenance (or health protection) refers to activities that preserve an individual's present state of health and that prevent disease or injury occurrence (Figure 7–1).

Anticipatory guidance includes teaching for families to promote provision of an environment for children to assist in meeting developmental milestones.

Health supervision is the provision of services that focus on disease and injury prevention (health maintenance), growth and developmental surveillance, and health promotion at key intervals during the child's life.

A medical home or **pediatric healthcare home** is the site of comprehensive healthcare by a pediatric healthcare professional to ensure optimal health (National Association of Pediatric Nurse Practitioners, 2002).

Screening is a procedure used to detect the possible presence of a health condition before symptoms are apparent. It is usually conducted on large groups of individuals at risk for a condition and represents the secondary level of prevention.

U.S. National Guidelines for Health Promotion

Bright Futures, Maternal and Child Health Bureau, Health Resources and Services Administration, Department of Health and Human Services [*Bright Futures* recently partnered with the American Academy of Pediatrics (AAP) for future editions of their recommendations. They are available at http://brightfutures.aap.org.]

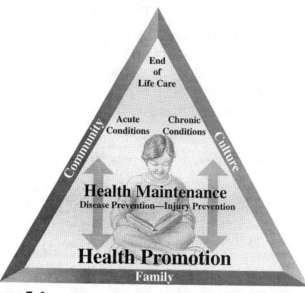

Figure 7–1 ■ The Bindler-Ball Continuum of Pediatric Healthcare for Children and Their Families. The outer bars represent the family, cultural, and community influences on the care that the child receives, either through the services sought by the family or the services provided in the community. Cultural influences include the family's decision to seek healthcare and follow recommendations, as well as the healthcare provider's cultural competence in caring for a child and family.

The inner categories represent the different types of healthcare needed by children. All children need health promotion and health maintenance services, represented by the base of the triangle. Notice the arrows representing the upward and downward movement between the levels of care as the child's condition changes.

Children may be healthy with episodic acute illnesses and injuries. Some children develop a chronic condition for which specialized healthcare is needed. A child's chronic condition may be well controlled, but acute episodes (e.g., with asthma) or other illnesses and injuries may occur, and the child also needs health promotion and health maintenance services to continue. Some children develop a life-threatening illness and ultimately need end-of-life care. A healthy child can also experience a catastrophic injury that causes death, and the family needs supportive end-of-life care.

Put Prevention into Practice, Office of Disease Prevention and Health Promotion, Public Health Service, Department of Health and Human Services (http://www.ahcpr.gov/clinic/ppipix.htm)

Guidelines for Adolescent Preventive Services, American Medical Association (http://www.ama-assn.org)

NEWBORN HEALTH PROMOTION AND HEALTH MAINTENANCE

Timing of Visits

During the hospital stay, the nurse provides ongoing physical assessment of the mother and newborn, whereas providing education and anticipatory guidance to prepare the mother to care for herself and her newborn after hospital discharge.

If the newborn is discharged from the hospital in less than 48 hours after birth, an experienced healthcare professional who is competent in newborn assessment should examine the newborn in the clinic or home setting within 48 hours of discharge (AAP, 2004).

For newborns discharged between 48 and 72 hours of age, the first follow-up visit should occur by 5 days of age.

General Observations

Welcome the family warmly.

Observe the family members that attend the visit and the interactions between them and with the new baby.

Apply information from observations to guide further questions and planned interventions.

Growth and Developmental Surveillance

For the healthy newborn, basic activities integrate surveillance of growth and development (Table 7–1), provide opportunities to work with the family, and promote the health of the newborn. These activities include

- First bath (to remove blood and amniotic fluid from the newborn's skin and prevent transmission of microorganisms to others)
- Umbilical cord care
- Vitamin K injection (to prevent vitamin K–deficiency bleeding)
- Eye prophylaxis (administration of ophthalmic antibiotic ointment to prevent gonococcal ophthalmia neonatorum)
- Physical assessment
- Feeding assessment
- Metabolic screen

Table 7–1 Newborn Growth and Developmental Milestones Observed in Health Promotion and Health Maintenance Visits

Growth	Weight: baby may lose up to one-tenth of birthweight in the first week of life; birthweight should be reattained by day 10; weight gain is approximately two-thirds of an ounce per day thereafter.
	Length increases by 1–1.5 in.
	Head circumference increases by approximately 1 in.
Vision	Focuses 8–12 in. away
	Eyes wander and may cross
	Prefers black and white or high-contrast patterns
	Prefers the human face to all other patterns
Hearing	Hearing is fully mature
	Recognizes some sounds
	May turn toward familiar sounds and voices

- Hepatitis B vaccination
- Hearing screen
- Maternal syphilis screen reviewed
- Other screening test results reviewed as indicated by maternal–newborn risk factors and state regulations, including screening for human immunodeficiency virus infection (AAP, 2004)
- Assessment of parental ability to adequately care for the newborn and to recognize and report signs of illness (Gilstrap & Oh, 2002)

Administer any needed medications/immunizations.

Perform physical assessment (see Chapter 3), including metabolic screening to include

- Classic phenylketonuria
- Primary congenital hypothyroidism
- Classic galactosemia
- Sickle cell anemia
- Classic congenital adrenal hyperplasia
- Biotinidase deficiency
- Maple syrup urine disease
- Homocystinuria
- Medium-chain acylcoenzyme A dehydrogenase deficiency (March of Dimes, 2004)

Perform gestational age examination (see Chapter 3).

Observe for expected developmental performance (see Table 7–1).

Teach parents about expected growth and developmental milestones and ways to encourage the newborn's development.

Nutrition

Measure weight, length, head circumference, and chest circumference, and compare them to expected norms.

Assess type and amount of all feedings.

Ask about wet diapers (six to eight daily usually indicate adequate hydration).

Encourage breastfeeding as the most beneficial form of infant feeding to include decreased incidence of
- Ear infections (otitis media)
- Allergies
- Diarrhea
- Vomiting
- Respiratory disease
- Meningitis and other infections

Teach proper mixing of formula, if used, and proper storage of breast milk.

Physical Activity

Newborn reflexes are strong and should be symmetric.

Hands are kept in tight fists and extremities flexed.

As the first month of life progresses, the baby straightens and lengthens.

Methods to encourage normal physical activity should be provided for parents
- Position baby on stomach for supervised play periods (Persing, Hector, Swanson, et al., 2003). Be sure to place the baby on back when tired and starting to fall asleep.
- Allow the baby free movement of arms and hands. If the baby is swaddled, allow the hands to be outside the blanket and positioned in midline (Shelov, 2002).
- Encourage appropriate toys, such as a mobile with contrasting colors and patterns; a plastic mirror; music boxes and exposure to soft music on the radio; a tape recorder or CD player; and soft toys with colors, patterns, and gentle sounds.
- Encourage switching positions when bottle feeding. Breastfeeding babies automatically feed from both sides. Parents who bottle feed may need to be reminded to promote this skill in their newborn.
- Beginning at birth, prevent flat spots on the newborn's head from supine positioning by nightly alternating the head position from

left to right during sleep and occasionally changing the orientation of the newborn in relation to the activity at the doorway of the room (Persing et al., 2003).

Oral Health

Perform oral assessment (see Chapter 3).

Instruct parents to avoid propping bottles and prolonged feedings.

Breast milk, formula, and water should be the only liquids provided.

Ask about plans for dental care and provide resources for use in the future if needed.

Mental Health

Establishing a sense of attachment is critical for the newborn's developing mental health.

Assess signs of attachment between baby and parents
- Parent looks at the newborn frequently
- Parent has specific questions and observations about the individual characteristics of the newborn
- Parent touches, massages, or gently rubs the newborn
- Parent attempts to soothe the newborn when the newborn is upset
- Newborn looks content
- Newborn signals needs
- Newborn feeds well
- Newborn responds to parent's attempts to soothe

Provide suggestions for parents of activities that will enhance the newborn's mental health
- Encourage your newborn to look at your face while feeding; imitate the baby's soft sounds and accommodate the baby's movements.
- Respond quickly to your baby's feeding cues, and avoid rigid feeding schedules; feeding times are unpredictable, especially in the first few months.
- Identify ways to soothe the crying newborn; babies cry for reasons other than hunger.
- Learn infant massage; for healthy infants, massage reportedly facilitates bonding, helps induce sleep in the baby, and makes parents feel relaxed while massaging their baby.
- Allow the baby to suck on fingers, hands, or a pacifier.
- Make eye contact with the baby, hold and rock the baby frequently, and read and sing to the baby. If you cannot think of

what to say to the baby, talk about your day, or talk about what is happening—for example, "Are you hungry now?" "Is that milk nice and warm?" "Do you hear that dog barking outside?" "You are very alert. I like it when you look at me that way."

- Be consistent and predictable in the way you respond to the newborn's needs.

(Adapted from Jellinek, Patel, & Froehle, 2002; Shelov, 2002)

Teach parents about the sleep and wake cycles of the baby so that they can engage the newborn during alert periods.

Newborn mental health relates directly to the parent's state.

Evaluate parents, and especially mothers, for adaptation, signs of depression, and stress.

Relationships

Family adaptation begins in the prenatal period and extends into the newborn period.

Perform assessment of risk and protective factors in family relationships (Table 7–2).

Evaluate for signs of domestic abuse, substance abuse, or child neglect or abuse.

Provide ideas for activities that promote family health and positive parent–newborn interaction

- Share newborn care activities. Recognize that you may do things differently than your partner, such as the way you change a diaper or give a bath, but, if the baby is cared for, safe, and secure, these differences in technique do not matter.
- Compliment one another on newborn caregiving strengths, such as the mother's ability to breastfeed and the partner's ability to calm the crying baby.
- Attend health supervision visits together as much as possible.
- Be sensitive to when your partner is overstressed and overtired. Ask how you can help, and then follow through with suggested activities. Sometimes listening is the most helpful thing you can do.
- Rest and take time for yourself. Make decisions about what must be done (paying bills, laundry, grocery shopping) and what could wait (traveling to visit grandparents, painting the house, cleaning closets). Accept help from family and friends.

Table 7–2   Risk and Protective Factors in Newborn and Family Relationships

Newborn Risk Factors	Newborn Protective Factors
Preterm birth, congenital disabilities, and chronic illness	Good health
Feeding and sleep problems	Normal eating, bowel, and sleep patterns
Fussing, crying, irritability, and difficulty consoling	Positive temperament
Diminished social interactions and responsiveness	Responds to parents' attention
Undernutrition, developmental delay	Normal growth and development

Parental Risk Factors	Parental Protective Factors
Baby unplanned and unwanted at birth; potential for neglect and/or rejection	Welcome baby at birth
Financial insecurity, homelessness, and lack of knowledge about how to care for newborn	Meet newborn's basic needs for food, shelter, clothing, and healthcare
Cannot promote strong nurturing environment owing to serious problems, such as abusive behavior, depression, mental illness, or substance abuse.	Provide a strong nurturing environment
Severe marital problems, absent parent, or frequent change of partners	Parents have strong relationship with one another, and share care of newborn
Lack of parenting skills, lack of parenting self-esteem, inability to cope with multiple roles, and inappropriate coping strategies	Strong self-esteem, developmental maturity, and knowledge of infant development
History of maltreatment as a child (risk increases with positive history)	No history of maltreatment as a child

- Discuss how you will raise your baby in a loving, supportive, and respectful environment.
- Discuss how you were raised and what you would like to be different in your new family. Learn about parenting strategies, and try out what feels comfortable for you.
- Keep in contact with family and friends. Maintain community ties that are important to you, such as social, religious, and cultural or recreational organizations or programs.
- Leave the baby with a trusted friend or family member, and take time to be alone once in a while. Talk about something other than the baby.
- Supervise siblings in their contacts with the newborn. Allow siblings to "help" care for the new baby in age-appropriate ways. Praise siblings for positive attention they give to the baby, and allow siblings to express their feelings about the new baby and changes in the family.

- Support one another in seeking and using community resources to strengthen parenting skills, such as classes and parenting groups.
- Cuddle, hold, and rock the baby as much as possible. Babies cannot be spoiled by too much attention.
- Take advantage of baby's time awake to play with baby. Singing, reading, and simply talking to the baby about what is happening provide developmental stimulation.

Injury and Disease Prevention

Assess parental knowledge of injury prevention strategies.

Promote healthy and safe habits by including teaching about proper and consistent use of an infant car seat and strategies to prevent falls, burns, choking, drowning, and suffocation (Table 7–3).

Table 7–3 Injury Prevention Topics for Newborns

Topic	Injury Prevention Teaching Topics
Car safety seat (AAP, 2004)	Choose an infant-only seat or a convertible seat suitable for an infant.
	Infant rides rear-facing until at least 1 year of age and >20 lb.
	The safest place for all children to ride is in the back seat. Never place a rear-facing car safety seat in the front seat with an active passenger airbag.
	Use a car safety seat every time the infant is in the car.
	Read and follow the manufacturer's instructions for the car safety seat and the vehicle owner's manual for installation information.
	Dress the infant in clothes that allow the straps to go between the legs. Never place blankets under the baby. Buckle the baby into the seat and place blankets over the baby.
	To make sure the car safety seat is installed correctly and the baby is positioned correctly, go to a car seat inspection station. A certified Child Passenger Safety (CPS) technician will assist you. Find a list of certified CPS technicians by state or zip code on the National Highway Traffic Safety Administration website at http://www.nhtsa.dot.gov/people/injury/childps/contacts. Find a car safety seat inspection station at http://www.nhtsa.dot.gov/people/injury/childps/cpsfitting or 1-866-SEAT-CHECK.
Shaken baby syndrome	Never shake a baby. Recognize that sometimes you will not be able to console your baby. Shaking a baby, even for only a few seconds, can cause serious brain damage and death. One of four shaken babies dies.
Crib	Use a safety approved crib. Slats should be no more than 2 3/8 in. apart. Mattress should be firm and fit snugly into the crib. Keep crib rails raised.

(continued)

Table 7–3 Injury Prevention Topics for Newborns (Continued)

Topic	Injury Prevention Teaching Topics
Co-sleeping	The AAP discourages co-sleeping because of the risk of sudden infant death syndrome (with overheating as a possible factor) and the danger of suffocation. Sleep with the baby nearby but not in the parental bed. If the parent must sleep with the baby, ensure that the infant is supine, separated from any soft surfaces such as pillows, and no blankets will cover the infant's head; beware of spaces between the mattress and the wall, headboard, or footboard; and do not sleep with the baby while under the influence of drugs or alcohol. The infant should never sleep in the same bed with siblings owing to the high risk of suffocation.
Baby toys	Use age-appropriate baby toys. Check toys for sharp edges or loose parts. Keep older siblings' toys out of baby's reach. Do not use toys with loops or string cords.
Drowning	Never leave baby alone in the bathtub. If you must turn your back on the baby or leave the room, take the baby out of the tub.
Suffocation	Keep plastic bags and wrappings away from baby (take the plastic bag off the crib mattress). Shake baby powder into your hand first then apply it so the baby does not inhale it. Do not allow a baby or sibling to play with a latex balloon. Keep small objects (e.g., safety pins, coins, and small toys) out of baby's reach. Do not attach pacifiers, medals, or other objects to the crib or to the baby's body with a string or cord. Do not put the crib near blinds, curtains, or anything with a hanging cord. Do not let baby wear clothing with strings near the neck (e.g., a sweatshirt hood that ties with a cord) or a headband that could slip down and wrap around baby's neck. Use a tight-fitting crib sheet that does not come loose when the corner is pulled.
Burns	Set the hot water heater thermostat lower than 120°F. Do not smoke or drink hot liquids while holding the baby. Do not microwave bottles of formula or breast milk due to uneven heating. Do not expose baby to direct sunlight.
Falls	Keep a hand on the baby while dressing or diaper changing on a surface other than on the floor. Never leave the baby unsupervised on any high surface, such as a bed, changing table, or sofa. Always keep one hand on the baby.
Pet safety	Keep some distance between the newborn and the pet until the pet's initial reaction to the new baby is assessed. Never leave the baby unsupervised with the family dog or cat or any animal capable of harming the newborn.

(continued)

Table 7-3   Injury Prevention Topics for Newborns (Continued)

Topic	Injury Prevention Teaching Topics
Sibling supervision	Never leave your baby alone with a young sibling. When young children hold the baby, seat the child on a large soft surface, such as the couch, and supervise closely. Watch siblings for aggressive behavior toward the newborn, such as hitting or biting. Siblings may take on a caregiving role and imitate adults; watch for "feeding" of nonfood items or choking hazards.
Fire safety	Install working smoke detectors on every floor of the house and in every sleeping area. Have a fire escape plan from your house and practice it.
Poisoning	Post the universal phone number for poison control near your telephone: 1-888-222-1222.
Gun safety	Keep any gun unloaded and locked up. Keep the ammunition locked up separately from the gun. Consider not keeping a gun in the household owing to safety hazards for family members.
In case of emergency	Know when and how to call your pediatric care provider. Know when it is appropriate to go to the emergency department. Take a first aid class and learn cardiopulmonary resuscitation for children and adults.

AAP, American Academy of Pediatrics.
Note: Adapted from American Academy of Pediatrics. (2004). Car safety seats: A guide for families 2004. Elk Grove Village, IL: American Academy of Pediatrics; S. F. Carbaugh. (2004). Understanding shaken baby syndrome. Advanced Neonatal Care, 4(2), 105–114; M. Green, & J. S. Palfrey (Eds.) (2002). Bright futures: Guidelines for health supervision of infants, children, and adolescents (2nd ed.). Arlington, VA: National Center for Education in Maternal and Child Health; S. P. Shelov (Ed.) (2002). Caring for your baby and young child: Birth to age 5. Elk Grove IL: American Academy of Pediatrics; and Safe Ride News Publications. (2004). Child restraints for newborn infants: A health care provider's guide. Seattle, WA: Safe Ride News Publications.

Be alert for the most common neonatal conditions that require extension of the newborn hospital stay or return to the hospital—conditions associated with bilirubin metabolism, prematurity (including respiratory distress), respiratory problems, infections, and birth defects (Owens, Thompson, Elixhauser, et al., 2003).

Integrate health maintenance activities for disease prevention into the visit

- Metabolic screening
- Hearing screening
- Eye examination
- Immunizations (hepatitis B is needed, with an additional injection of hepatitis B immune globulin if the mother is hepatitis B surface antigen–positive)

- Prevention of secondhand smoke exposure
- Sudden infant death syndrome risk reduction
- Formula safety
- Handwashing
- Minimizing the newborn's exposure to disease by avoiding infant exposure to large crowds, especially in cold and flu season; covering coughs and sneezes and using good handwashing technique; alerting baby's caregiver if newborn is exposed to varicella, pertussis, or other serious communicable disease

INFANT HEALTH PROMOTION AND HEALTH MAINTENANCE
General Observations

Who is bringing the baby in for care?

What are interactions like between the adults present or adults, other siblings, and the baby?

Is the baby awake or sleeping?

If awake, is the baby's body posture and alertness appropriate for age and developmental level?

Does the infant look well nourished and cared for?

Do the parents appear adequately rested, dressed, and of expected mental status?

Instruct parents to contact a provider if the child has

- Temperature ≥100.4°F (38.0°C)
- Seizure
- Skin rash, purplish spots, petechiae
- Change in activity or behavior that makes the parent uncomfortable
- Unusual irritability, lethargy
- Failure to eat
- Vomiting
- Diarrhea
- Dehydration
- Cough

(Green & Palfrey, 2002)

Growth and Developmental Surveillance

Measure length, weight, and chest and head circumference.

Plot findings on growth grids and evaluate percentiles (see Chapter 3).

Perform physical assessment (see Chapter 3).

Ask parents about care
- Skin, nails, bathing
- Nutritional intake
- Elimination patterns
- Sleep patterns
- Activity levels and developmental milestones
- Illnesses or health conditions

Recognize types of infant sleep
- Drowsy—flaccid posture, eyes slowly opening and closing, random movements
- Rapid eye movement or active sleep—body activity, eye movement with eyes open or closed, irregular respirations, sucking motions
- Non–rapid eye movement or quiet sleep—little body activity, eyes quiet, regular sucking motions, little motion

Recognize normal sleep patterns
- Birth–3 months—16 hours daily in five periods of 30 minutes to 3 hours; by 4–6 weeks of age, a consistent sleep pattern should emerge
- 3–6 months—14 hours daily with a longer sleep at night and two to three naps
- 6–12 months—12–14 hours daily with a longer sleep at night and one to two naps
  (Data from Green & Palfrey, 2002)

Provide teaching to promote healthy sleep patterns
- Place the baby to sleep in a quiet and darkened room.
- Have similar bedtime routines each night.
- Provide a consistent transitional object, such as a favorite blanket, each night.
- Put the baby to bed while still awake rather than after falling asleep nursing so he or she becomes accustomed to getting to sleep without nursing.
- Do not try to awaken the baby in non–rapid eye movement (quiet) sleep.
- Establish a regular sleep routine and time; routine may involve some cuddling and rocking time but should not be vigorous, stimulating play.
- For the baby who has trouble going to sleep, remain in the room for a few minutes but do not establish eye contact; place a hand on the abdomen or chest or gently hold flailing arms and legs.
  (Green & Palfrey, 2002; Jellinek et al., 2002; Mindell, 2003)

Perform recommended screening (Table 7–4).

Table 7–4   Screening during Infant Health Promotion and Health Maintenance Visits

Age	Recommended Screening Tests
1 month	Vision (follow objects, red reflex)
	Hearing (response to sound; screening by machine if not completed in the hospital)
	Physical examination with special attention to skin problems, hip dysplasia, foot position, and range of motion; mouth, abdomen, cardiac abnormality, tearing of eyes, neurologic (including child abuse), and anthropometric measurements
	Developmental milestones
	Dietary screening and stool/urine pattern assessment
	Review immunization record
2 months	As above
4 months	As above
	Vision (add cover-uncover test for strabismus)
6 months	As above
	Vision (add ability to follow object bilaterally, corneal light reflex)
	Physical examination with special attention to muscle tone, extremities, appearance of first teeth, tympanic membrane, and testicle descent for males
9 months	As above
	Lead exposure and levels if appropriate
	Anemia
	Physical examination with special attention to symmetry of movement
12 months	As above
	Tuberculosis test if indicated
	Physical examination with special attention to condition of teeth

Note: Data from M. Green, & J. S. Palfrey (Eds.) (2002). Bright futures: Guidelines for health supervision of infants, children, and adolescents (2nd ed.). Arlington, VA: National Center for Education in Maternal and Child Health.

Recognize growth and developmental milestones (Table 7–5).

Nutrition

Evaluate amount and type of feedings (breast and/or bottle).

Evaluate intake of table and finger foods.

Combine results of length and weight measurement with nutritional intakes.

Hematocrit taken during infancy, usually at 9–12 months to rule out iron deficiency anemia.

Table 7–5 Developmental Milestones Observed in Infant Health Promotion and Health Maintenance Visits

Age	Developmental Milestones
1 month	Responds to sound by startle or increased alertness Follows objects and human face with eyes Has periods of alertness and restfulness Comforted by touch or feeding by parent Has symmetrical movements and generally has arms and legs flexed Lifts head momentarily when prone
2 months	Above characteristics Makes noises, such as cooing, in response to interaction with adult Smiles Lifts head, neck, upper chest when prone Has increasing head control when held in sitting position
4 months	Increasing cooing and babbling Smiles, laughs, makes other noises during interactions Supports self on hands when prone Rolls front to back Touches objects and grasps rattle placed near hand
6 months	Uses sounds in repeated speech, such as bababa, dadadada Interested in surroundings and toys When pulled to sitting has no head lag Sits with support Grasps objects easily and places in mouth Transfers objects from one hand to other Bears weight on legs when held in standing position
9 months	Understands simple words and uses more sounds in babbling Responds to name Enjoys interactive games with parent Moves when placed on floor by crawling, creeping, or rolling repeatedly Sits without support Stands holding on to support Plays with toys Feeds self readily with fingers and tries to use cup
12 months	Has one or more words Imitates sounds readily Increasing interactions and interest in surroundings Follows directions, such as saying or waving bye Pulls to standing, walks a few steps holding on Well-developed pincer grasp Able to drink from cup

Table 7–6 Nutrition Teaching for Infant Health Promotion and Health Maintenance Visits

Age	Nutrition Teaching
1 month	Support breastfeeding efforts. Teach correct formula types and preparation if used. Teach burping and rate of feeding information. Suggest water during hot weather or if family wants to use a bottle at baby's bedtime. Encourage families to view feedings as social interactions; emphasize importance of holding the infant and not propping bottles.
2 months	Continue above. Review fluid needs of infants. Reinforce food safety for partially used bottles of breast milk or formula. Use warm water for heating bottles rather than microwave to avoid burning. Warn against feeding honey in the first year of life. Begin cleaning of infant gums daily. Provide information about any supplements needed (e.g., iron for premature infant, vitamin D for babies not exposed to adequate sunlight).
4 months	Continue above. Discuss introduction of first foods between 4 and 6 months, and surveillance for symptoms of allergy or intolerance. Discuss changing food patterns such as increasing amounts and decreasing numbers of daily milk feedings.
6 months	Continue above. Reinforce proper introduction of new foods, to include rice cereal, fruits, and vegetables. Discuss any unusual food reactions observed. Introduce cup for drinking. Introduce soft finger foods. Serve juice only in a cup and limit to no more than 6 oz. daily. Caution about common choking foods and items. Provide information about fluoride supplement if water supply is not fluoridated.
9 months	Continue above. If mother does not continue to breastfeed, teach family to use iron-fortified formula for the first year of life. Encourage self-feeding of finger foods, integrating common foods for the family. Introduce source of protein such as tofu, cheese, mashed beans, and slivers of meats.

(continued)

Table 7–6 Nutrition Teaching for Infant Health Promotion and Health Maintenance Visits (Continued)

Age	Nutrition Teaching
12 months	Continue above. Support mother who wishes to continue breastfeeding beyond 1 year of age. Encourage cups for all feedings other than breast.

Perform teaching to enhance nutrition (Table 7–6)

- Support breastfeeding.
- Ensure use of breast or iron-fortified formula.
- Teach recommended introduction of foods
  - Begin at 4–6 months.
  - Introduce one food at a time and wait 4–5 days before next food.
  - Start with rice cereal or other rice source; then vegetables and fruits; then meat, tofu, and other protein sources; and then finger foods by 7–9 months.

Physical Activity

Observe developmental milestones.

Ask parents about opportunities for crawling, reaching for toys, and other physical activity in daily routines.

Evaluate risk and protective factors for physical activity; plan interventions that enhance protective factors and alleviate risks (Table 7–7).

Table 7–7 Risk and Protective Factors Regarding Physical Activity in Infancy

Risk Factors	Protective Factors
Premature birth Delayed developmental milestones Limited stimulation by family or other care providers Lack of knowledge by family about infant's physical activity needs Limited community resources for families with infants	Meets developmental milestones at expected ages Has contact with parents, siblings, and others for significant time each day A supportive environment with room to play safely; stimulating surroundings Physically active family Family knowledge about infant's physical activity needs Community programs that promote physical activity in infants and information for families

Note: Data from K. Patrick, B. Spear, K. Holt, & D. Sofka (Eds.) (2001). Bright futures in practice: Physical activity. Arlington, VA: National Center for Education in Maternal and Child Health.

Perform teaching to enhance health

- Frequent and supervised play opportunities are needed.
- Holding the infant in various positions, helping the older infant to stand, and providing positive feedback for the infant's accomplishments are encouraged.
- Toys should be placed near child to encourage movement.
- Participation in parent–infant playgroups provides stimulation for the child, provides social interaction with other infants, and increases the parent's knowledge of the child's abilities.
- Discussion of the next fine and gross motor skills anticipated. (Patrick, Spear, Holt, et al., 2001)

Oral Health

Count number of teeth.

Ask about teething patterns and discomfort.

Teach healthy oral health and hazards of bottles at bedtime.

Ask about accessibility to dental care, and provide resources as needed.

Mental and Spiritual Health

The baby's mental health is related to early experiences; inborn characteristics, such as temperament and resilience; and relationships with caregivers.

Children who feel secure and have nurturing environments usually grow as expected and perform milestones at usual times.

Slow growth and delayed development are sometimes related to feeding disorder of infancy and early childhood.

Stranger anxiety is manifested by crying when exposed to new people and indicates expected attachment to parents; common in second half of the first year of life.

Also in the second half of the first year of life, infants may exhibit **separation anxiety** by inconsolable crying and other signs of distress when parents are not present.

Self-regulation is the process of dealing with feelings, learning to soothe self, and focusing on activities for increasing periods of time. Infants learn early how to comfort and calm themselves.

Observe and ask about how parents provide comfort to the crying baby. Suggestions to enhance comforting measures include

- Offer a breastfeeding or bottle feeding, especially if the last feeding was more than 2 hours earlier.

- If feeding was recent, hold the baby in a sitting position and rub or pat the back to help expel gastric gas.
- Change the diaper if wet or soiled.
- Place a hand on the abdomen and feel for movement. If movement or passing gas is present, hold the baby against the chest, walk slowly, and pat the back.
- Swaddle the baby securely in a blanket and hold horizontally while rocking.
- Hold the baby on your lap, secure the hands in yours, and talk softly.
- Never shake or throw the baby, no matter how long the crying. Call your healthcare provider for suggestions if you feel like nothing works, and you are very frustrated.

Relationships

Social relationships are foundational to the psychosocial health of infants.

Temperament characteristics of the infant interact with the environment and other people. Common patterns of temperament include
- Easy (moderate activity, easy to console, regular sleep and eating patterns)
- Slow to warm up (slow adaptation to new events and people or to changes in environment and schedule)
- Difficult (high activity, difficult to console, irregular sleep and eating patterns)

Assess social skills
- Smiling
- Cooing and other sounds, words
- Response to siblings and other children
- Sleep patterns
- Childcare arrangements, playgroups

Suggest activities to parents that foster infant relationship formation
- Encourage parents to hold, read to, and talk to babies. Positively reinforce these behaviors when observed.
- Point out the infant's abilities to respond to faces and voices, to smile and laugh, and to reflect the mood of adults in the home.
- Review sleep patterns and make recommendations for methods to plan bedtime routines.
- Be sure that parents have resources to turn to when needing assistance with infant care or other household responsibilities.

Evaluate problems in relationships

- **Domestic violence** is a situation in which parents or adult care providers commit violent acts toward one another. Assess for domestic violence, and refer to appropriate resources.
- **Child abuse** interferes with the formation of healthy relationships. See mental health chapter (Chapter 25) for assessment and interventions related to child abuse.

Injury and Disease Prevention

Car seats for infants

Review the family's routines for transporting an infant by car at every health supervision visit. Recommendations for infants from birth to 1 year, or 2–22 lb, include

- Use only "infant-only" or rear-facing convertible seat.
- The seat must always be placed in the back seat in the rear-facing position.
- Harness straps should be at or below shoulder level.
- Be sure to follow guidelines for every trip, no matter how short.
- Have car seat and car checked at examiner station and evaluated for correct technique.
- If car seat is changed between two or more cars, it should be checked for proper installation in each car.
  [Guidelines from National Highway Traffic Safety Administration (http://www.nhtsa.dot.gov)]

Perform safety teaching (Table 7–8).

Table 7–8   Injury Prevention Topics for Infancy by Age

Age	Injury Prevention Teaching Topics
1 month	Infant car safety seat.
	Put baby to sleep on back.
	Avoid loose bedding and toys in crib.
	Avoid tobacco use in the environment.
	Provide adult supervision of the baby at all times by trusted individuals.
	Test bath water temperature and never leave baby alone in the bath.
	Never place baby on high objects, such as counter, table, or bed; always keep one hand on the baby during activities like diaper changes to prevent falling.
	Wash hands correctly and often, especially before feeding or holding infant, and after providing hygiene care.
	Avoid contact with persons with communicable diseases.
	Have smoke alarms, and avoid fire hazards.

(continued)

Table 7-8 Injury Prevention Topics for Infancy by Age (Continued)

Age	Injury Prevention Teaching Topics
1 month (*continued*)	Learn infant cardiopulmonary resuscitation and airway obstruction removal. Never shake the baby. Have plans for emergency care.
2 months	As above. Use only recommended playpens or cribs and keep sides up. Avoid moldy environments. Keep baby toys cleaned. Avoid direct sunlight for the baby. Keep sharp and small objects out of baby's environment. Keep hot water heater lower than 120°F. Review emergency plan with all care providers.
4 months	As above. Get all poisonous substances out of baby's view and reach; install locks to keep them inaccessible. Do not use latex balloons or plastic bags near the baby.
6 months	As above. If an infant-only car seat was used, switch to rear-facing convertible safety seat (intended for babies up to 40 lb) when baby is 20–30 lb or 26 in. Empty containers of water immediately after use; be sure pools or other bodies of water are locked and not accessible to baby. Use sunscreen, hat, and long sleeves when baby is in the sun. Keep heavy and sharp objects out of reach; check that all poisons are locked away, including in homes visited; keep pet food and cosmetics out of reach. Do not drink hot liquids or eat soup while holding the baby. Have poison control number by phones and programmed into cell phones. Be alert for dangers of hot curling irons and other appliances. Have electrical cords out of reach and not hanging down. Have home and environment checked for lead hazards. Lower infant crib mattress if still in upper position. Install gates and guards on stairs and windows. Never use an infant walker.
9 months	As above. Crawl on the floor and look for hazards at baby's eye level. Pad sharp corners on tables and other furniture. Watch for tables, chairs, and other devices the baby may use for climbing to unsafe places.

(continued)

Table 7–8 Injury Prevention Topics for Infancy by Age (Continued)

Age	Injury Prevention Teaching Topics
12 months	As above.
	Change to forward facing car safety seat if baby is at least 20 lb; install correctly and have installation checked; place in back seat and never in front seat with a passenger air bag.
	Start teaching the child to wash hands frequently, showing how.
	Provide own personal items, such as clothing and blankets, to child care providers; wash often.
	Change batteries in home smoke alarms and check system.
	Turn handles to back of stove; use back rather than front burners; watch for hot liquids.
	Check care provider setting for safety hazards.
	Remember that responsible adults should always supervise your infant, not other children.
	Peruse home once again for hazards now that the child is more active, climbing, and walking.

Note: Adapted from M. Green, & J. S. Palfrey (Eds.) (2002). Bright futures: Guidelines for health supervision of infants, children, and adolescents (2nd ed.). Arlington, VA: National Center for Education in Maternal and Child Health.

Administer needed immunizations (Table 7–9).

TODDLER AND PRESCHOOLER HEALTH PROMOTION AND HEALTH MAINTENANCE
General Observations

Observe for signs of independence and reliance on parents.

Look at independence from adults in ambulation.

Does the parent respond to the child's questions?

Table 7–9 Routine Immunizations Recommended during Infancy

Immunization	Age Recommended
Hepatitis B	After birth up to 2 months (No. 1)
	1–4 months (No. 2)
	6–18 months (No. 3)
Diphtheria, tetanus, pertussis	2, 4, and 6 months (three doses)
Haemophilus influenzae type b (HIB)	2, 4, and 6 months [three doses; third dose is not needed if PRP-OMP (PedvaxHIB or Comvax) are used for primary series]
Inactivated poliovirus	2, 4, and 6–18 months (three doses)
Pneumococcal	2, 4, and 6 months (three doses)

PRP-OMP, polyribosylribitol phosphate–outer membrane protein.

Were age-appropriate toys or activities brought to the visit to help occupy the child while waiting?

Is the child observant of the environment and alert?

Direct greetings or questions to the child to evaluate stranger anxiety and ability to understand simple commands or questions.

What verbal skills are observed?

Comment positively about a child's traits, and encourage parents to share thoughts about the child.

Recognize that the mental health of the parents influences the environment in which the child is growing and learning, so inquire about how the family is adjusting to the growing child, and ask about the health and development of other children.

Growth and Developmental Surveillance
Measure head circumference until approximately 2 years of age.

Measure recumbent length (until approximately 2–3 years) or standing height (once the child can stand well) and weight.

Calculate body mass index, and place all measurements on growth grids (see Chapter 4).

Perform physical assessment (see Chapter 3). Engage child by games, and leave intrusive procedures until last. Perform needed surveillance tests (Table 7–10).

Ask about daily life and care, such as sleeping and eating patterns, bowel movements, dental care, skin care, play patterns and toys, social interactions, and illnesses that have occurred.

Perform developmental surveillance (Table 7–11).

Instruct parents about developmental progression, and perform anticipatory guidance for skills to be learned by the child soon.

Nutrition
Analyze growth patterns.

Perform nutritional assessment and dietary recall.

Ask about weaning and introduction of foods; all major food groups should be present in the diet.

Ask specific questions about dietary intake.

Perform nutrition teaching to enhance health. Topics may include dietary needs of young children, limitation of fast-food intake, food

Table 7–10 Screening during Toddler and Preschooler Health Promotion and Health Maintenance Visits

Age	Recommended Screening Tests
15 months	Vision
	Hearing
	Anemia (if not previously done)
	Tuberculosis (if at risk)
	Teeth present and condition
	Physical examination with special attention to skin, gait, bruising, and other signs of possible abuse
	Developmental milestones
	Dietary screening
	Review immunization record
18 months	As above
2–3 years	As above
	Language development
	Lead exposure risk
	Hyperlipidemia risk
3–4 years	As above
	Blood pressure
	Behavioral abnormalities
4–5 years	As above
	Dental malocclusion problems

Note: Adapted from M. Green, & J. S. Palfrey (Eds.) (2002). Bright futures: Guidelines for health supervision of infants, children, and adolescents (2nd ed.). Arlington, VA: National Center for Education in Maternal and Child Health.

preparation and safety, avoidance of foods that can cause choking, and importance of family meals. See Table 7–12.

Physical Activity

Evaluate type and amount of physical activity.

Assess motor development and coordination.

Suggestions for the family may include setting guidelines to limit television and other screen activities to a maximum of 2 hours daily to facilitate adequate physical activity time; children should not have a television and computer in their bedrooms. See Table 7–13 for risk and protective factors regarding physical activity.

Oral Health

Evaluate teeth for condition and number. By approximately 2 years of age, the toddler has a full set of 20 teeth. The first primary tooth is lost at approximately 6 years of age.

Table 7–11 Developmental Milestones Observed during Health Promotion and Health Maintenance Visits of Toddlers and Preschoolers

Age	Developmental Milestones
12 months	Walking alone or with help Enjoys social games and interactions Speaks one to three words and understands simple commands Drinks from cup and feeds self
15 months	Walks by self, crawls or walks up stairs Stacks two blocks Points to one or more body parts Increasingly interactive Explores environment
18 months	Walks with ease Pushes or pulls toy Stacks three or more blocks Uses spoon to eat, spilling often Follows directions and uses 15–20 words
2–3 years	Goes up and down steps Kicks ball Scribbles and draws lines on paper Imitates words and actions of adults
3–4 years	Jumps Rides tricycle Draws precise lines on paper; attempts to imitate circle, line, and cross Always feeds self Dresses self, although sometimes clothes are backward Has friends and plays with others
4–5 years	Recites rhymes and songs States name Draws a rudimentary person Builds tower of blocks and bridges with blocks Throws ball overhand

Inquire about dental visits. By 1 year of age, the child should have made a first visit to the dentist with continuing visits every 6 months.

Observe for caries or poor dental health. **Early childhood caries** is defined as one or more decayed, missing, or filled tooth surfaces in a child younger than 5 years of age (American Academy of Pediatric

Table 7–12   Nutrition Teaching for Toddler and Preschooler Health Promotion and Health Maintenance Visits

Age	Nutrition Teaching
1 year	Support mother who continues to breastfeed. Wean child from bottle by substituting cup. If beginning to use cow's milk, use whole milk. Limit juice to 4–6 oz. daily; offer water several times daily. Encourage safety measures—use high chair with strap, secure child and use caution in grocery carts, and do not allow foods to be eaten in car. Provide information on choking and airway obstruction removal training. Provide food and water safety guidelines. Be sure all major food groups have been introduced. Limit high-fat and high-sugar foods. Review amounts of food commonly consumed and frequency of feedings. Review use of fluoride if water supply is not fluoridated.
2 years	Encourage total removal of bottle if still in use. Ensure that all foods common to family have been offered. Offer child-sized eating utensils. Child can change to low-fat or skim milk if family desires. Limit milk to two servings daily. Teach parents methods for dealing with temper tantrums over food—make food available at meal and snack times only, do not force intake, and offer a variety of foods. Teach that child may have days of very low intake due to slowing growth rate.
3 years	Teach normal intake and decreasing number of snacks. Engage child in food preparation and pouring liquids from small pitcher. Recognize that **food jags** (periods when only one or two foods are eaten) are common. Recognize importance of the social nature of eating; expect child to sit for a short period at meals with family. Meals and snacks should not be eaten while watching television.
4 years	Encourage involving child in snack selection and preparation. Start to teach food groups and importance of nutrition for the body. Alter intake as appropriate depending on weight and body mass index. Dairy products consumed should all be low or reduced fat.

Table 7–13 Risk and Protective Factors Regarding Physical Activity in Toddlerhood and Preschool

Risk Factors	Protective Factors
Limited stimulation by family or other care providers	Expected developmental progression
Long work hours by parents	Daily contact with other young children
Parents who have little physical activity on a daily basis	Easily engaged socially with others
Limited social time with other children	Eagerness to try new physical activity
Limited access to balls, slides, balance beams, tricycles, and other materials that foster physical activity	Access to balls, slides, balance beams, tricycles, and other materials that foster physical activity
Adequate safety gear for activities is not available	Adequate safety gear that properly fits child is available
Reluctance to try new physical activity	Family members engage in daily physical activity
Television or other screen activities are engaged in for >2 hours daily	Family members spend time daily in physical activity with child
Developmental delay	Family understands motor developmental milestones and importance of physical activity in childhood
Slow development of social skills	Television and other screen activities are limited to ≤2 hours daily
Lack of knowledge by family about child physical activity needs	Neighborhood contains access to child care that integrates physical activity
Limited community resources for child care and physical activity	Neighborhood is safe and contains lawns, parks, and other facilities
Unsafe neighborhood and lack of lawns, parks, and other facilities	

Note: Adapted from K. Patrick, B. Spear, K. Holt, & D. Sofka (Eds.) (2001). Bright futures in practice: Physical activity. Arlington, VA: National Center for Education in Maternal and Child Health.

Dentistry, 2000). Refer the child with early childhood caries for dental care. Assist the family without dental insurance to locate dental programs for young children.

What is the source of your drinking water? Do you know if it is fluoridated? If not, does your child take fluoride? How much? How often?

Describe how your child's teeth get brushed and how often? Do you use toothpaste? What type? How much? Is it hard for you to afford toothbrushes?

How much juice or sweetened drinks does your child have each day? Is a bottle or cup used for drinking? How many sweet foods, such as candy, gum, cookies, cake, and doughnuts, are eaten daily?

Teach the child and family dental care techniques, and provide access to toothpaste, a toothbrush, and referrals for care as needed.

Provide teaching as needed about fluoride, healthy food intake, and weaning from bottle.

Mental and Spiritual Health

Do parents communicate readily with the child?

Are interactions generally warm, caring, and loving, or are there constant criticisms of behavior?

Does the parent seem willing to point out the child's accomplishments, or have trouble making any positive statements about the child?

Does the child appear at ease with the parent? Is the child at ease in the healthcare setting? (Toddlers often still have some stranger anxiety and may show discomfort, while preschoolers are more often eager and excited to meet you.)

The child's sense of self and mental status are related to new accomplishments. Inquire about toilet training, tooth brushing, choosing clothes and getting dressed, using crayons, or other developmental tasks.

Ask about how the parent deals with the child who is having a temper tantrum or showing other undesirable behaviors. Reinforce positive ways of helping the child set limits for self and make suggestions when parents need assistance.

Ask about sleep patterns. Most toddlers have established regular sleeping patterns with occasional night awakenings. They sleep approximately 10–12 hours at night with one or two daytime naps. The preschooler sleeps approximately 9–11 hours and may have one or no naps each day (Murray & Zentner, 2001).

Relationships

Families with members who handle stress well and have healthy lifestyle patterns offer security for the young child.

Ask how things are going for the family in general. Inquire about siblings and whether there are any issues of concern that might influence the toddler or preschooler.

Ask about discipline techniques and whether there has been violence in the family or neighborhood.

Identify strengths in the family
- Family time together each day
- Parents proud of child's accomplishments and knowledgeable about developmental progression
- Childcare center personnel and family members interact regularly to plan consistent approaches for the toddler and preschooler
- Teen mother of toddler enrolled in high school continuation program with childcare component

Identify risks to health
- Mother has been diagnosed with depression
- Uncle in home uses street drugs
- Child awakens with night terrors
- Child was recently in a serious car accident
- Teen mother is estranged from own family and has few goals and resources

Observe play patterns
- Toddlers often engage in parallel play, or side-by-side play.
- Preschoolers begin associating with other children in play and engage in dramatic play.

Assess language and communication ability, temperament, and social interactions with others.

Suggest activities that can assist in the child's development of social skills
- Talk with and read to the child daily.
- Ensure interactions with other children and adults.
- Consider a preschool as opportunity to socialize and learn interactional skills.
- Understand the child's temperament, and structure the environment to maximize learning within the child's characteristics.

Injury and Disease Prevention
Car seats for toddlers and preschoolers
- Car safety needs reinforcing as the types of seats change when the child reaches 20 and then 40 lb. Be certain that children from 20 to 40 lb
  - Use a convertible forward-facing seat that has been placed in the back seat
  - Have harness straps at or above the shoulders

- Children more than 40 lb should be placed in a belt-positioning booster seat
  - In the back seat
  - That uses both lap and shoulder belts
  - With the lap belt low and tight across the lap/upper thigh area and shoulder belt snug across the chest and shoulder
- Recommend that parents have their car seat checked by a childcare inspector. Give them the addresses of the closest inspection stations, which you can locate by going through the National Highway Traffic Safety Administration (http://www.nhtsa.dot.gov).

Assess safety hazards, and perform safety teaching (Table 7–14).

Administer needed immunizations (Table 7–15).

Table 7–14   Disease and Injury Prevention Topics for Toddlers and Preschoolers by Age

Age	Injury Prevention Teaching Topics
15 months	Wash adult and toddler hands frequently.
	Clean toys with soap and water regularly.
	Provide child's own bedding for childcare setting, and wash weekly.
	Use forward-facing car safety seat if child is 20 lb; install correctly and have installation checked; place in back seat and never in front seat with a passenger air bag.
	Empty containers of water immediately after use; be sure pools or other bodies of water are locked and not accessible.
	Use sunscreen, hat, and long sleeves in the sun.
	Keep heavy and sharp objects out of reach; check that all poisons are locked away, including in homes visited; keep pet food and cosmetics out of reach.
	Have poison control number by phones and programmed into cell phones.
	Be alert for dangers of hot curling irons and other appliances.
	Have electrical cords out of reach and not hanging down.
	Keep water temperature from being too hot to touch.
	Have home environment checked for lead hazards.
	Secure the child in shopping carts.
	Do not let child have access to alcoholic drinks.
	Remember that responsible adults should always supervise your child, not other children.
	Know cardiopulmonary resuscitation (CPR), airway obstruction removal, and other first aid.

(continued)

Table 7–14   Disease and Injury Prevention Topics for Toddlers and Preschoolers by Age (Continued)

Age	Injury Prevention Teaching Topics
18 months	As above.
	Bolt heavy objects that might be pulled down securely to the wall.
	Be cautious of the toddler near machinery in the yard, such as lawn mowers and farm equipment.
	Use a helmet on the child when taking on the back of a bicycle.
	Check batteries in home smoke alarms and check system.
	Ask care providers about discipline methods; do not allow corporal punishment.
2–3 years	As above.
	When the child is 40 lb, switch to a belt-positioning booster seat, using vehicle lap and shoulder belt; place in rear seat.
	Teach handwashing after toileting and other activities.
	Clean potty chair thoroughly.
	Keep guns unloaded and locked away in a different locked place than ammunition; have trigger locks installed.
	Teach how to cross streets.
	Provide a helmet for riding tricycles.
	Check playgrounds for safety hazards and hard surfaces under equipment.
3–4 years	As above.
	Do not let child play unsupervised.
	Know CPR, airway obstruction removal, and other first aid for the child who has become a preschooler.
4–5 years	As above.
	Continue teaching safety skills to the child.
	Continue supervising when near streets and water sources.
	Teach safety around strangers (never go with a stranger; find a trusted person like parent or police).

Note: Adapted from M. Green, & J. S. Palfrey (Eds.) (2002). Bright futures: Guidelines for health supervision of infants, children, and adolescents (2nd ed.). Arlington, VA: National Center for Education in Maternal and Child Health.

Table 7–15 Routine Immunizations Recommended during Toddlerhood and Preschool Age

Immunization	Age Recommended
Hepatitis B	6–18 months (administer No. 3 if series not completed during infancy)
Diphtheria, tetanus, pertussis	15–18 months (No. 4) 4–6 yrs (No. 5)
Haemophilus influenzae type b	12–15 months (No. 4 or will be No. 3 for PRP-OMP type that requires only three doses for whole series)
Inactivated poliovirus	4–6 years (No. 4)
Measles, mumps, rubella	12–15 months (No. 1)
Varicella	12–18 months (only 1 dose needed at this age)
Pneumococcal	12–15 months (No. 4)

PRP-OMP, polyribosylribitol phosphate–outer membrane protein.
Note: Schedule may need to be adapted if child did not receive all recommended immunizations during infancy. See Centers for Disease Control and Prevention and American Academy of Pediatrics for recommended catch-up schedules (http://www.cdc.gov and http://www.aap.org).

Ask about occurrence of acute diseases, and reinforce with teaching as needed.

Evaluate any chronic conditions, refer to resources as needed, and adjust health promotion visit to meet the child's needs.

SCHOOL-AGE CHILD HEALTH PROMOTION AND HEALTH MAINTENANCE
General Observations

The child should walk showing symmetry and ease of movement, follow instructions about where to go and taking off shoes for weighing, and demonstrate clear language skills with parent or healthcare personnel.

Observe whether the child brought a book, toy, or some other object to the visit.

How are the parents interacting with the child? What types of speech tones are used?

Is there mutual respect, or are parents and the child ignoring each other or having disagreements?

Does the child communicate readily and at age level?

Is the child appropriately dressed? Adequately nourished? Well rested and alert?

Ask the child to describe a typical day to obtain clues about daily life.

Growth and Developmental Surveillance

Measure height and weight, calculate body mass index, and evaluate percentiles on growth grids.

Perform physical assessment (see Chapter 3). Explain what you are doing and why: "I'm listening to your heart with this stethoscope and counting how many times it beats in a minute. Have you heard your heart? When have you noticed it beating hard?"

Concentrate on skills that influence performance in school. Vision, hearing, muscular strength, and coordination are examples of areas that impact school performance.

Inquire about injuries, illnesses, and health practices.

Perform recommended screening tests (Table 7–16).

Direct observations, history questions, and questionnaires that parents complete are methods for developmental surveillance. See Table 7–17 for expected developmental milestones during school age.

Perform teaching to enhance sleep patterns, knowledge of normal growth and development patterns, and use of community resources.

Table 7–16   Screening during School-Age Health Promotion and Health Maintenance Visits

Age	Recommended Screening Tests	
5 years	Vision Hearing Lead exposure risk Anemia	Hyperlipidemia risk Blood pressure Urinalysis Tuberculosis (if at risk)
6–8 years	Vision Hearing Lead exposure risk	Hyperlipidemia risk Blood pressure Tuberculosis (if at risk)
8–10 years	Vision Hearing Hyperlipidemia risk	Blood pressure Tuberculosis (if at risk)
10–12 years	Vision Hearing Hyperlipidemia risk	Blood pressure Tuberculosis (if at risk)

Note: Adapted from M. Green, & J. S. Palfrey (Eds.) (2002). Bright futures: Guidelines for health supervision of infants, children, and adolescents (2nd ed.). Arlington, VA: National Center for Education in Maternal and Child Health.

Table 7–17 **Developmental Milestones Observed during Health Promotion and Health Maintenance Visits of School-Age Children**

Age	Developmental Milestones
5 years	Independent in bathroom and dressing activities Ties shoes, buttons Runs well, jumps, may skip, balances on one foot 10 seconds Pours fluids well, uses hands to catch ball Prints some letters, first name Draws triangle, square, three- to five-part person Knows full name, address, phone
6–8 years	Skilled in physical activities, such as running, skipping, jumping, hopping Learns to ride bicycle Can cut, paste, write all letters Reads
8–10 years	Has increasingly longer periods of concentration for both physical activity and school or other quiet activity Can throw objects far and with accurate aim Increased coordination Develops hobbies, such as model building, musical instrument, video production, building with wood, needle work
10–12 years	Fine and gross motor skills similar to adult in ability Writes well, adept at computer use Some clumsiness may develop as prepubertal growth spurt begins

Nutrition

Recognize that children are increasingly independent in food choices. They may come home alone and prepare snacks. Vending machines are often available at schools.

Evaluate nutritional patterns because habits are being formed that will impact nutrition and health in general in the years to come. Good choices help to promote health—to maintain weight at a recommended level, provide nutrients for adequate growth and activity, and prevent onset of some chronic diseases. On the other hand, poor choices can lead to being overweight and its accompanying problems—lack of adequate calcium and resultant osteoporosis, eating disorders, or lack of energy for brain growth and optimal performance in school.

Integrate some questions for the parent and child into the visit that provide clues about diet.

Plan nursing interventions to enhance knowledge about foods, family participation in good nutritional practices, and access to healthy foods.

Physical Activity

Observe developmental milestones and coordination.

Ask about participation in school and community sports and other types of physical activity.

Evaluate risk and protective factors for physical activity; plan interventions that enhance protective factors and alleviate risks (Table 7–18).

Table 7–18   **Risk and Protective Factors Regarding Physical Activity in School-Age Children**

Risk Factors	Protective Factors
Limited role modeling of daily physical activity by parents and other family members	Expected developmental skill level
	Feels self confident in ability and physical appearance
Limited facilities in the neighborhood to encourage activity, such as parks, skate board facilities, rinks, and ball courts	Willing to try new activities
	Sets goals for learning physical skills
	Parents exercise daily and exercise with the child some of this time in setting the child can see
Inadequate financial resources to join clubs or pay for organized sports	
School cuts to physical education programs and recess	Parents set expectation that everyone in family will choose a physical activity and engage in it regularly
School tryouts for sports that eliminate all but the best players in certain sports	Schools provide physical education each day with a variety of offerings; student gets to choose and set goals for some of activities
Reluctance to try new activity	Schools schedule recess or physical activity breaks twice daily
Worry about competence and physical appearance	Sports teams are leveled so that all students desiring to play a particular sport, such as soccer, are able to do so
Television viewing or other screen activities for >2 hours daily	Adequate safety gear that properly fits child is available
Developmental delay and special needs	Neighborhood provides access to parks, skate board facilities, rinks, ball courts, and other facilities
	Family has adequate financial resources to pay for health club or organized sports
	Television viewing and other screen activities limited to ≤2 hours daily

Note: Adapted from K. Patrick, B. Spear, K. Holt, & D. Sofka (Eds.) (2001). Bright futures in practice: Physical activity. Arlington, VA: National Center for Education in Maternal and Child Health.

Perform teaching to enhance health

- Encourage participation of parents and siblings in physical activity to serve as role models.
- Help the child to identify interests for activity, and refer to community resources as needed.
- Encourage parent participation in schools to urge for daily physical education for all children.
- Assist in planning and adapting activities for the child who has a physical disability.

Oral Health

Evaluate number and condition of primary and secondary teeth.

Evaluate oral care and access to dental professionals.

Assess intake of snacks with sugar/carbohydrates.

Reinforce teaching for dental hygiene—brushing, flossing, and care of braces.

Refer to dental professionals if needed.

Mental and Spiritual Health

Assess the child's self-concept and all of its facets by observing the child and asking questions that provide clues to the child's view of self. Ask about school activities, sports, interests, and what the family does together. Observe for prepubertal physical growth and development. Ask about exposure to screen (television, game) activities and violence in the neighborhood, family, or school. Ask the child whether bullying occurs at school.

Be observant for and ask parents about any concerns that might signal mental illness—high levels of stress, unusual reactions to events, mood swings, anxiety, depression, eating disorder.

Perform teaching as needed
- Expected body changes
- Need for friends and meaningful activities
- Continuing need for adequate rest and sleep

Relationships

The family remains an important anchor while peers become increasingly important to self-identity.

Ask about family members and peers with whom the child interacts regularly.

Ask children about how they handle disagreements.

Consider the child's temperament, and work with the family to adapt the environment to best support individual characteristics (i.e., a quiet study place for a child who has difficulty studying, several activities for the child who thrives on socializing with others).

Suggest activities to enhance relationships

- Encourage regular family activities.
- Ensure parents know families of friends and where the child is spending time.
- Foster the parent's active involvement in the child's school.

Injury and Disease Prevention

Evaluate correct use of car safety system for age and size.

Ask about injuries that have occurred, and adapt teaching to address prevention.

Examine safety risks and perform safety teaching (Table 7–19).

Table 7–19   Injury Prevention Topics for School-Age Children

Age	Injury Prevention Teaching
5–8 years	Use a booster seat, properly positioned in the back seat of the car; use lap and shoulder belts.
	Never place the child in a front car seat with a passenger air bag.
	Be sure the child knows how to swim and works on these skills regularly.
	Protect the child with sunscreen when outside.
	Check smoke alarms, and keep them in proper function.
	Have an escape plan in case of fire in the home.
	Keep poisons, electrical appliances, and fire starters locked.
	Keep firearms unloaded and locked; store ammunition in separate locked location; have trigger locks installed on guns; keep dangerous knives locked.
	Provide protective gear for bicycling and other activities, and insist that it be worn.
	Teach safety precautions for bicycling and other activities.
	Teach safety with strangers.
	Provide list of people a child can approach if feeling threatened by touch or other experience.
	Choose care providers carefully; occasionally pick up child earlier than expected; ask policies about discipline and do not leave child with someone who uses corporal punishment.
	Be sure the child knows emergency numbers, names, and plans.

(continued)

Table 7–19   Injury Prevention Topics for School-Age Children (Continued)

Age	Injury Prevention Teaching
5–8 years (continued)	Review carefully any hazardous event that has occurred with the child, and summarize what was done correctly and how response could be improved.
	Limit screen time to 2 hours daily; do not allow violent games or viewing.
	Review behavior with strangers regularly such as not getting in cars and not engaging in phone or internet conversations.
8–10 years	Continue to reinforce other teaching described above, including the child in teaching fully, and enlarging responsibility to the child with increasing age.
	Car booster seat used until child sits upright against back seat with bent knees over edge of seat; insist on use of lap and shoulder belts.
	Do not place child in front seat of car with a passenger air bag.
	Do not allow child to operate power tools or machinery.
10–12 years	Continue to reinforce teaching described above.
	Parents and child should attend class on cardiopulmonary resuscitation and airway obstruction removal.
	Avoid high noise levels, such as when listening to music through earphones.

Note: Adapted from M. Green, & J. S. Palfrey (Eds.) (2002). Bright futures: Guidelines for health supervision of infants, children, and adolescents (2nd ed.). Arlington, VA: National Center for Education in Maternal and Child Health.

Be sure the child uses helmet and other safety gear for sports.

Evaluate for signs of disease or problems, such as frequent illness, bruising, fatigue, pain, vision or hearing problems, headaches, lack of coordination, or changes in school or other performance.

Immunizations are generally up to date for school-age children. However, some children may have missed earlier doses due to illness or missed healthcare visits. Evaluate the immunization record to be sure it meets all recommendations. Some of the most common immunization needs at this time are

- Hepatitis B (whole series or a missed third shot)
- Hepatitis A (if in state with recommendation for immunization)
- Tetanus-diphtheria, polio, or measles-mumps-rubella (if booster dose was not given before school entry)
- Varicella, if not given earlier and the child has not had the disease
- Certain vaccines for children at high risk, such as pneumococcal, influenza, meningococcal

Evaluate the general health and condition of children with chronic healthcare needs.

Intervene to perform necessary screening for disease, and teach to promote health.

ADOLESCENT HEALTH PROMOTION AND HEALTH MAINTENANCE
General Observations
As you call the adolescent back for care, observe whether parents or friends are present, or if the teen is alone. Watch to see if a parent or friend is present and if that person comes with the teen when called. If someone comes with the teen, be alert that you may need to provide some private time by asking the other person to wait outside for a moment. Reassure the parents that you will talk with them about any of their concerns and questions. Provide them with an opportunity to ask questions and get information also.

Be alert, quiet, and sensitive in working with adolescents. Initial observations guide the interaction with the teen. Someone who appears nervous needs a confident reassuring approach. Provide privacy for issues that may be sensitive, such as weighing the overweight teen or providing information on birth control.

Observe clothing, hygiene, nutritional status, appearance of being rested or fatigued, and social skills.

Growth and Developmental Surveillance
Measure height and weight, calculate body mass index, and evaluate percentiles on growth grids.

Perform physical assessment (see Chapter 3). Some particular parts of the examination to include for teens are scoliosis screening; sexual maturity rating (Tanner stages); breast examination; testing for sexually transmitted diseases (among those sexually active); pelvic examination and pap smear (for sexually active females); hematocrit for anemia annually in menstruating adolescents; hearing screening at 12, 15, and 18 years; blood pressure annually; lipid screening for those with family history of early heart disease or other risk factors; and tuberculosis screening for those in high-risk areas. See Table 7–20 for a summary of health assessments.

Sexually active teens should be screened annually for

- Chlamydia
- Gonorrhea
- Trichomoniasis

Table 7–20   Screening during Health Promotion and Health Maintenance Visits of Adolescents

Age	Recommended Mental Health/Behavioral Screening	Recommended Physical Health Screening Tests
11–14 years	Use of tobacco and alcohol History of abuse Unsatisfactory school performance History of depression or other mental health problems History of violence or risk taking History of multiple personal or family stresses Loneliness or lack of friends	Vision Hearing Anemia Lipids Blood pressure Urinalysis Tuberculosis (if at risk) Pap smear (for sexually active females) Breast examination Sexually transmitted disease risks
15–17 years	As above	As above
18–21 years	As above Difficulty with job	As above Offer pelvic examination for all females even if not sexually active

Note: Adapted from M. Green, & J. S. Palfrey (Eds.) (2002). Bright futures: Guidelines for health supervision of infants, children, and adolescents (2nd ed.). Arlington, VA: National Center for Education in Maternal and Child Health.

- Human papilloma virus
- Herpes simplex virus
- Bacterial vaginosis

Teens should be screened for syphilis and/or human immunodeficiency virus/acquired immunodeficiency syndrome if requesting testing or meeting any of these criteria:

- History of sexually transmitted infections
- More than one sexual partner in past 6 months
- Intravenous drug use
- Sexual intercourse with a partner at risk
- Sex in exchange for drugs or money
- Homelessness
- Males—sex with other males
- Syphilis—residence in areas where disease is prevalent
- Human immunodeficiency virus/acquired immunodeficiency syndrome—blood or blood product transfusion before 1985
  (From Green & Palfrey, 2002)

Integrate questions pertinent to the adolescent years and teaching throughout the health promotion/health maintenance visit.

Nutrition

Although nutrition is important, a fast lifestyle and focus on eating with peers can provide dietary challenges; high-caloric and -fat intake and inadequate calcium, iron, and zinc are frequent.

Perform nutritional assessments and identify teaching needs.

Plan interventions that involve teaching
- Getting five fruits and vegetables daily
- Including whole grain products to replace refined products whenever possible
- The importance of eating three meals each day, including breakfast and lunch
- Eating together as a family several times weekly, which enhances quality food intake
- How to plan menus and prepare foods for balanced intake
- Limiting refined sugar and high-fat intake (e.g., soft drinks and fried foods) to maintain weight at recommended level
- Including two to three servings of dairy products daily to enhance bone formation and decrease chance of osteoporosis as an adult
- Using resources for treatment of eating disorders if they are identified

Physical Activity

Physical activity decreases as youth progress through the adolescent years.

Inquire about frequency and length of moderate and vigorous exercise, including school- and community-based sports, as well as other activities.

Ask whether the school requires daily physical activity.

Identify risk and protective factors for physical activity (Table 7–21).

Teach importance of 20–60 minutes of moderate to vigorous physical activity daily for mental and physical health.

Assist the teen to identify meaningful activity that can be performed regularly.

Oral Health

Ask about oral hygiene practices.

Examine number and condition of teeth.

Table 7–21   Risk and Protective Factors Regarding Physical Activity in Adolescence

Risk Factors	Protective Factors
Lives in isolated setting with little opportunity for contact with other teens	Has opportunities for participation in physical activity at home, at school, and in the community
Has a developmental disability that impairs physical movement	Likes physical activity
Does not like physical activity	Has exercised during all of childhood, often with parents
Has a pattern and history of low activity levels	Knowledgeable about benefits of activity; committed to maintaining exercise patterns
Is overweight	
Does not feel competent in most sports	Has many friends living close who participate in physical activity
Limited financial resources to pay registration fees or buy protective gear for sports	Youth and parents agree to a limit of 2 hours daily of screen time
Family members who have little physical activity	Availability of financial and other resources for sports gear and protective equipment
Parents who are not active in school sports and committees	Parents participate in regular physical activity and encourage the adolescent to do so also
Parents who do not like physical activity and have had low levels while their teen was growing up	Neighborhood and community provide physical activity options
Parents who have little time or facilities for exercise or always exercise at a club out of view of their family	Public policies maintain parks, green spaces, biking trails, and playgrounds
Lack of youth and parent knowledge about physical activity needs and benefits	Programs are available for adolescents with developmental disabilities or other healthcare needs
Lack of neighborhood programs for physical activity promotion	
Presence of neighborhood hazards and unsafe areas	

Note: Adapted from M. Green, & J. S. Palfrey (Eds.) (2002). Bright futures: Guidelines for health supervision of infants, children, and adolescents (2nd ed.). Arlington, VA: National Center for Education in Maternal and Child Health.

Reinforce need for daily brushing and flossing and dental appointments every 6 months.

Fluoride supplements may be discontinued by approximately 14 years.

Refer for dental care if resources are needed.

Mental and Spiritual Health

Self-concept, self-esteem, and self-regulation remain key to mental health formation.

Ask about meaningful activities and about disappointments and how they were handled.

Evaluate body image and sexuality.

Ask about discipline and interactions with parents.

Encourage parents to
- Gradually increase the teen's independence. If there is success with growing responsibility, the teen may be ready for more. If the teen misuses independence (perhaps by staying out too late, having a party at home without parents present, lying about location on an evening out), there should be clear limits and loss of privilege.
- Be willing to talk with and hear the teen's story. On the other hand, do not be talked out of consequences for the teen's bad decisions.
- Recognize that driving a car, staying out late, and other activities are not a given. They are privileges for responsibility displayed.
- Comment on a teen's behavior rather than making belittling comments about them as a person.
- Realize that the teen is establishing independence and that the relationship will change. Be consistent and loving as your adolescent tries out and learns about limits and the self.

Evaluate for signs of depression, substance abuse, or other mental health problems. See Table 7–22 for common signs. Refer teen for treatment when needed.

Many teens do not get recommended hours of sleep. Make the following recommendations:
- Try to keep to similar hours for sleeping so your body is accustomed to them.
- Avoid caffeine in the late afternoon and evening.

Table 7–22 Signs of Depression and Substance Abuse in Adolescents

Depression	Substance Abuse
Changes in behavior, school performance, sleep, and appetite	Changes in behavior, school performance, sleep, and appetite
Physical complaints	Accidents and other unexplained events
Loss of interest in usual activities	Lack of responsibility
Difficulty in motivating self and setting goals	Labile mood and attitude
Change in friends	Hopelessness
Feelings of worthlessness	Depression
Consideration of death or suicide	Feelings of ambivalence
	A variety of physical changes depending on the substance

Note: Adapted from M. Jelinek, B. P. Patel, & M. C. Froehle (Eds.) (2002). Bright futures in practice: Mental health (Vols. I & II). Arlington, VA: National Center for Education in Maternal and Child Health.

- Do homework early, and relax a bit before going to bed.
- Plan 1 day each weekend to simply relax and have few demands on your time.

Ask about meaning in life, and refer to spiritual resources as needed.

Relationships

Parents are sources of guidance and reassurance, while increasingly close ties emerge with friends.

Assess type and quality of relationships with friends.

Ask about family relationships.

Be alert for signs of domestic abuse.

Some helpful tips for adolescents include

- Most teens get frustrated with their parents at times; list some things you like and some you don't like about your family.
- Be sure to focus complaints on specific issues like wanting a later curfew rather than telling your parents they don't know anything.
- Most parents, like kids, want to know what they do right; tell your parents occasionally things that are going well or that you appreciate.
- Talk to your parents; if you don't feel you can, find another adult you respect, like an older sibling, a teacher, counselor, or clergy.

Injury and Disease Prevention

Injury is the greatest health hazard for adolescents, so injury prevention must be integrated into every health contact with youth.

The major hazard is automobile crashes. Inquire about seat belt use and driving practices.

Motorcycles, four-wheelers, boats, jet skis, farm machinery, and tools are other sources of injury. Ask about the youth's exposure, and teach about avoiding alcohol and drug use, use of safety gear and precautions to be employed.

Review the teen's activities and injury hazards, such as falls, burns, accidental shooting, extreme sports, and date violence.

Teach about hazards and protective measures.

Teens are generally healthy and may be seen only rarely in health-care. Some common problems include

- Acne and skin infections
- Body piercing and tattooing
- Sports overuse injuries

- Constipation and diarrhea
- Dental problems

Other observations may signal more serious health concerns and need to be referred for further evaluation. Some examples include

- Scoliosis
- Anemia
- Excessive tiredness
- Bruising
- Sexually transmitted diseases
- Eating disorder
- Abuse or severe bullying

Perform teaching about disease prevention measures, such as weight control, avoidance of smoking, and use of sunscreen (Table 7–23).

Table 7–23   Injury Prevention Topics for Adolescents

Topic	Teaching
Driving	Always wear seat and shoulder belt.
	Do not drink and drive or ride with others who do.
	Do not talk on a cell phone as you drive.
	Do not drive when you are tired.
	Drive with parents or other adults for several months in winter driving conditions if you live where there is snow, ice, or heavy rains.
	Keep your car in good repair.
Sun	Wear sunscreen.
	Limit time outside especially early in summer.
Machinery	Learn how to use power tools correctly.
	Always have someone near when you use tools or machinery.
Emergency care	Learn first aid, cardiopulmonary resuscitation, and airway obstruction removal.
Water safety	Learn to swim well.
	If you supervise younger children near water, never leave them alone, even for a minute.
Fires	Do not play with fire.
	Follow guidelines to avoid igniting gasoline.
	Test smoke alarms in your house every 6 months, and change batteries annually.

(continued)

Table 7–23   Injury Prevention Topics for Adolescents (Continued)

Topic	Teaching
Firearms	Know and follow rules to keep firearms locked with ammunition locked in a separate place.
	Never take out a gun to show a friend unless your parent is also present.
	Take firearm safety classes if you hunt or target shoot.
Hearing	Avoid loud music especially for long periods and through ear phones.
Sports	Wear protective gear recommended for your sport.
Abuse	Report any abuse to an adult you trust.
	Date with other couples whenever possible, and report date rape.
	Do not drink or take drugs.

Note: Adapted from M. Green, & J. S. Palfrey (Eds.) (2002). Bright futures: Guidelines for health supervision of infants, children, and adolescents (2nd ed.). Arlington, VA: National Center for Education in Maternal and Child Health.

Many adolescents have not had immunizations since approximately school-entry time, so their record should be carefully reviewed. Some questions to ask to determine immunizations needed by adolescents include

- When was the last tetanus-diphtheria booster? It is recommended every 10 years if no wounds have required an update in the interim. So, if the child received it at age 5 years, a booster is needed at 15 years.
- Was a second measles-mumps-rubella administered? A second dose may not have been routine when teens were younger, so they may need it now.
- Is hepatitis A common in your state? If so, the teen needs to get that vaccine.
- Has the youth had hepatitis B vaccine? This is important for all youth, and some may not have received it as infants.
- Did the youth have a clear history of varicella disease? If not, the vaccine is needed.

8. Immunization Schedules

RECOMMENDED CHILDHOOD IMMUNIZATION SCHEDULE—UNITED STATES, JULY–DECEMBER, 2005

Vaccines are listed under the routinely recommended ages. Bars indicate range of acceptable ages for vaccination. Shaded bars indicate *catch-up vaccination* (Centers for Disease Control and Prevention, National Immunization Program).

Recommended Childhood and Adolescent Immunization Schedule UNITED STATES • 2005

Vaccine ▼ / Age ▶	Birth	1 month	2 months	4 months	6 months	12 months	15 months	18 months	24 months	4–6 years	11–12 years	13–18 years
Hepatitis B[1]	HepB #1	HepB #2			HepB #3						HepB Series	
Diphtheria, Tetanus, Pertussis[2]			DTaP	DTaP	DTaP		DTaP	DTaP		DTaP	Td	Td
Haemophilus influenzae type b[3]			Hib	Hib	Hib	Hib						
Inactivated Poliovirus			IPV	IPV	IPV	IPV				IPV		
Measles, Mumps, Rubella[4]						MMR #1				MMR #2	MMR #2	
Varicella[5]						Varicella				Varicella	Varicella	
Pneumococcal Conjugate[6]			PCV	PCV	PCV	PCV	PCV		PCV	PPV	PPV	
Influenza[7]						Influenza (Yearly)				Influenza (Yearly)	Influenza (Yearly)	
Hepatitis A[8]										Hepatitis A Series	Hepatitis A Series	

. . . . . . Vaccines below red line are for selected populations . . . . . .

This schedule indicates the recommended ages for routine administration of currently licensed childhood vaccines, as of December 1, 2004, for children through age 18 years. Any dose not administered at the recommended age should be administered at any subsequent visit when indicated and feasible. ▨ Indicates age groups that warrant special effort to administer those vaccines not previously administered. Additional vaccines may be licensed and recommended during the year. Licensed combination vaccines may be used whenever any components of the combination are indicated and other components of the vaccine

are not contraindicated. Providers should consult the manufacturers' package inserts for detailed recommendations. Clinically significant adverse events that follow immunization should be reported to the Vaccine Adverse Event Reporting System (VAERS). Guidance about how to obtain and complete a VAERS form is available at www.vaers.org or by telephone, 800-822-7967.

▨ Range of recommended ages   ▨ Only if mother HBsAg(−)
▨ Preadolescent assessment   ▨ Catch-up immunization

DEPARTMENT OF HEALTH AND HUMAN SERVICES
CENTERS FOR DISEASE CONTROL AND PREVENTION

The Childhood and Adolescent Immunization Schedule is approved by:
Advisory Committee on Immunization Practices www.cdc.gov/nip/acip
American Academy of Pediatrics www.aap.org
American Academy of Family Physicians www.aafp.org

1. **Hepatitis B (HepB) vaccine.** All infants should receive the first dose of HepB vaccine soon after birth and before hospital discharge; the first dose may also be administered by age 2 months if the mother is hepatitis B surface antigen (HBsAg) negative. Only monovalent HepB may be used for the birth dose. Monovalent or combination vaccine containing HepB may be used to complete the series. Four doses of vaccine may be administered when a birth dose is given. The second dose should be administered at least 4 weeks after the first dose, except for combination vaccines which cannot be administered before age 6 weeks. The third dose should be given at least 16 weeks after the first dose and at least 8 weeks after the second dose. The last dose in the vaccination series (third or fourth dose) should not be administered before age 24 weeks.

   Infants born to HBsAg-positive mothers should receive HepB and 0.5 mL of hepatitis B immune globulin (HBIG) at separate sites within 12 hours of birth. The second dose is recommended at age 1–2 months. The final dose in the immunization series should not be administered before age 24 weeks. These infants should be tested for HBsAg and antibody to HBsAg (anti-HBs) at age 9–15 months.

   Infants born to mothers whose HBsAg status is unknown should receive the first dose of the HepB series within 12 hours of birth. Maternal blood should be drawn as soon as possible to determine the mother's HBsAg status; if the HBsAg test is positive, the infant should receive HBIG as soon as possible (no later than age 1 week). The second dose is recommended at age 1–2 months. The last dose in the immunization series should not be administered before age 24 weeks.

2. **Diphtheria and tetanus toxoids and acellular pertussis (DTaP) vaccine.** The fourth dose of DTaP may be administered as early as age 12 months, provided 6 months have elapsed since the third dose and the child is unlikely to return at age 15–18 months. The final dose in the series should be given at age ≥4 years. **Tetanus and diphtheria toxoids (Td)** is recommended at age 11–12 years if at least 5 years have elapsed since the last dose of tetanus and diphtheria toxoid-containing vaccine. Subsequent routine Td boosters are recommended every 10 years.

3. ***Haemophilus influenzae* type b (Hib) conjugate vaccine.** Three Hib conjugate vaccines are licensed for infant use. If PRP-OMP (PedvaxHIB® or ComVax® [Merck]) is administered at ages 2 and 4 months, a dose at age 6 months is not required. DTaP/Hib combination products should not be used for primary immunization in infants at ages 2, 4, or 6 months but can be used as boosters after any Hib vaccine. The final dose in the series should be administered at age ≥12 months.

Section II: Nursing Care in the Community/Hospital

4. Measles, mumps, and rubella vaccine (MMR). The second dose of MMR is recommended routinely at age 4–6 years but may be administered during any visit, provided at least 4 weeks have elapsed since the first dose and both doses are administered beginning at or after age 12 months. Those who have not previously received the second dose should complete the schedule by age 11–12 years.

5. Varicella vaccine. Varicella vaccine is recommended at any visit at or after age 12 months for susceptible children (i.e., those who lack a reliable history of chickenpox). Susceptible persons aged ≥13 years should receive 2 doses administered at least 4 weeks apart.

6. Pneumococcal vaccine. The heptavalent **pneumococcal conjugate vaccine (PCV)** is recommended for all children aged 2–23 months and for certain children aged 24–59 months. The final dose in the series should be given at age ≥12 months. **Pneumococcal polysaccharide vaccine (PPV)** is recommended in addition to PCV for certain high-risk groups. See *MMWR* 2000;49(RR-9):1-35.

7. Influenza vaccine. Influenza vaccine is recommended annually for children aged ≥6 months with certain risk factors (including, but not limited to, asthma, cardiac disease, sickle cell disease, human immunodeficiency virus [HIV], and diabetes), healthcare workers, and other persons (including household members) in close contact with persons in groups at high risk (see *MMWR* 2004;53[RR-6]:1-40). In addition, healthy children aged 6–23 months and close contacts of healthy children aged 0–23 months are recommended to receive influenza vaccine because children in this age group are at substantially increased risk for influenza-related hospitalizations. For healthy persons aged 5–49 years, the intranasally administered, live, attenuated influenza vaccine (LAIV) is an acceptable alternative to the intramuscular trivalent inactivated influenza vaccine (TIV). See *MMWR* 2004;53(RR-6):1-40. Children receiving TIV should be administered a dosage appropriate for their age (0.25 mL if aged 6–35 months or 0.5 mL if aged ≥3 years). Children aged ≤8 years who are receiving influenza vaccine for the first time should receive 2 doses (separated by at least 4 weeks for TIV and at least 6 weeks for LAIV).

8. Hepatitis A vaccine. Hepatitis A vaccine is recommended for children and adolescents in selected states and regions and for certain high-risk groups; consult your local public health authority. Children and adolescents in these states, regions, and high-risk groups who have not been immunized against hepatitis A can begin the hepatitis A immunization series during any visit. The 2 doses in the series should be administered at least 6 months apart. See *MMWR* 1999;48(RR-12):1-37.

CATCH-UP SCHEDULE FOR CHILDREN AGED 4 MONTHS THROUGH 6 YEARS

Vaccine	Minimum Age for Dose 1	Minimum Interval Between Doses				
		Dose 1 to Dose 2	Dose 2 to Dose 3	Dose 3 to Dose 4	Dose 4 to Dose 5	
Diphtheria, Tetanus, Pertussis	6 wks	**4 weeks**	**4 weeks**	**6 months**	**6 months**[1]	
Inactivated Poliovirus	6 wks	**4 weeks**	**4 weeks**	**4 weeks**[2]		
Hepatitis B[3]	Birth	**4 weeks**	**8 weeks** (and 16 weeks after first dose)			
Measles, Mumps, Rubella	12 mo	**4 weeks**[4]				
Varicella	12 mo					
***Haemophilus influenzae* type b**[5]	6 wks	**4 weeks** if first dose given at age <12 months **8 weeks (as final dose)** if first dose given at age 12–14 months **No further doses needed** if first dose given at age ≥15 months	**4 weeks**[6] if current age <12 months **8 weeks (as final dose)**[6] if current age ≥12 months and second dose given at age <15 months **No further doses needed** if previous dose given at age ≥15 mo	**8 weeks (as final dose)** This dose only necessary for children aged 12 months–5 years who received 3 doses before age 12 months		
Pneumococcal Conjugate[7]	6 wks	**4 weeks** if first dose given at age <12 months and current age <24 months **8 weeks (as final dose)** if first dose given at age ≥12 months or current age 24–59 months **No further doses needed** for healthy children if first dose given at age ≥24 months	**4 weeks** if current age <12 months **8 weeks (as final dose)** if current age ≥12 months **No further doses needed** for healthy children if previous dose given at age ≥24 months	**8 weeks (as final dose)** This dose only necessary for children aged 12 months–5 years who received 3 doses before age 12 months		

CATCH-UP SCHEDULE FOR CHILDREN AGED 7 YEARS THROUGH 18 YEARS

Vaccine	Minimum Interval Between Doses		
	Dose 1 to Dose 2	Dose 2 to Dose 3	Dose 3 to Booster Dose
Tetanus, Diphtheria	4 weeks	6 months	**6 months[8]** if first dose given at age <12 months and current age <11 years **5 years[8]** if first dose given at age ≥12 months and third dose given at age <7 years and current age ≥11 years **10 years[8]** if third dose given at age ≥7 years
Inactivated Poliovirus[9]	4 weeks	4 weeks	IPV[2,9]
Hepatitis B	4 weeks	8 weeks (and 16 weeks after first dose)	
Measles, Mumps, Rubella	4 weeks		
Varicella[10]	4 weeks		

Children and Adolescents Catch-up Schedules UNITED STATES · 2005

Footnotes

1. **DTaP.** The fifth dose is not necessary if the fourth dose was administered after the fourth birthday.

2. **IPV.** For children who received an all-IPV or all-oral poliovirus (OPV) series, a fourth dose is not necessary if third dose was administered at age ≥4 years. If both OPV and IPV were administered as part of a series, a total of 4 doses should be given, regardless of the child's current age.

3. **HepB.** All children and adolescents who have not been immunized against hepatitis B should begin the HepB immunization series during any visit. Providers should make special efforts to immunize children who were born in, or whose parents were born in, areas of the world where hepatitis B virus infection is moderately or highly endemic.

4. **MMR.** The second dose of MMR is recommended routinely at age 4–6 years but may be administered earlier if desired.

5. **Hib.** Vaccine is not generally recommended for children aged ≥5 years.

6. **Hib.** If current age <12 months and the first 2 doses were PRP-OMP (PedvaxHIB® or ComVax® [Merck]), the third (and final) dose should be administered at age 12–15 months and at least 8 weeks after the second dose.

7. **PCV.** Vaccine is not generally recommended for children aged ≥5 years.

8. **Td.** For children aged 7–10 years, the interval between the third and booster dose is determined by the age when the first dose was administered. For adolescents aged 11–18 years, the interval is determined by the age when the third dose was given.

9. **IPV.** Vaccine is not generally recommended for persons aged ≥18 years.

10. **Varicella.** Administer the 2-dose series to all susceptible adolescents aged ≥13 years.

For additional information about vaccines, including precautions and contraindications for immunization and vaccine shortages, please visit the National Immunization Program Web site at www.cdc.gov/nip or call
800-CDC-INFO / 800-232-4636
(English or Spanish)

Recommendations for Immunization of Children and Adolescents with Primary and Secondary Immune Deficiencies

Category	Specific Immunodeficiency	Vaccine Contraindications	Effectiveness and Comments
Primary			
B-lymphocyte (humoral)	X-linked and common variable agammaglobulinemia	OPV,[a] vaccinia, and live bacteria; consider measles and varicella	Effectiveness of any vaccine dependent on humoral response is doubtful; IGIV interferes with measles and possibly varicella response.
	Selective IgA deficiency and selective subclass IgG deficiency	OPV,[a] other live vaccines seem to be safe, but caution is urged	All vaccines probably effective. Vaccine response may be attenuated.
T-lymphocyte (cell-mediated and humoral)	Severe combined	All live vaccines[b,c]	Effectiveness of any vaccine dependent on humoral or cellular response is doubtful.
Complement	Deficiency of early components (C1, C4, C2, C3)	None	All routine vaccines probably effective. Pneumococcal and meningococcal vaccines recommended.
	Deficiency of late components (C5–C9), properdin, factor B	None	All routine vaccines probably effective. Meningococcal vaccine recommended.
Phagocytic function	Chronic granulomatous disease Leukocyte adhesion defect Myeloperoxidase deficiency	Live bacterial vaccines[c]	All routine vaccines probably effective. Inactivated influenza vaccine should be considered to decrease secondary infection

(continued)

Recommendations for Immunization of Children and Adolescents with Primary and Secondary Immune Deficiencies (Continued)

Category	Specific Immunodeficiency	Vaccine Contraindications	Effectiveness and Comments
Secondary			
	HIV/AIDS	OPV,[a] vaccinia, BCG; withhold MMR and varicella in severely immunocompromised children	MMR, varicella, and all inactivated vaccines, including influenza, may be effective.[d]
	Malignant neoplasm, transplantation, immunosuppressive or radiation therapy	Live viral and bacterial, depending on immune status[b,c]	Effectiveness of any vaccine depends on degree of immune suppression.

AIDS, acquired immunodeficiency syndrome; BCG, bacille Calmette–Guérin; IgA, immunoglobulin A; IgG, immunoglobulin G; IGIV, immunoglobulin intravenous; HIV, human immunodeficiency virus; MMR, measles-mumps-rubella; OPV, oral poliovirus.

[a]OPV vaccine no longer is recommended for routine use in United States.

[b]Live viral vaccines: MMR, OPV, varicella, vaccinia (smallpox). Smallpox vaccine is not recommended for children.

[c]Live bacterial vaccines: BCG and Ty21a *Salmonella typhi* vaccine.

[d]HIV-infected children should receive immunoglobulin after exposure to measles and may receive varicella vaccine if CD4+ lymphocyte count = 25%.

Note: From Committee on Infectious Diseases. (2003). Redbook. Elk Grove Village, IL: American Academy of Pediatrics, with permission.

Suggested Intervals between Immune Globulin Administration and Measles Immunization (Measles-Mumps-Rubella or Monovalent Measles Vaccine)

Indication for Immunoglobulin	Route	Dose Units or mL	Dose mg IgG/kg	Interval, Month[*]
Tetanus (as TIG)	IM	250 Units	Approximately 10	3
Hepatitis A prophylaxis (as IG)				
Contact prophylaxis	IM	0.02 mL/kg	3.3	3
International travel	IM	0.06 mL/kg	10	3
Hepatitis B prophylaxis (as HBIG)	IM	0.06 mL/kg	10	3
Rabies prophylaxis (as RIG)	IM	20 Units/kg	22	4
Measles prophylaxis (as IG)				
Standard	IM	0.25 mL/kg	40	5
Immunocompromised host	IM	0.50 mL/kg	80	6
Varicella prophylaxis (as VZIG)	IM	125 Units/10 kg (maximum 625 Units)	20–39	5
RSV prophylaxis (palivizumab monoclonal antibody)	IM	—	15 mg/kg	None
Blood transfusion				
Washed RBCs	IV	10 mL/kg	Negligible	0
RBCs, adenine-saline added	IV	10 mL/kg	10	3
Packed RBCs	IV	10 mL/kg	20–60	5
Whole blood	IV	10 mL/kg	80–100	6
Plasma or platelet products	IV	10 mL/kg	160	7

(continued)

Suggested Intervals between Immune Globulin Administration and Measles Immunization (Measles-Mumps-Rubella or Monovalent Measles Vaccine) (Continued)

Indication for Immunoglobulin	Route	Dose Units or mL	Dose mg IgG/kg	Interval, Month*
Replacement (or therapy) of immune deficiencies (as IGIV)	IV	—	300–400	8
ITP (as IGIV)	IV	—	400	8
RSV-IGIV	IV	—	750	9
ITP	IV	—	1,000	10
ITP or Kawasaki syndrome	IV	—	1,600–2,000	11

HBIG, hepatitis B immunoglobulin; IG, immunoglobulin; IgG, immunoglobulin G; IGIV, immunoglobulin intravenous; ITP, immune (formerly termed "idiopathic") thrombocytopenic purpura; MMR, measles-mumps-rubella; RBCs, red blood cells; RIG, rabies immunoglobulin; RSV, respiratory syncytial virus; RSV-IGIV, respiratory syncytial virus IGIV; TIG, tetanus immunoglobulin; VZIG, varicella-zoster immunoglobulin.

*These intervals should provide sufficient time for decreases in passive antibodies in all children to allow for an adequate response to measles vaccine. Physicians should not assume that children are fully protected against measles during these intervals. Additional doses of IG or measles vaccine may be indicated after exposure to measles.

Note: From Committee on Infectious Diseases. (2003). Redbook. Elk Grove Village, IL: American Academy of Pediatrics, with permission.

National Childhood Vaccine Injury Act
Vaccine Injury Table, 2005

Vaccine	Adverse Event	Time Interval
Tetanus toxoid–containing vaccines (e.g., DTaP, Tdap, DTP-Hib, DT, Td, TT)	Anaphylaxis or anaphylactic shock	0–4 hr
	Brachial neuritis	2–28 days
	Any acute complication or sequela (including death) of above events	Not applicable
Pertussis antigen–containing vaccines (e.g., DTaP, Tdap, DTP, P, DTP-Hib)	Anaphylaxis or anaphylactic shock	0–4 hr
	Encephalopathy (or encephalitis)	0–72 hr
	Any acute complication or sequela (including death) of above events	Not applicable
Measles, mumps, and rubella virus–containing vaccines in any combination (e.g., MMR, MR, M, R)	Anaphylaxis or anaphylactic shock	0–4 hr
	Encephalopathy (or encephalitis)	5–15 days
	Any acute complication or sequela (including death) of above events	Not applicable
Rubella virus–containing vaccines (e.g., MMR, MR, R)	Chronic arthritis	7–42 days
	Any acute complication or sequela (including death) of above event	Not applicable
Measles virus–containing vaccines (e.g., MMR, MR, M)	Thrombocytopenic purpura	7–30 days
	Vaccine-strain measles viral infection in an immunodeficient recipient	0–6 months
	Any acute complication or sequela (including death) of above events	Not applicable
Polio live virus–containing vaccines (OPV)	Paralytic polio	
	In a non-immunodeficient recipient	0–30 days
	In an immunodeficient recipient	0–6 months
	In a vaccine associated community case	Not applicable
	Vaccine-strain polio viral infection	
	In a non-immunodeficient recipient	0–30 days
	In an immunodeficient recipient	0–6 months
	In a vaccine-associated community case	Not applicable

(continued)

National Childhood Vaccine Injury Act
Vaccine Injury Table, 2005 (Continued)

Vaccine	Adverse Event	Time Interval
Polio live virus–containing vaccines (*continued*)	Any acute complication or sequela (including death) of above events	Not applicable
Polio inactivated virus–containing vaccines (e.g., IPV)	Anaphylaxis or anaphylactic shock	0–4 hr
	Any acute complication or sequela (including death) of above event	Not applicable
Hepatitis B antigen–containing vaccines	Anaphylaxis or anaphylactic shock	0–4 hr
	Any acute complication or sequela (including death) of above event	Not applicable
Haemophilus influenzae (type b polysaccharide conjugate vaccines)	No condition specified for compensation	Not applicable
Varicella vaccine	No condition specified for compensation	Not applicable
Rotavirus vaccine	No condition specified for compensation	Not applicable
Vaccines containing live, oral, rhesus-based rotavirus	Intussusception	0–30 days
	Any acute complication or sequela (including death) of above event	Not applicable
Pneumococcal conjugate vaccines	No condition specified for compensation	Not applicable
Any new vaccine recommended by the Centers for Disease Control and Prevention for routine administration to children, after publication by Secretary, HHS of a notice of coverage		

DT, diphtheria-tetanus; DTaP, diphtheria, tetanus, and acellular pertussis; DTP, diphtheria, tetanus, and pertussis; DTP-Hib, DTP-*Haemophilus influenzae* type b; HHS, Department of Health and Human Services; IPV, inactivated poliovirus vaccine; M, measles; MMR, measles-mumps-rubella; MR, measles-rubella; OPV, oral polio vaccine; P, pertussis; R, rubella; Td, tetanus-diphtheria; Tdap, tetanus, diphtheria, acellular pertussis vaccine; TT, tetanus toxoid.
Note: Effective date: July 1, 2005.
Note: From Health Resources and Services Administration. (2005). National Childhood Vaccine Injury Act vaccine injury table. http://www.hrsa.gov/osp/vicp/table.htm, accessed 7/30/2005, with permission.

VACCINE ADVERSE EVENT REPORTING SYSTEM

To report an adverse event, download the reporting form from www.vaers.org. The report can be submitted by internet or by fax.

Approaches to the Evaluation and Immunization of Internationally Adopted Children

Vaccine	Recommended Approach	Alternative Approach
Hepatitis B	Serologic testing for hepatitis B surface antigen	—
Diphtheria and tetanus toxoids and acellular pertussis (DTaP)	Immunize with DTaP, with serologic testing for specific IgG antibody to tetanus and diphtheria toxins in the event of a severe local reaction to first dose	Children whose records indicate receipt of three or more doses: serologic testing for specific IgG antibody to diphtheria and tetanus toxins before administering additional doses or administer a single booster dose of DTaP, followed by serologic testing after 1 month for specific IgG antibody to diphtheria and tetanus toxins with reimmunization as appropriate
Haemophilus influenzae type b	Age-appropriate immunization	—
Poliovirus	Immunize with inactivated poliovirus vaccine (IPV)	Serologic testing for neutralizing antibody to poliovirus types 1, 2, and 3 (limited availability) or administer single dose of IPV followed by serologic testing for neutralizing antibody to poliovirus types 1, 2, and 3
Measles-mumps-rubella (MMR)	Immunize with MMR or obtain measles antibody, and, if positive, give MMR for mumps and rubella protection	Serologic testing for IgG antibody to vaccine viruses indicated by immunization record
Varicella	Age-appropriate immunization of children who lack reliable history of previous varicella disease or serologic evidence of protection	—
Pneumococcal	Age-appropriate immunization	—

IgG, immunoglobulin G.
Note: From Centers for Disease Control and Prevention. (2002). General recommendations on immunization. Recommendations of the Advisory Committee on Immunization Practices and the American Academy of Family Physicians. Morbidity and Mortality Weekly Report Recommendation Reports, 51(RR-2), 1–35.

9. PEDIATRIC DOSAGE CALCULATIONS

I. Principles of Pediatric Dosages
   A. Solutions
      1. Intravenous (IV) flow rates are most frequently calculated in microdrops in pediatrics. For all companies, 60 microdrops = 1 mL of solution. Note the number of drops (gtt) required to administer 1 mL of IV fluid using tubing manufactured by different companies.

Company	Number of Drops (gtt/1 mL)
Baxter	10
Lifeline	10
Travenol	10
Abbot	15
Braun/McGaw	15
All companies	60 microgtt (mcgtt) = 1 mL

Flow rate is calculated using the following formula:

$$\text{Drops/minute} = \frac{\text{Total volume ordered} \times \text{gtt/mL}}{\text{Total infusion time (minutes)}}$$

For example, if 250 mL of fluid were to be administered by microdrop over 3 hours, the drops per minute would be calculated as follows:

$$\text{Drops/minute} = \frac{250 \times 60}{180}$$

$$= \frac{15,000}{180}$$

$$= 83.3$$

The IV flow rate in this example would be adjusted to administer 83 drops/minute.

      2. When microdrip tubing is used, because 60 drops = 1 mL and there are 60 minutes in an hour, the

formula to use is drops/minute = mL/hour. For example, if a child needed 250 mL to be delivered in 6 hours, the problem would be calculated as follows:

$$\frac{250 \text{ mL}}{6 \text{ hours}} = 41.67 \text{ mL/hour}$$

Therefore, the rate is set at 42 drops/minute.

3. IV pumps are generally used in pediatrics. Regulation of dosage is easier and safer with use of these pumps. Pumps usually calculate the required flow rate in milliliters per hour. So, if 500 mL of IV fluid needed to be delivered in 8 hours

$$\frac{500 \text{ mL}}{8 \text{ hours}} = 62.5 \text{ mL/hour}$$

Therefore, the pump would be set at 62 or 63.

II. Dosage Calculations
  A. A certain number of milligrams of a drug is specified for each kilogram of body weight. This is commonly written as *mg/kg*.
  B. A certain number of milligrams of a drug is specified for each square meter of body surface area. This is commonly written as *mg/m²*.
  C. Rules for calculation of pediatric dosages using adult doses and considering the age or weight of the child have sometimes been used in the past. These are not considered safe or accurate and should not be used.

III. Guidelines for Medication Administration
  A. Before giving any medication to a child, ask yourself these questions:
    1. How will the drug be absorbed, metabolized, and excreted?
    2. How will the child's illness and developmental physiology influence the absorption, metabolism, and excretion of the drug?
    3. Is the child taking other drugs that will interact or compete with this drug for use and excretion?
    4. What dose should be given?
    5. What are the child's pulse, temperature, respiratory rate, blood pressure, skin color and condition, fluid status, and behavior? (Document in the medical record.)

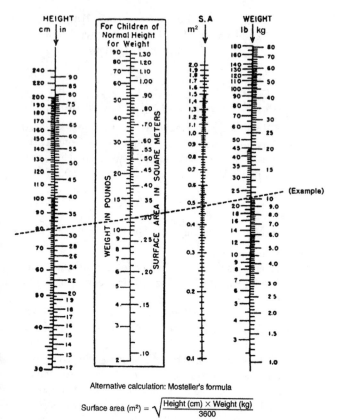

HEIGHT
cm | in

For Children of
Normal Height
for Weight

S.A
m²

WEIGHT
lb | kg

(Example)

Alternative calculation: Mosteller's formula

$$\text{Surface area (m}^2) = \sqrt{\frac{\text{Height (cm)} \times \text{Weight (kg)}}{3600}}$$

Figure 9–1 ■ The body surface area is indicated at the intersection of a straight line connecting the height and weight column with the surface area column; if the patient is roughly average size, it is determined by the weight alone (enclosed area). Adapted from Behrman, R. E., Kliegman, R. M., & Jenson, T. B. (Eds.). (2004). Nelson textbook of pediatrics (17th ed.). Philadelphia: W. B. Saunders; and Briars, G., & Bailey, B. (1994). Surface area estimation: Pocket calculator v nomogram. Archives of Disease in Children, 70, 246.

   B. After giving any medication to a child, ask these questions:
   1. What time, route, amount, and site (for injections) were used for medication administration? (Document in the medical record.)
   2. What pertinent physical findings, such as changes in condition, lack of expected results, side effects, or unusual effects of the drug, are observed? (Document in the medical record.)

3. Would it be useful to obtain blood levels of the drug for establishing the therapeutic dose?
4. How can results of this therapy be shared with other health professionals?

C. Confirm correct drug and dose with every medication given, and properly document procedure.

1. Always check dosage prescribed against safe dosage ranges. Nurses are liable legally for any drug they administer. Use the Five Patient Rights of Medication Administration (see below).

2. Identify each child carefully to avoid giving a medication to the wrong child. In the hospital, check identification bands, and, in the office or outpatient setting, have the parent or child provide verbal identification. Verify allergy history.

3. Use the Five Patient Rights of Medication Administration. Nurses should follow these five "Rights" when administering medications to help prevent errors:
   a. The Right drug
   b. In the Right dose
   c. To the Right patient
   d. At the Right time
   e. By the Right route

4. After administration, use a sixth "Right," which is correct documentation. Document the drug, dose, time, route, and site, as well as the name and title of the person who administered the medication. Check the child's response to the medication, and document the response as needed.

5. In patient-specific documentation, including clinical documentation, order forms, progress notes, and consultation and operative reports; certain abbreviations should not be used because of the potential problem of misinterpretation. Additional recommendations about abbreviations to avoid can be found on the Joint Commission on Accreditation of Healthcare Organization's Web site (http://www.jcaho.org) and on the ISMP Medication Safety Alert Web site (http://www.ismp.org).

6. The American Academy of Pediatrics has adopted a policy statement titled *Prevention of Medication Errors in the Pediatric Inpatient Setting*. The statement lists recommendations regarding hospital-wide system actions

Abbreviation to Avoid	Preferred Term
U	Unit
IU	International unit
QD	Daily
QOD	Every other day
Trailing zero (X.0 mg)	Omit a zero by itself after a decimal point (X mg)
Lack of leading zero (.X mg)	Always use a zero before a decimal point (0.X mg)
MS, MSO_4, $MgSO_4$	Morphine sulfate or magnesium sulfate in words.

Note: From Joint Commission on Accreditation of Healthcare Organizations. http://www.jcaho.org/accredited+organizations/06_goal2_faqs.pdf, accessed 7/27/2005, with permission.

and guidelines, prescriber actions and guidelines, prescriber education and communication, pharmacy action and guidelines, nursing actions and guidelines, nursing education and communication, patients, and families. The nursing actions and guidelines follow:

- Check medication calculations with another professional member of the healthcare team.
- Confirm patient identity before administration of each dose.
- Be familiar with medication ordering and dispensing systems.
- Verify drug orders before medication administration.
- Unusually large or small volumes or dosage units for a single patient dose should be verified.
- When a patient, parent, or caregiver questions whether a drug should be administered, listen attentively, answer questions, and double-check the medication order.
- Remain familiar with the operation of medication administration devices and the potential for error with such devices, particularly patient-controlled analgesia or infusion pumps.

Note: Data from Committee on Drugs and Committee on Hospital Care. (2003). Prevention of medication errors in the pediatric inpatient setting. Pediatrics, 112, 431–436.

10. Pain Assessment Tools

TOOLS FOR NONVERBAL CHILDREN
Neonatal Infant Pain Scale

The neonatal infant pain scale is designed to measure procedural pain in preterm and full-term neonates up to 6 weeks after birth. The neonate's facial expression, cry quality, breathing patterns, arm and leg position, and state of arousal are observed (Table 10–1).

FLACC Behavioral Pain Assessment Scale

The FLACC is designed to measure acute pain in infants and young children after surgery, and it can be used until the child is able to self-report pain with another pain scale. See Table 10–2 for scoring and interpretation (Merkel, Voepel-Lewis, Shayevitz, et al., 1997).

TOOLS FOR VERBAL CHILDREN
Assessing Readiness to Use a Pain Scale

The child must understand the basic concept of a little or a lot of pain well enough to tell the nurse. The correct response to either of the items below indicates the child has the conceptual understanding to use a numeric scale (Merkel, 2002).

- Ask the child, "Which number is larger, five or nine?" Then ask, "Which number is smaller, seven or four?"
- Ask the child to place several blocks or pieces of paper of different sizes in a row from biggest to smallest.

Oucher Scale

Use the Oucher Scale that is the best match for the ethnicity of the child (Figure 10–1). After determining that the child has an understanding of number concepts, teach the child to use the scale. Point to each photograph, and explain that the bottom picture is "no hurt," the second picture is a "little hurt," the third picture is "a little more hurt," the fourth picture is "even more hurt," the fifth picture is "a lot of hurt," and the sixth picture is "the biggest or most hurt you could ever have." The numbers beside the photos can be used to score the amount of pain the child reports.

Table 10–1 Neonatal Infant Pain Scale

Characteristic	Scoring Criteria
Facial Expression	
0 = Relaxed muscles	Restful face with neutral expression
1 = Grimace	Tight facial muscles; furrowed brow, chin, and jaw
	(At low gestational ages, infants may have no facial expression)
Cry	
0 = No cry	Quiet, not crying
1 = Whimper	Mild moaning, intermittent cry
2 = Vigorous cry	Loud screaming, rising, shrill, and continuous
	(Silent cry may be scored if infant is intubated, as indicated by obvious facial movements)
Breathing Patterns	
0 = Relaxed	Relaxed, usual breathing pattern maintained
1 = Change in breathing	Change in drawing breath: irregular, faster than usual, gagging, or holding breath
Arm Movements	
0 = Relaxed/restrained (with soft restraints)	Relaxed, no muscle rigidity, occasional random movements of arms
1 = Flexed/extended	Tense, straight arms; rigid; or rapid extension and flexion
Leg Movements	
0 = Relaxed/restrained (with soft restraints)	Relaxed, no muscle rigidity, occasional random movements of legs
1 = Flexed/extended	Tense, straight legs; rigid; or rapid extension and flexion
State of Arousal	
0 = Sleeping/awake	Quiet, peaceful sleeping; or alert and settled
1 = Fussy	Alert and restless or thrashing; fussy

Note: From J. Lawrence, D. Alcock, D. P. McGrath, et al. (1993). The development of a tool to assess neonatal pain. Neonatal Network, 12(6), 61, with permission.

Visual Analogue Scale

The Visual Analogue Scale or numeric scale is a single horizontal or vertical line anchored with descriptors of pain at each end. This tool often has marks at equal intervals to provide a numeric dimension to the tool. A 10-cm line is usually the standard, with a mark and number at each cm. Teach the child to use the tool by pointing to the side of the line that is no pain and the worst possible pain. Ask the child to make a mark along the line that best matches the amount of pain felt.

Table 10–2 FLACC Behavioral Pain Assessment Scale

Categories	Scoring		
	0	1	2
Face	No particular expression or smile	Occasional grimace or frown; withdrawn, disinterested	Frequent to constant frown, clenched jaw, quivering chin
Legs	Normal position or relaxed	Uneasy, restless, tense	Kicking or legs drawn up
Activity	Lying quietly, normal position, moves easily	Squirming, shifting back and forth, tense	Arched, rigid, or jerking
Cry	No cry (awake or asleep)	Moans or whimpers, occasional complaint	Crying steadily, screams or sobs; frequent complaints
Consolability	Content, relaxed	Reassured by occasional touching, hugging, or being talked to; distractible	Difficult to console or comfort

How to Use the FLACC

In patients who are awake: observe for 1–5 minutes or longer. Observe legs and body uncovered. Reposition patient or observe activity. Assess body for tenseness and tone. Initiate consoling interventions if needed.

In patients who are asleep: observe for 5 minutes or longer. Observe body and legs uncovered. If possible, reposition the patient. Touch the body, and assess for tenseness and tone.

Face
- ▶ Score 0: a relaxed face, makes eye contact, or shows interest in surroundings
- ▶ Score 1: a worried facial expression with eyebrows lowered, eyes partially closed, cheeks raised, and mouth pursed.
- ▶ Score 2: deep furrows in the forehead, closed eyes, an open mouth, and deep lines around nose and lips.

Legs
- ▶ Score 0: muscle tone and motion in the limbs are normal.
- ▶ Score 1: increased tone, rigidity, or tension and intermittent flexion or extension of the limbs.
- ▶ Score 2: hypertonicity, the legs are pulled tight, exaggerated flexion or extension of the limbs, and tremors.

Activity
- ▶ Score 0: moves easily and freely and shows normal activity or restrictions.
- ▶ Score 1: shifts positions; appears hesitant to move; demonstrates guarding, a tense torso, or pressure on a body part.
- ▶ Score 2: in a fixed position, rocking; or demonstrates side-to-side head movement or rubbing of a body part.

(continued)

Table 10–2   FLACC Behavioral Pain Assessment Scale   (Continued)

Cry

- ► Score 0: no cry or moan, awake or asleep.
- ► Score 1: occasional moans, cries, whimpers, or sighs.
- ► Score 2: frequent or continuous moans, cries, or grunts.

Consolability

- ► Score 0: calm and does not require consoling.
- ► Score 1: responds to comfort by touching or talking in 30 seconds to 1 minute.
- ► Score 2: requires constant comforting or is inconsolable.

Interpreting the Behavioral Score

Each category is scored on the 0–2 scale, which results in a total score of 0–10.

0 = Relaxed and comfortable	**4–6** = Moderate pain
1–3 = Mild discomfort	**7–10** = Severe discomfort or pain or both

FLACC is the acronym for five categories assessed: face, legs, activity, cry, and consolability. Note: From S. I. Merkel, T. Voepel-Lewis, J. R. Shayevitz, & S. Malviya. (1997). The FLACC: A behavioral scale for scoring postoperative pain in young children. Pediatric Nursing, 23(3), 293–297, with permission. The FLACC scale was developed by Sandra Merkel, MS, RN, Terri Voepel-Lewis, MS, RN, and Shobha Malviya, MD, at C. S. Mott Children's Hospital, University of Michigan Health System, Ann Arbor, MI.

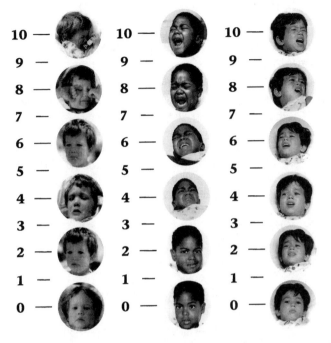

Figure 10–1 ■ From Caucasian version of the Oucher, developed and copyrighted by Judith E. Beyer, RN, PhD, 1983; African-American version of the Oucher, developed and copyrighted by Mary J. Denyes, RN, PhD, and Antonio M. Villarruel, RN, PhD, 1990; and Hispanic version of the Oucher, developed and copyrighted by Antonio M. Villarruel, RN, PhD, 1990, with permission.

11. POISON CONTROL INFORMATION

EMERGENCY MANAGEMENT FOR POISONING

1. Stabilize the child. Assess ABCs (airway, breathing, and circulation). Provide ventilatory and oxygen support.

2. Perform a rapid physical examination, start an intravenous infusion, draw blood for toxicology screen, and apply a cardiac monitor.

3. Obtain a history of the ingestion, including substance ingested, where child was found, by whom, position, when found, how long unsupervised, history of depression or suicide, allergies, and any other medical problems.

4. Reverse or eliminate the toxic substance using the appropriate method:

   - *Antidotes and agonists*
     - Mucomyst (for acetaminophen poisoning)
     - Narcan (for opioid overdose)
     - Flumazenil (Romazicon; for benzodiazepine overdose)

   - *Gastric lavage*
     - A gastric tube is inserted through the mouth.
     - Normal saline solution is instilled and aspirated until the return is clear. This is reserved for children with central nervous system depression, diminished or absent gag reflex, or unwillingness to cooperate with other measures.
     - Contraindicated in children who have ingested alkaline corrosive substances, because insertion of the tube may cause esophageal perforation.

   - *Activated charcoal*
     - Used in children who have ingested acids to decrease continued damage and potential perforation of stomach and intestines.
     - Given to absorb and remove any remaining particles of toxic substances.
     - Usual dosage administration is 1 g/kg of body weight.
     - A commercial preparation of activated charcoal is administered orally or through a gastric tube.

- Available as a ready-to-drink solution in an opaque container.
- May be mixed with apple juice or soda, if protocol allows, to encourage consumption.
- A covered cup and straw are used for oral ingestion to prevent the child from seeing the black liquid and to minimize spillage.
- Activated charcoal is administered only after the child has stopped vomiting, because aspiration of charcoal is damaging to lung tissue.
- Should not be administered for ingestion of caustic substances or hydrocarbons.

- *Cathartics*
  - Hasten excretion of a toxic substance, and minimize absorption.
  - The most commonly used cathartic is magnesium sulfate.

  Note: The use of syrup of ipecac is no longer recommended because it may not remove all poison and can be harmful in some situations. Encourage parents to remove it from their homes.

5. Other measures depend on the child's condition, the nature of the ingested substance, and the time since ingestion. May include diuresis, fluid loading, cooling or warming measures, anticonvulsive measures, antiarrhythmic therapy, hemodialysis, or exchange transfusions.
6. The child's total condition is constantly evaluated to maintain airway, breathing, and circulation. Therapeutic management is adjusted as needed to treat evolving condition.
7. Consider the emotional status of the family. Provide information about the child, involve the child in care when possible, and arrange for support persons and services to be available to the child.

Clinical Manifestations of Commonly Ingested Toxic Agents

Type	Sources	Clinical Manifestations	Clinical Therapy
Corrosives (strong acids and alkaline products that cause chemical burns of mucosal surfaces)	Batteries Household cleaners Clinitest tablets Denture cleaners Bleach Toilet bowl cleaners	Severe burning pain in mouth, throat, or stomach; swelling of mucous membranes; edema of lips, tongue, and pharynx (respiratory obstruction); violent vomiting; hemoptysis; drooling; inability to clear secretions; signs of shock, anxiety, and agitation	Do not induce vomiting! Dilute toxin with water to prevent further damage. Give activated charcoal.
Hydrocarbons (organic compounds that contain carbon and hydrogen; most are distillates of petroleum)	Gasoline Kerosene Furniture polish Lighter fluid Paint thinners	Gagging Choking Coughing Nausea Vomiting Alteration in sensorium (lethargy) Weakness Respiratory symptoms of pulmonary involvement, tachypnea, cyanosis, retractions, grunting	Do not induce vomiting! (Aspiration of hydrocarbons places child at high risk for pneumonia.) Use gastric lavage if severe central nervous system and respiratory impairment are present. Use of activated charcoal is controversial. Provide supportive care. Decontaminate skin by removing clothing and cleansing skin.
Acetaminophen	Many over-the-counter products	Nausea Vomiting Sweating	Induce vomiting or perform gastric lavage, depending on amount ingested.

		Administer charcoal or NAC (concentrated form of Mucomyst), which binds with the metabolite, preventing absorption and protecting the liver.
	Pallor Hepatic involvement (pain in upper right quadrant, jaundice, confusion, stupor, coagulation abnormalities)	
Salicylate	Products containing aspirin	Depends on amount ingested. Induce vomiting. Administer IV sodium bicarbonate, fluids, and vitamin K.
	Nausea Disorientation Vomiting Dehydration Diaphoresis Hyperpnea Hyperpyrexia Bleeding tendencies Oliguria Tinnitus Convulsions Coma	
Mercury	Broken thermometers Chemicals Paints Pesticides Fungicides	Similar to that for lead poisoning (see following table).
	Tremors Memory loss Insomnia Weight loss Diarrhea Anorexia Gingivitis	

(continued)

Clinical Manifestations of Commonly Ingested Toxic Agents (Continued)

Type	Sources	Clinical Manifestations	Clinical Therapy
Iron	Multiple vitamin supplements	Vomiting Hematemesis Diarrhea Bloody stools Abdominal pain Metabolic acidosis Shock Seizures Coma	Induce vomiting. Administer IV fluids and sodium bicarbonate. Deferoxamine chelation therapy.

Clinical Manifestations of Lead Poisoning

Mild Toxicity (10–15 mcg/dL)	Moderate Toxicity (16–69 mcg/dL)	Severe Toxicity (≥70 mcg/dL)
Myalgia or paresthesia	Arthralgia	Paresis or paralysis
Mild fatigue	General fatigue	Encephalopathy may lead abruptly to seizures, changes in consciousness, coma, and death
Irritability, lethargy	Difficulty concentrating	
Occasional abdominal discomfort	Muscular exhaustibility	
	Tremor	Lead line (blue–black) on gingival tissue
	Headache	
	Diffuse abdominal pain	Colic (intermittent, severe, abdominal cramps)
	Vomiting	
	Weight loss	
	Constipation	
	Anemia	

Note: Adapted from Agency for Toxic Substances and Disease Registry. (1990). Lead toxicity. Case studies in environmental medicine (p. 11). Atlanta: Agency for Toxic Substances and Disease Registry.

12. EMERGENCY ASSESSMENT OF THE CHILD

INITIAL IMPRESSION

Make a quick initial impression of the severity or urgency of the child's condition using visual and auditory clues to make a rapid judgment.

Appearance

Alert, making eye contact and interacting with parent or caregiver, interested in toys or objects

Spontaneous movement, good muscle tone

Consolability

Quality of speech or cry

Breathing Effort

Observe for nasal flaring, retractions, and head bobbing.

Listen for abnormal airway sounds, such as stridor, wheezing, grunting, snoring, or muffled or hoarse speech.

Observe for tripod positioning, sitting with the head and neck extended, or refusal to lie down.

Circulation of the Skin

Observe the color of the skin and mucous membranes.

Inspect the mucous membranes. In children of darker skin, the mucous membranes are usually pink, regardless of skin color.

Next Steps

Analyze information from appearance, breathing effort, and circulation of skin to evaluate the child's physiologic stability. The greater the number of abnormal findings present, the more serious the child's condition.

When an emergency condition exists, alter the sequence of assessment to identify the presence of a life-threatening condition.

- Airway—e.g., if the airway is obstructed, no oxygen can enter the child's system.
- Breathing—e.g., if there is lung damage, the child may be unable to ventilate and support gas exchange.

- Circulation—e.g., hemorrhage may reduce blood volume and circulation to the brain and other vital organs.

Interrupt assessment as soon as a potential life-threatening physiologic condition is identified to provide the needed care.

Resume assessment when the physiologic condition is stabilized.

Reassess the physiologic status of the airway, breathing, and circulation every 5 minutes.

ASSESSING THE ABCs (AIRWAY, BREATHING, AND CIRCULATION)

Airway Assessment

Is the infant or child crying or talking?

Are there any airway sounds?

Could the tongue be blocking the airway?

Does the chest rise?

Airway Management

Open the airway in cases of airway obstruction.

Perform a chin lift or a jaw thrust to lift the tongue out of the pharynx.[1]

Insert an oropharyngeal airway to maintain the airway in an unconscious child.[1]

Suction secretions and blood.

Insert an endotracheal tube to maintain and secure the airway.[1]

Use a bag valve mask or perform rescue breathing with a pocket mask, and give two slow breaths if the chest does not rise.[1]

Reposition the child's head with the chin lift or jaw thrust if the head does not rise, and give two slow breaths again.

Initiate procedures for removing a foreign body obstruction if the chest still does not rise.[1]

Breathing Assessment

What is the effort associated with breathing?

---

[1]This technique and others mentioned in this chapter can be found in the Skills Manual (Bindler & Ball, 2003).

What is the respiratory rate, and how does it compare with the expected rate for age?

What sounds are heard when auscultating the chest?

Are there any penetrating chest injuries? Are there any rib fractures? Are there any marks on the chest indicating injury?

Breathing Management

Provide high-concentration oxygen. Use a nonrebreather mask (a face mask with a reservoir bag) that enables delivery of 60–90% oxygen at a flow rate of 12–15 L/minute when the mask maintains a tight seal on the face.[1]

Assist ventilation with a resuscitation bag connected to oxygen when the child has minimal or no respiratory effort. Use only enough pressure and air volume to make the chest rise.[1]

Assist with insertion of a nasogastric or orogastric tube to keep the stomach deflated and to reduce the risk for vomiting.[1]

Cover any open chest wound with an occlusive dressing, taped on three sides.

Assist with chest-tube insertion when a pneumothorax is present.[1]

Circulatory Assessment

What is the circulation to the skin?

What is the capillary refill time?

Is there any bleeding or potential internal bleeding? How much blood has been lost?

Is the child possibly dehydrated?

What is the heart rate?

What is the child's blood pressure?

Circulation Management

When bradycardia is present, provide oxygen, and assist ventilation as described under Breathing Management.

Attach a cardiorespiratory monitor. Monitor the heart rate during interventions to see whether the heart rate increases and stabilizes.[1]

Establish an intravenous (IV) line to provide emergency medications. Alternatively, small amounts of some medications can be administered down the endotracheal tube.

Initiate cardiac compressions if no pulse can be palpated or the pulse rate is less than 60 beats/minute in an infant or child with poor tissue perfusion.[1]

Assist with defibrillation of the infant or child with ventricular fibrillation or pulseless ventricular fibrillation. Place the appropriate size pads or electrodes to the child's chest so that the heart is between them. A starting dose of 2 J/kg is recommended, increasing to 4 J/kg if ventricular fibrillation persists after the first shock (American Heart Association, 2002).[1]

Control bleeding with direct pressure using a gloved hand, and elevate the body part if it is safe to do so. Apply pressure to an arterial pressure point proximal to the injury to slow the flow of bleeding in cases of hemorrhage.

When hypovolemic shock is present, quickly administer 20 mL/kg of lactated Ringer's or normal saline. Reassess the heart rate, capillary refill, and responsiveness for the next 5–15 minutes to determine the child's response and the need for additional IV fluid, albumin, or blood. Give additional fluids or blood until the circulatory system is stabilized.

Disability (Neurologic) Assessment

What is the infant's or child's level of responsiveness using the AVPU (alert/verbal/painful/unresponsive) scale? What is the Glasgow Coma Scale score?

Check the pupils for size, symmetry, and reactivity to light.

Has the child had a seizure?

Is the child moving spontaneously? Is the child flaccid? Is any abnormal posturing present?

Disability Management

If the child has a brain injury, ensure oxygenation with assisted ventilation at the appropriate respiratory rate for the infant or child. Hyperventilate only for an acute elevation in intracranial pressure or signs of brainstem herniation (asymmetric or fixed dilated pupils, bradycardia, hypertension, and irregular respirations) (American Heart Association, 2002).

Administer a benzodiazepine medication if the child has had a seizure.

If spinal cord injury is suspected, immobilize the head in neutral position, and prevent movement of other parts of the body.

Exposure Assessment

Perform a rapid inspection of the entire body, when the child's condition is stabilized, to identify any additional injuries.

Check for the presence of pulses in extremities distal to the injury.

Stabilize in place any object impaling a part of the body.

Assess the child's pain level.

Exposure Management

Keep the child warm with heat lamps and warmed IV fluids to maintain a neutral temperature.

HISTORY

Obtain an abbreviated history of the event leading to the emergency. The acronym for this history is SAMPLE:

Signs and symptoms—onset and nature of the symptoms

Allergies—any known allergies

Medications—names and doses of prescribed and over-the-counter medications, including aerosol medications and complementary therapies

Past medical problems—any significant health conditions, hospitalizations, and immunizations

Last food or liquid—when the infant or child last ate or had liquids, including bottle or breastfeeding

Events leading to the injury or illness—progression of illness over time, activities contributing to injury

13. INFECTIOUS AND COMMUNICABLE DISEASES

CHICKENPOX (VARICELLA)
Epidemiology
Caused by varicella-zoster, human herpesvirus 3. Wild virus cases and breakthrough cases occur in vaccinated children.

Transmitted by direct mucous membrane contact by the virus primarily through airborne spread of secretions and direct lesion contact. Incubation period is 14–21 days.

Communicable 5 days before the onset of the rash to a maximum of 6 days after the appearance of the first group of vesicles, when all lesions have crusted over.

Clinical Manifestations
Acute onset of mild fever, malaise, anorexia, headache, mild abdominal pain, and irritability; occur before eruption of lesions.

Itchy; begins as a macule on an erythematous base, progresses to a papule, then to a clear, fluid-filled vesicle. Eruption lasts 1–5 days. Lesions of all stages present. Crusts may remain for 1–3 weeks. A more severe rash with eczema or sunburn.

Lesions begin on the trunk, scalp, and face and spread to the rest of the body. Ulcerative lesions on mucous membranes may lead to decreased fluid intake and dehydration.

Clinical Therapy
Supportive medical management for healthy children.

Oral and intravenous acyclovir for immunocompromised patients, for adolescents, and for children with chronic cutaneous and pulmonary diseases treated with chronic salicylate therapy or oral or aerosol corticosteroids (American Academy of Pediatrics, 2003).

Varicella-zoster immunoglobulin is given, up to 4 days after exposure, to newborns of infected mothers or to immunocompromised children with no history of immunization or chickenpox.

Immunize children after 12 months of age. The vaccine can be given within 72 hours of exposure to prevent or reduce severity of the disease.

Complications

Secondary infection, cellulitis, lymphadenitis, local abscesses, sepsis, encephalitis, pneumonia, thrombocytopenia, hepatitis, glomerulonephritis, arthritis, meningitis, and Reye syndrome.

Significant illness or death to immunocompromised children. The disease is more severe when steroids have been given during the incubation period (Arvin, 2002).

Nursing Management
Assessment

Observe for complications such as drowsiness, meningeal signs, respiratory distress, and dehydration. Disorientation and restlessness may indicate viral encephalitis.

Monitor for acyclovir side effects: nausea, vomiting, diarrhea, abdominal pain, as well as allergic skin reactions or headache. Monitor renal function.

Implementation

Use airborne and contact precautions.

Isolate all children admitted to the hospital with a history of recent varicella exposure.

Isolate the child treated at home from medically fragile children, immunocompromised children or adults, and women early in pregnancy. Notify the school or childcare facility of the child's illness.

Give nonaspirin antipyretics to control fever.

Reduce itching with oral antihistamines, oatmeal and Aveeno baths, or Caladryl lotion. Keep the child's fingernails short and clean.

Change bed linens frequently.

ERYTHEMA INFECTIOSUM (FIFTH DISEASE)
Epidemiology

Caused by human parvovirus B19.

Transmitted by respiratory secretions and blood. Incubation period is 6–14 days.

Most communicable before the onset of symptoms.

Clinical Manifestations

Flu-like illness (headache, chills, malaise, nausea, body ache) that lasts 2–3 days.

A week later, a fiery-red rash appears on the cheeks and circumoral pallor.

In 1–4 days, a lace-like symmetric, erythematous, maculopapular rash appears on the trunk and limbs, spreading proximal to distal. The palms and soles are spared.

During the third stage, lasting 1–3 weeks, the rash fades but reappears if the skin is irritated or exposed to sunlight. The rash may be mildly pruritic.

Clinical Therapy
No treatment; recovery spontaneous

Complications
Transient aplastic crisis in children with hemolytic conditions; may need blood transfusion.

Immunodeficient patients may develop a chronic infection that can be treated with intravenous immunoglobulin therapy (American Academy of Pediatrics, 2003).

Nursing Management
Isolate the child with aplastic crisis or when immunosuppressed. Use standard and droplet precautions.

Control fever with nonaspirin antipyretics.

Use antipruritics or oatmeal or Aveeno baths if the rash is pruritic.

Encourage rest and offer frequent fluids. Provide quiet diversionary activities.

Keep children out of direct sunlight if possible. Provide protective, light, loose clothing if exposure to sunlight cannot be avoided.

The immune-competent child may attend school or day care.

Explain the three stages of rash development to parents.

HAEMOPHILUS INFLUENZAE TYPE B
Epidemiology
Caused by coccobacilli *Haemophilus influenzae* bacterium, which has several serotypes and can be encapsulated or nonencapsulated.

Transmitted by direct person-to-person contact or droplet inhalation. Unknown incubation period.

Communicable for 3 days from onset of symptoms.

Clinical Manifestations

Starts with a viral upper respiratory infection. The organism passes through the mucosal barrier to directly invade the bloodstream.

Several severe invasive illnesses may result: meningitis, epiglottitis, pneumonia, septic arthritis, cellulitis, and sepsis (in infants). Other illnesses include sinusitis, otitis media, bronchitis, and pericarditis.

Clinical Therapy

Treatment includes antibiotic therapy. Intravenous antibiotics should be given for severe infections; others can be treated orally.

Rifampin may be given to unprotected household contacts (not pregnant women).

Immunize infants, beginning at 2 months of age.

Complications

Severe sequelae and death may occur in young infants from meningitis, epiglottitis, sinusitis, pneumonitis, and cellulitis.

Nursing Management

Use droplet precautions until 24 hours after the initiation of antibiotics.

Administer nonaspirin antipyretics to help the child feel more comfortable.

Perform nursing care measures specific to the illness.

Inform family members that rifampin turns urine and other body fluids orange, and it will cause stains.

LYME DISEASE
Epidemiology

Caused by *Borrelia burgdorferi*, a spirochete.

Transmitted by a tick bite. The tick must feed for 36 hours to transmit the disease. Incubation period is 3–32 days after the infected tick bites. A rash in 48 hours is an allergic reaction or infection, not Lyme disease.

Not contagious from person to person. Infection does not induce immunity.

Clinical Manifestations

A flat or raised red area that progresses to partial clearing in the center, with a bull's eye appearance, usually at least 5 cm in diameter. May look like a bruise in dark-skinned patients. Spontaneously resolves within 4 weeks.

Stage 1 symptoms, lasting 5–21 days, include malaise, fatigue, headache, stiff neck, mild fever, and muscle and joint aches.

Stage 2 (early disseminated), 1–4 months after the bite: pain and swelling of the joints (commonly the knee), facial palsy, meningitis, and atrioventricular block.

Stage 3 (late disseminated), months later: Lyme arthritis and central nervous system changes.

Clinical Therapy
Antibiotics for 2 weeks: amoxicillin or cefuroxime axetil for children 8 years of age or younger and doxycycline or tetracycline for children older than age 8 years

Complications
Recurrent arthritis, central nervous system changes, or carditis; treated for 4 weeks with intravenous ceftriaxone, cefotaxime, or penicillin G

Nursing Management
Use standard precautions if the child is hospitalized.

Educate parents about need to take all medications and to avoid sun exposure if doxycycline is used.

Encourage the use of nonaspirin analgesics and antipyretics.

Promote rest and discourage vigorous activities, as the child may tire easily.

Educate parents and children to avoid areas that are heavily tick-infested and wear protective clothing, to check for ticks (especially hidden in hair) after every outing and remove ticks as soon as possible, and to clean the area with soap and water.

Tell parents to mark the date of tick bite on the calendar and monitor the child's health for flu-like symptoms over the next 30 days. Encourage them to seek medical attention promptly if symptoms develop.

MEASLES (RUBEOLA)
Epidemiology
Caused by *Morbillivirus*, a member of the paramyxovirus group.

Maternal immunity is active in the infant until the age of approximately 12–15 months.

Transmitted by airborne, respiratory droplets and contact with infected persons. Incubation period is approximately 8–12 days.

Communicable during the prodromal phase until 2–4 days after the rash appears.

Clinical Manifestations

Prodromal phase of 3–5 days, with high fever, conjunctivitis, coryza, cough, anorexia, and malaise.

Koplik's spots (small, irregular, bluish white spots on a red background) appear on the buccal mucosa approximately 2 days before and after the onset of the rash.

Characteristic red, blotchy, maculopapular rash becomes confluent; usually appears 2–4 days after onset of prodromal phase; begins on the face and spreads to the trunk and extremities. Symptoms gradually subside in 4–7 days.

Other symptoms include anorexia, malaise, fatigue, and generalized lymphadenopathy.

Clinical Therapy

Treatment is supportive. Antibiotics for bacterial secondary infections.

Prevention is by vaccine. Immunoglobulin, administered up to 6 days after exposure, may help prevent the disease in susceptible persons.

Complications

Diarrhea, otitis media, bronchopneumonia, bronchitis, laryngotracheobronchitis, and encephalitis.

Children who are malnourished, medically fragile, and immunosuppressed have most complications.

Nursing Management

Assess lungs carefully, as pneumonia is a common complication.

Maintain airborne precautions during the contagious period. If the child is home, limit visitors to those immunized or immune.

Use a cool-mist vaporizer to help clear respiratory passages. Suction nose and oral cavity very gently as necessary.

Give nonaspirin antipyretics for fever, antipruritics for itching, and antitussives may be ordered to control coughing.

Maintain fluid intake. Offer cool liquids frequently in small amounts. Blended, pureed, and mashed foods are most easily tolerated.

Keep skin clean and dry. No soaps should be used.

Keep lights dim, and cover windows if the child has photophobia.

Maintain bed rest. Elevate the head of the bed. Keep the room cool with good air circulation. Provide light, nonirritating blankets. Provide diversional activities.

MONONUCLEOSIS
Epidemiology
Caused by Epstein-Barr virus, a member of the herpesvirus group.

Transmitted by direct contact with infected oropharyngeal and genital tract secretions or by blood transfusion. Incubation period is 10–50 days. The virus is shed for up to 18 months after recovery, and the infected individual becomes a lifelong carrier (American Academy of Pediatrics, 2003).

The virus can be reactivated during periods of immunosuppression.

Clinical Manifestations
Young children may be irritable but otherwise asymptomatic.

A maculopapular rash may be seen in a few cases.

Malaise, headache, anorexia, abdominal pain, fatigue, and fever for 2–3 days, followed by lymphadenopathy and a sore throat. Hepatosplenomegaly may occur. Pain from swelling of the tonsils and lymph nodes may be significant.

Syndrome lasts 2–3 weeks and is self-limited. Weakness and lethargy may continue for several months.

Clinical Therapy
No specific treatment.

Corticosteroids to control tonsillar swelling and pain when there is impending airway obstruction, massive splenomegaly, myocarditis, or hemolytic anemia.

Antibiotics (ampicillin and amoxicillin) should be avoided, as a non-allergic rash often develops (American Academy of Pediatrics, 2003).

Complications
Encephalitis, aseptic meningitis, Guillain-Barré syndrome, splenic rupture, respiratory failure, and thrombocytopenia; are rare.

In immunodeficient children, fatal infections or lymphomas can develop.

Nursing Management
Use standard precautions. Children are usually treated at home.

Give nonaspirin antipyretics and analgesics for fever and sore throat. Offer warm salt water for gargling. Offer soft foods and encourage fluids.

Teens should avoid kissing until the fever has been gone several days.

Maintain bed rest during acute phase.

Contact sports should be avoided until the liver and spleen are normal, usually in approximately 4 weeks.

Children and adolescents can return to school when the fever is gone and the sore throat has resolved.

MUMPS (PAROTITIS)
Epidemiology
Caused by *Rubulavirus*, in the paramyxovirus family.

Maternal antibodies disappear in infants at the age of 12–15 months.

Transmitted by contact with respiratory secretions. The incubation period is 12–25 days.

Communicable for 7 days before parotid swelling until 9 days after swelling subsides.

Clinical Manifestations
Malaise, low-grade fever, earache, headache, pain with chewing, decreased appetite and activity, bilateral or unilateral parotid gland swelling. Parotid swelling peaks at approximately the third day.

Meningeal signs (stiff neck, headache, and photophobia) in approximately 15% of patients.

Clinical Therapy
Therapy is supportive, focused on symptom relief.

Prevention is with vaccination.

Complications
Orchitis may occur in postpubertal males; sterility is relatively rare (American Academy of Pediatrics, 2003).

Oophoritis, pancreatitis, aseptic meningoencephalitis, and unilateral permanent deafness.

Nursing Management
Assess for headache, stiff neck, vomiting, and photophobia (meningeal irritation).

Use standard and droplet precautions. Avoid exposure to immuno-compromised individuals and susceptible persons.

Give nonaspirin analgesics and antipyretics to control fever and pain. Give steroids if ordered.

Encourage fluid intake. Avoid foods and beverages that increase salivary flow (citrus, spices, and candies) because they cause pain. Offer soft and blended foods; chewing and swallowing are painful.

Apply warm or cool compresses, whichever is preferred, to the parotid area.

Provide scrotal supports if testicular swelling occurs.

Keep children out of school or day care until 9 days after parotid swelling begins. Encourage diversional activities.

PERTUSSIS (WHOOPING COUGH)
Epidemiology
Caused by *Bordetella pertussis*.

It is transmitted by respiratory droplets and direct contact with discharge from the respiratory membranes. Incubation period is 7–21 days (commonly 7–10 days).

Pertussis is communicable beginning approximately 1 week after exposure until 5–7 days after starting antibiotic therapy. It is most contagious before the paroxysmal cough stage.

Clinical Manifestations
Catarrhal stage: nasal congestion, a runny nose, low-grade fever, and a mild nonproductive cough lasting approximately 2 weeks.

Paroxysmal stage: spasms of paroxysmal coughing followed by inspiration, stridor, or "whooping" that may last 1–4 weeks. May be accompanied by flushing, cyanosis, vomiting, and profuse drainage from the nose, eyes, and mouth. Dehydration from decreased oral intake.

Young infants do not manifest the "whooping"; they present with frequent apnea.

Convalescent stage: up to 6 weeks when paroxysms gradually subside.

Clinical Therapy
Treatment with antibiotics (erythromycin and other macrolides) and corticosteroids, if ordered.

Supportive care.

Prevention is by vaccination beginning early in infancy. A new vaccine has been approved for preteens and adolescents.

Complications
Pneumonia, atelectasis, otitis media, encephalopathy, seizures, and death.

Highest rate of mortality and complications in infants younger than 1 year.

Nursing Management
Use droplet precautions until 5–7 days after the initiation of antibiotics.

Closely monitor respirations and oxygen saturation. The smaller the child, the greater the risk for respiratory distress and apnea. Remain with the child during coughing spells, when hypoxic and apneic episodes are most likely. Give oxygen if ordered. Have emergency equipment available.

Provide humidification. Gentle suctioning may be necessary.

Give nonaspirin antipyretics for fever.

Encourage frequent rest periods.

Monitor for dehydration. Encourage fluids. Sucking may trigger the coughing spell. Intravenous hydration if oral intake not tolerated.

Allow the child to eat desired foods in small frequent feedings.

Teach parents to watch for signs of respiratory failure and dehydration if the child is managed at home. Provide emotional support to parents.

ROSEOLA (EXANTHEM SUBITUM, SIXTH DISEASE)
Epidemiology
Caused by herpesvirus type 6.

Transmitted by respiratory secretions of healthy individuals. Incubation period is 5–15 days. Lifelong persistent infection and virus shedding in healthy individuals (American Academy of Pediatrics, 2003).

Clinical Manifestations
Sudden, high fever up to 40.5°C (105°F) for 3–8 days, but the child does not appear toxic (normal appetite and behavior).

A characteristic pale pink, discrete, maculopapular rash starts on the trunk and spreads to the face, neck, and extremities after the fever stage. The rash can last for 1–2 days.

Normal appetite.

Clinical Therapy
There is no treatment other than supportive care.

Complications
Children may have febrile seizures during high fever stage.

Encephalopathy may develop in rare cases.

Nursing Management
Use standard precautions.

Give nonaspirin antipyretics to control fever. Encourage fluids.

Observe for seizure activity during the acute febrile periods.

Reassure parents that the rash will disappear in a few days.

RUBELLA (GERMAN MEASLES)
Epidemiology
Caused by an RNA virus, a member of the family Togaviridae, genus *Rubivirus*.

Transmitted by droplet spread, direct contact with infected persons, or contact with articles soiled by nasal secretions. Incubation period is 14–21 days (most commonly 16–18 days).

Communicable from approximately 7 days before until approximately 4 days after the onset of the rash.

Clinical Manifestations
Mild disease with a characteristic pink, nonconfluent, maculopapular rash that appears on the face, progresses to the neck, trunk, and legs, and disappears in the same order.

Prodromal symptoms of low-grade fever, headache, malaise, coryza, sore throat, anorexia, and Forschheimer spots (discrete, erythematous pinpoint or larger lesions on the soft palate) are seen 1–5 days before the rash.

Generalized lymphadenopathy involving the postauricular, suboccipital, and posterior cervical areas is common up to 7 days before the rash.

Many cases are asymptomatic.

Clinical Therapy
Treatment is supportive.

Prevention is through immunization, particularly of females of child-bearing age.

Complications

Rare arthritis in adolescents, encephalitis, and congenital rubella syndrome

Nursing Management

Maintain standard and droplet precautions.

Give nonaspirin analgesics and antipyretics for any pain and fever.

Provide food and beverage choices. Encourage fluids.

Provide quiet activities.

Exclude children from childcare or school for 7 days after onset of rash. Notify school and childcare facility of child's illness. Isolate from pregnant women.

STREPTOCOCCUS A
Epidemiology

Caused by various M-protein groups of group A alpha- and beta-hemolytic streptococci. Different strains are associated with pharyngeal and pyodermal infections.

Transmitted by contact with respiratory secretions for pharyngitis or skin lesions for pyoderma. Incubation period for pharyngeal infection is usually 2–5 days and for pyodermal infection is usually 7–10 days.

Communicable for weeks in untreated pharyngeal infections.

Clinical Manifestations

Pharyngeal infection: abrupt onset with a sore throat, dysphagia, malaise, high fever, chills, headache, abdominal pain, anorexia, and vomiting. A beefy red pharynx with exudate (strep throat) and tender cervical nodes. Palatal petechiae may be seen.

Group A streptococci respiratory tract infection: serous rhinitis and respiratory illness with moderate fever, irritability, and anorexia.

Scarlet fever: a characteristic erythematous, sandpaper rash appearing 12–48 hours after onset of symptoms, starting on the neck and spreading to the trunk and extremities. In 3–4 days, the rash begins to fade and the tips of the toes and fingers begin to peel. The classic strawberry tongue is seen on day 4 or 5.

Pyodermal infection: lesions (impetigo) that are honey-colored crusts at the site of open lesions.

Clinical Therapy

Diagnosis is by a rapid strep test or a culture of secretions from the pharynx and tonsils.

Antibiotic treatment is with penicillin V or erythromycin if the child is allergic to penicillin.

Uncomplicated impetigo is treated with mupirocin ointment.

Complications

Acute otitis media, sinusitis, peritonsillar or retropharyngeal abscess, cervical lymphadenitis, acute rheumatic fever, acute glomerulonephritis, toxic shock syndrome, bacteremia, and necrotizing fasciitis or myositis

Nursing Management

Maintain droplet precautions for pharyngeal infections and contact precautions for skin lesions for 24 hours after beginning antibiotics.

Promote bed rest during the febrile stage. Give nonaspirin antipyretics to control fever. Teach parents important signs of a worsening condition.

For pharyngeal infections, offer warm salt water for gargling, a soft diet, and nonacidic beverages. Encourage fluids. Provide cool, clear liquids. Swallowing may be difficult.

Explain to parents the importance of the child's taking antibiotics for the full number of days prescribed.

Encourage other family members with sore throats to have throat cultures taken.

For impetigo, teach the parents to wash the skin, remove crusts, and apply antibiotic ointment. Monitor vital signs, especially temperature. Administer antibiotics as ordered.

14. Alterations in Fluid and Electrolyte Function

FLUID VOLUME IMBALANCES
Extracellular Fluid Volume Deficit (Dehydration)
Description and Etiology

Extracellular fluid volume deficit occurs when there is not enough fluid in the extracellular compartment (intravascular and interstitial).

Common causes are vomiting, diarrhea, nasogastric suction, hemorrhage, burns, use of radiant warmers for newborns, and excessive exercise in hot weather, all of which result in loss in sodium-containing body fluid.

Three types of extracellular fluid volume deficit may occur:

- **Isotonic dehydration (or isonatremic dehydration)** occurs when fluid loss is not balanced by intake and the loss of water and sodium is in proportion.
- **Hypotonic dehydration (or hyponatremic dehydration)** occurs when fluid loss is characterized by a proportionately greater loss of sodium than water.
- **Hypertonic dehydration (or hypernatremic dehydration)** occurs when water loss is proportionately greater than sodium loss.

Clinical Manifestations

Clinical manifestations include changes in vital signs, urinary output, skin, mucous membranes, fontanels (for infants), and behavior (Table 14–1).

The degree of variation is associated with degree of dehydration (Table 14–2).

Diagnostic Tests

Serum electrolytes, creatinine, and glucose levels, and elevated blood urea nitrogen (more than 25 mg/dL) and serum bicarbonate (more than 17 mEq/L) are useful to identify moderate and severe diarrhea.

Normal serum sodium is 132–141 mEq/L for infants and children and 131–144 mEq/L for newborns (Table 14–3).

Serum sodium may or may not be normal; in isotonic dehydration, water and sodium are lost in equal relative amounts, so sodium levels are normal. In hypotonic dehydration, serum

Table 14–1 Clinical Manifestations of Extracellular Fluid Volume Deficit

Etiology	Clinical Manifestations
Decreased fluid volume	Weight loss
	Sunken fontanel (infant)
Inadequate circulating blood volume to offset the force of gravity when in upright position	Postural blood pressure drop (older children)
	Dizziness
Decreased intravascular volume	Increased small-vein filling time
	Delayed capillary refill time
	Flat neck veins when supine (older children)
Inadequate circulation to the brain	Dizziness, syncope
Inadequate circulation to the kidneys	Oliguria
Cardiac reflex response to decreased intravascular volume	Thready, rapid pulse
Decreased interstitial fluid volume	Decreased skin turgor

sodium levels are low, and in hypertonic dehydration serum sodium levels are elevated.

Clinical Therapy

Treatment of extracellular fluid volume deficit is administration of fluid containing sodium by oral rehydration therapy (Box 14–1) or by intravenous fluids (Box 14–2).

Choice of treatment depends on degree of dehydration and type of fluid lost.

Nursing Management

Prevention of dehydration is the major aim; teach parents of all newborns and infants how to identify the problem because this age group is most at risk for dehydration and the signs are hardest to detect.

When a child is admitted to a facility with dehydration, weigh the child with the same scale as previous weighs and without clothing, and if the child is hospitalized, continue with daily weighs.

Calculate weight loss to identify degree of dehydration.

Carefully measure intake and output, urine specific gravity, level of consciousness, pulse rate and quality, skin turgor, mucous membrane moisture, quality and rate of respirations, and blood pressure (compare the blood pressure when the child is supine with the pressure when the child is sitting with legs hanging down or standing because if the child is dehydrated, the sitting or standing blood pressure is lower than the supine blood pressure).

Table 14–2 Severity of Clinical Dehydration

Clinical Assessment	Mild	Moderate	Severe
Percent of body weight lost	Up to 5% (40–50 mL/kg)	6–9% (60–90 mL/kg)	10% or more (100+ mL/kg)
Level of consciousness	Alert, restless, thirsty	Irritable or lethargic (infants and very young children); alert, thirsty, restless (older children and adolescents)	Lethargic to comatose (infants and young children); often conscious, apprehensive (older children and adolescents)
Blood pressure	Normal	Normal or low; postural hypotension (older children and adolescents)	Low to undetectable
Pulse	Normal	Rapid	Rapid, weak to nonpalpable
Skin turgor	Normal	Poor	Very poor
Mucous membranes	Moist	Dry	Parched
Urine	May appear normal	Decreased output (<1 mL/kg/hr); dark color; increased specific gravity	Very decreased or absent output
Thirst	Slightly increased	Moderately increased	Greatly increased unless lethargic
Fontanel	Normal	Sunken	Sunken
Extremities	Warm; normal capillary refill	Delayed capillary refill (>2 sec)	Cool, discolored; delayed capillary refill (>3–4 sec)
Respirations	Normal	Normal or rapid	Changing rate and pattern

Obtain samples of urine and blood as needed for laboratory tests.

Give 1–3 teaspoons of fluid every 10–15 minutes when beginning oral rehydration; for the first 2–4 hours of treatment, 50 mL of fluid for each kilogram of the child's weight should be the target intake.

Cereals, starches, soups, fruits, and vegetables are generally allowed, but avoid simple sugars, which can worsen diarrhea because of osmotic effects, including soft drinks (if used, they should be diluted with equal parts of water), undiluted juice, Jell-O, and sweetened cereal.

Table 14-3 Normal Serum Values for Electrolytes in Infants and Youth*

	Newborn	Infant and Child
Sodium	131–144 mmol/L	132–141 mmol/L
Potassium	Premature 4.5–7.2 mmol/L Term 3.2–5.7 mmol/L	3.3–4.7 mmol/L
Calcium	Premature 3.5–4.5 mEq/L (1.7–2.3 mmol/L) Term 4–5 mEq/L (2–2.5 mmol/L)	4.4–5.3 mEq/L (2.2–2.7 mmol/L)
Magnesium	1.3–2.7 mg/dL (0.5–1.1 mmol/L)	1.6–2.7 mg/dL (0.7–1.1 mmol/L)

*Laboratories may have slightly different levels of normal depending on assays performed. Always consult the normal values for your particular laboratory.

Box 14-1 Oral Rehydration Therapy Guidelines

Calculate the specific amounts required for individual children based on the guidelines below and instruct parents in terminology they understand. Provide measuring devices, with proper amounts marked.

- Children with diarrhea and no dehydration should be continued on age-appropriate diets.
- For mild dehydration, give 50 mL/kg oral rehydration therapy in first 4 hours in addition to replacing fluids lost in stool and emesis. (Measure emesis and give 10 mL/kg of fluid for each diarrheal stool.)
- Start slowly, administering 3–5 mL in a small cup or spoon every few minutes. Increase amounts gradually if no vomiting occurs.
- Recommend or provide samples of oral rehydration therapy solutions. Suggest ready-to-feed or powdered forms for choice by parents.
- For moderate dehydration, give 100 mL/kg oral rehydration therapy in first 4 hours in addition to replacing fluids lost as described above.
- For severe dehydration, the child is hospitalized and treated with intravenous fluids. When hydrated adequately or concurrently with intravenous rehydration, begin oral rehydration therapy with 50–100 mL/kg of fluid in 4 hours and stool replacement as described above.
- Recalculate fluid needs after first 4 hours and adjust as needed. If the child is not taking increased fluids and not otherwise improving by this time, contact healthcare provider.
- When rehydration is complete, resume normal diet.

Note: Adapted from Provisional Committee on Quality Improvement, Subcommittee on Acute Gastroenteritis (1996). Practice parameter: the management of acute gastroenteritis in young children. Pediatrics, 97, 424–436.

Section III: Body Systems

Box 14–2   Calculation of Intravenous Fluid Needs

1. First, calculate the maintenance fluid needs of the child, according to the following guidelines:

Usual Weight	Maintenance Amount
Up to 10 kg	100 mL/kg/24 hr
11–20 kg	1,000 mL + (50 mL/kg for weight above 10 kg)/24 hr
>20 kg	1,500 mL + (20 mL/kg for weight above 20 kg)/24 hr

2. Next, calculate replacement fluid for that lost.

Percent of lost weight × 10 = mL/kg

3. Finally, calculate continued losses and add to the total maintenance and replacement needs.

Note: These fluid needs are for normal children who have a problem causing dehydration. In special circumstances, such as very-low-birth-weight infants, or children with problems such as renal disease, the maintenance amounts need to be adjusted. Consult with specialists treating the child and specialized references to learn about fluid needs in these situations.

When intravenous fluids are used, calculate the fluid order to determine that the amount of fluid corresponds with the diagnosed dehydration state and maintenance fluid needs of the child.

Approximately half of the 24-hour total maintenance and replacement needs are given to a dehydrated child in the first 6–8 hours of intravenous fluids, with a slower rate infused for the remainder of the 24 hours; during the first 1–3 hours, the infusion rate may be highest to rapidly expand the vascular space.

Rapid infusion of 20–30 mL/kg intravenously over 1–2 hours is sometimes used in outpatient settings, followed or accompanied by oral fluids.

Play with the toddler and preschool child frequently and use diversionary methods as necessary to distract the child from the intravenous line.

Instruct all parents to keep oral rehydration fluids at home for use when instructed.

Instruct parents in signs of worsening dehydration so that additional care is sought when needed.

Extracellular Fluid Volume Excess

Extracellular fluid volume excess occurs when there is too much fluid in the extracellular compartment (intravascular and interstitial); the imbalance is also called *saline excess* or *extracellular volume overload.*

If the disorder occurs by itself (without saline disturbance), the serum sodium concentration is normal; there is simply too much extracellular fluid, even though it has a normal concentration.

An overload of fluid in the blood vessels and interstitial spaces can cause clinical manifestations such as bounding pulse, distended neck veins in children (not usually evident in infants), hepatomegaly, dyspnea, orthopnea, and lung crackles.

Edema is the sign of overload of the interstitial fluid compartment; in an infant, edema is often generalized, whereas edema in children with extracellular fluid volume excess occurs in the dependent parts of the body.

Edema occurs if the balance of forces is altered so that excess fluid either enters or leaves the interstitial compartment through (1) increased blood hydrostatic pressure, (2) decreased blood colloid osmotic pressure, (3) increased interstitial fluid osmotic pressure, or (4) blocked lymphatic drainage.

Clinical therapy for extracellular fluid volume excess, such as diuretics to remove fluid from the body, focuses on treating the underlying cause of the disorder.

Nursing Management

Administer medical therapy as prescribed and monitor for any complications of the therapy, such as hypokalemia, associated with many diuretics.

If edema is present, provide careful skin care and protection for edematous areas; teach parents how to provide skin care and perform position changes at home.

Elevation of an area of localized edema helps to reduce the swelling.

If a child has a long-term condition such as chronic renal failure that predisposes to extracellular fluid volume excess, a dietary sodium restriction may be prescribed; teach parents how to manage sodium restriction.

Measure weight and edematous parts daily.

Intake and output are a necessary part of the daily assessment.

Administer intravenous fluids carefully to avoid complications.
- Use small bags of fluid, so if the fluid were to infuse quickly, the amount infused would be limited.

- Apply caution when infusing solutions containing sodium such as normal saline (0.9% NaCl), Ringer's solution, and lactated Ringer's solution.
- Always use infusion pumps when available so that the rate is programmed and monitored.
- Check and double-check the machine after setting to be sure it has been properly programmed.
- Have another nurse check your calculation of rates and total fluid to be infused until you are certain of your skill in this area.
- Remember that even mechanical pumps can have faulty performance; check the intravenous line, bag, and rate frequently.

ELECTROLYTE IMBALANCES
Hypernatremia

Hypernatremia is a condition of increased osmolality of the blood; body fluids are too concentrated, containing excess sodium relative to water.

Serum sodium level of more than 144 mmol/L in children (141 mmol/L in newborns) is diagnostic of hypernatremia.

Hypernatremia results from conditions that cause the body to lose relatively more water than sodium or to gain relatively more sodium than water.

An infant or child who has hypernatremia is generally thirsty, and urine output is small unless the hypernatremia is caused by diabetes insipidus.

A decreased level of consciousness manifested by confusion, lethargy, or coma results from shrinking of the brain cells, and seizures can occur when hypernatremia occurs rapidly or is severe.

Specific gravity or urine is concentrated in hypernatremia and dilute in hyponatremia.

Hypernatremia is treated by intravenous administration of hypotonic fluid, or fluid that is more dilute than normal body fluid.

If a child is dehydrated, isotonic fluids (those with the osmolality of body fluids) may be ordered first to replenish the volume, followed by hypotonic fluid to correct the osmolality.

Teaching can prevent many cases of hypernatremia.

Be sure the breastfeeding mother has instruction and resources about lactation before discharge after delivery.

Children with delayed development are at risk for hypernatremia because they may not be able to recognize thirst or obtain fluids when dehydrated; teach parents about the child's fluid requirements.

Parents should be cautioned to keep salt out of reach, because eating handfuls of salt has caused hypernatremia.

Teach parents to offer extra fluids during hot weather.

When a child is hospitalized for hypernatremia, monitor serum sodium level, and measure intake and output and urine specific gravity.

Watch for rebound hyponatremia while monitoring the fluid replacement.

Implement safety interventions such as raised bed rails for protection.

Ensure adequate rest and introduce developmentally appropriate activities when the child is alert.

Hyponatremia

In hyponatremia, the osmolality of the blood is decreased, so the body fluids are too dilute, containing excess water relative to sodium.

Serum sodium level below 135 mmol/L in children (133 mmol/L in newborns) is diagnostic of hyponatremia.

Hyponatremia results from conditions that cause gain of relatively more water than sodium or loss of relatively more sodium than water.

The child with hyponatremia has a decreased level of consciousness that results from swelling of brain cells and can be manifested as anorexia, headache, muscle weakness, decreased deep tendon reflexes, lethargy, confusion, or coma.

If hyponatremia arises rapidly or is extreme, seizures may occur; hyponatremia is a frequent cause of seizures in infants younger than 6 months of age.

Nausea and vomiting also occur in some children.

Serum sodium is the major diagnostic test.

Antidiuretic hormone levels and 24-hour urinary output are helpful in diagnosing diabetes insipidus as the cause of hyponatremia.

Hyponatremia is commonly treated by restricting the intake of water; this therapy allows the kidneys to correct the imbalance by excreting excess water from the body.

If a child is having seizures from hyponatremia, intravenous hypertonic fluid (more concentrated than body fluid) may be administered to rapidly increase body fluid concentration; the child must be monitored carefully because this therapy can easily cause rebound hypernatremia.

Nurses can prevent hyponatremia in hospitalized children by using normal saline instead of distilled water for irrigations and by avoiding tap water enemas.

The nurse monitors serum sodium level of children with hyponatremia and measures intake and output.

If an infant with hyponatremia has normal antidiuretic hormone levels and other causes have been ruled out, careful questioning about proper preparation of formula and feeding practices is needed.

Frequent assessment of responsiveness is necessary to monitor the response to therapy.

Hyperkalemia

Hyperkalemia is an excess of potassium in the blood, reflected by a level of more than 5.8 mmol/L in children or of more than 5.2 mmol/L in newborns.

Hyperkalemia is caused by conditions that involve increased potassium intake, shift of potassium from cells into the extracellular fluid, and decreased potassium excretion.

Renal insufficiency, increased potassium intake, shift of potassium from cells to extracellular fluid, and medications such as potassium-sparing diuretics and others containing potassium are common causes of hyperkalemia.

Clinical manifestations of hyperkalemia are related to muscle dysfunction and are manifested by hyperactivity of gastrointestinal smooth muscle, with resultant intestinal cramping and diarrheal weak skeletal muscles; general weakness progressing to flaccid paralysis; lethargy; and dysfunction of cardiac muscle resulting in cardiac arrhythmias such as tachycardia and potentially progressing to heart failure and cardiac arrest, abnormalities in the electrocardiogram including a prolonged QRS complex, a peak in T waves, atrioventricular block, and ventricular tachycardia (Nechyba & Gunn, 2002).

The major diagnostic test is serum potassium; normal levels for premature infants are 4.5–7.2 mmol/L, full-term newborns have levels from 3.7 to 5.2 mmol/L, and children have levels from 3.5 to 5.8 mmol/L.

Hyperkalemia is primarily treated by management of the underlying condition that caused the imbalance.

Potassium can be removed from the body by peritoneal dialysis or hemodialysis, by potassium-wasting diuretics, or with a cation-exchange resin (Kayexalate) that is administered orally or rectally.

Medical treatments that drive potassium ions into cells are intravenous calcium and bicarbonate, intravenous insulin, and glucose.

Any child who is receiving an intravenous infusion that contains potassium is at risk for hyperkalemia, so nurses assess for normal urine output before administering intravenous potassium solutions.

Intravenous solutions to which potassium has been added should be mixed thoroughly by gentle turning of the solutions before they are connected to the infusion tubing.

Ensure that infusions of blood or packed red blood cells are fresh, especially for the child receiving multiple transfusions; for all neonates, use a cardiac monitor during infusion of these products to watch for arrhythmias.

Once a child is diagnosed as hyperkalemic, ensure that any infusions with added potassium are stopped.

Several corrective infusions may need to be managed, including glucose, bicarbonate, and calcium gluconate; maintain the infusion at the ordered rate and monitor the child's condition frequently.

On diagnosis of hyperkalemia, an electrocardiogram is performed and a cardiac monitor applied; monitor for any changes in cardiac status and for cardiac arrhythmias, and report abnormal rate and character of pulse as well as shortness of breath.

Because the child is weak, side rails should be raised; position the child carefully; assist the child with activities requiring leg muscle strength, such as climbing into bed or pushing up in bed.

Encourage quiet activities with frequent rest periods, considering both the child's developmental level and the degree of muscle involvement.

Document and report any change in muscle weakness.

Adequate caloric intake is necessary to prevent tissue breakdown and the resultant potassium release from cells, so offer the child nourishing snacks if appetite is decreased; restrict potassium-rich foods.

If the child has chronic renal failure or another condition that decreases aldosterone secretion, parents and the child need to be taught to restrict foods that are high in potassium—for example, most oral rehydration solutions, including Pedialyte, as well as cola drinks, contain potassium and should not be used to provide fluid for the child.

Instruct parents to check with the care provider and pharmacist before giving even over-the-counter products to the child, as some of these medications contain potassium.

Management of renal failure at home with frequent visits for dialysis and other treatments can be challenging.

Hypokalemia
Description and Etiology
Hypokalemia occurs when the serum potassium concentration is too low; total body potassium level may be decreased, normal, or even increased when the serum level is low, depending on the cause of the imbalance.

Serum potassium levels below 3.5 mmol/L in children (3.7 mmol/L for newborns) are diagnostic of hypokalemia.

Hypokalemia is caused by conditions that involve increased potassium excretion, decreased potassium intake, shift of potassium from the extracellular fluid into cells, and loss of potassium by an abnormal route.

- Increased potassium excretion is a major cause of hypokalemia in children; in addition to diuretics and other medications, causes of increased urinary potassium excretion are osmotic diuresis (glucose present in urine), hypomagnesemia, increased aldosterone (hyperaldosteronism, congestive heart failure, nephrotic syndrome, cirrhosis), and increased cortisol (Cushing's disease and syndrome).
- Eating large amounts of black licorice increases renal excretion of potassium.
- Diarrhea causes potassium to be excreted in the feces and is a major cause of the imbalance in developing countries.
- Loss of potassium by an abnormal route occurs through vomiting.
- Nasogastric suctioning and intestinal decompression can cause potassium loss.
- Decreased potassium intake leads to hypokalemia slowly, or more rapidly if combined with increased excretion or loss of potassium.
- Hospitalized children may be placed on "nothing by mouth" status and receive prolonged intravenous therapy without potassium.
- Adolescents concerned about weight loss or those with anorexia nervosa may embark on diets low in potassium and may take medications that induce diuresis or diarrhea.

- Shift of potassium from the extracellular fluid into cells occurs in alkalosis and hypothermia (unintentional or induced for surgery).
- Hyperalimentation often causes hypersecretion of insulin, which also shifts potassium into cells.

Hypokalemia can also be caused by several medications, including the following:
- Beta-adrenergic agonists
- Insulin
- Potassium-wasting diuretics
- Parenteral penicillins
- Glucocorticoids
- Aminoglycoside antimicrobials
- Systemic antifungals
- Antineoplastics
- Laxatives

Clinical Manifestation and Diagnostic Tests

Because the ratio of intracellular to extracellular potassium determines the responsiveness of muscle cells to neural stimuli, clinical manifestations of hypokalemia involve muscle dysfunction.

Gastrointestinal smooth muscle activity is slowed, leading to abdominal distention, constipation, or paralytic ileus.

Skeletal muscles are weak and unresponsive to stimuli, and weakness may progress to flaccid paralysis.

The respiratory muscles may be impaired; cardiac arrhythmias can occur.

Polyuria results from changes in the kidney caused by hypokalemia.

Mild muscle fatigue occurs with potassium levels of less than 3.5 mmol/L, muscle necrosis at levels less than 2.5 mmol/L, and flaccidity and respiratory problems at levels less than 2 mmol/L (English, 2002).

Serum measurement of potassium is the major laboratory test; see normal values in Table 14–3.

Clinical Therapy

Clinical therapy of hypokalemia focuses on replacement of potassium while treating the cause of the imbalance; potassium replacement may be given intravenously or orally.

Nursing Management

Monitor serum potassium levels.

Observe for muscle weakness, which is frequently detected first in the legs.

Muscle weakness may affect the respiratory muscles; monitor respirations and assess the child frequently to determine the need for assisted ventilation.

Cardiac monitoring is important for continued assessment of hypokalemia-associated arrhythmias.

Assess for diminished bowel sounds and polyuria.

A hypokalemic child who is able to eat should be given a high-potassium diet; teach parents (and the child if old enough) which foods are high in potassium and how to incorporate them into the daily diet.

Children who have no oral intake for a period of time should receive intravenous fluids that contain potassium; calculate the dosage to ensure accuracy, and be sure that the infusion runs on schedule.

Maintain patency of intravenous infusions with potassium to avoid infiltration, which can cause painful tissues; consult the hospital formulary for dilution and administration guidelines.

Monitor urine output.

A hypokalemic child who is receiving digitalis needs careful surveillance for digitalis toxicity, which is manifested as anorexia, nausea, vomiting, and bradycardia (take the pulse rate and rhythm regularly).

Ensure adequate fluids and fiber in the diet; monitor and record the number of stools and report inadequate stools.

Keep side rails up; assist the child as needed to move into and out of bed; use supportive pillows to position the child properly.

Reposition the child frequently to preserve skin integrity of limbs that are not moved regularly.

Perform passive range of motion if the child is not moving.

The adolescent who is trying to lose weight and not consuming a nutritious diet needs dietary teaching; refer teens who are anorexic or bulimic for mental health counseling.

Teach parents how to give potassium supplements, if prescribed; liquid or powdered potassium supplements can be mixed with juice or sherbet to improve the bitter taste.

Hypercalcemia

Hypercalcemia refers to a plasma excess of calcium [more than 5.3 mEq/L (2.7 mmol/L) in children or 5 mEq/L (2.5 mmol/L) in newborns]; because so much calcium is stored in the bones, however, the serum levels of calcium may not reflect body stores.

Hypercalcemia is caused by conditions that involve increased calcium intake or absorption, shift of calcium from bones into the extracellular fluid, and decreased calcium excretion.

- Hypercalcemia due to increased calcium intake or absorption may occur if an infant is fed large amounts of chicken liver (source of vitamin A) or is given megadoses of vitamin D or vitamin A or if a child or adolescent consumes large amounts of calcium-rich foods concurrently with antacids (milk-alkali syndrome).
- Infants with very low birth weight can develop hypercalcemia if they have inadequate phosphorus intake, as bone phosphorus and calcium will be resorbed.
- Hypercalcemia may also occur when children receiving total parenteral nutrition are given doses of calcium that are too high.
- Most cases of hypercalcemia in children are due to a shift of calcium from bones into the extracellular fluid; the excessive amounts of parathyroid hormone produced in hyperparathyroidism cause calcium withdrawal from bones; prolonged immobilization also causes withdrawal of calcium from bones.
- Hypercalcemia also occurs with many types of malignancies such as leukemias.
- Familial hypercalcemia and infantile hypercalcemia are rare congenital disorders.
- Thiazide diuretics (e.g., thiazide and hydrochlorothiazide) decrease calcium excretion in the urine and may contribute to development of hypercalcemia.

Signs and symptoms of hypercalcemia include constipation, anorexia, nausea, and vomiting; fatigue and skeletal muscle weakness, confusion, lethargy, and decreased attention span are common, and polyuria/polydipsia may develop.

Renal calculi may form due to the high calcium levels; severe hypercalcemia may cause cardiac arrhythmias and arrest.

Neonates with hypercalcemia have flaccid muscles and exhibit failure to thrive.

Hypercalcemia is treated by increasing fluids and administering the diuretic furosemide (Lasix) to increase excretion of calcium in the urine; treatment to decrease intestinal absorption of calcium involves effective use of glucocorticoids; bone resorption can be decreased by administration of glucocorticoids and calcitonin; phosphate is sometimes given to treat hypercalcemia, but it may cause dangerous precipitation of calcium phosphate salts in body.

Severe hypercalcemia may need to be treated with dialysis.

Nursing Management

Nursing assessment of a child with hypercalcemia includes monitoring serum calcium levels, level of consciousness, gastrointestinal function, urine volume, specific gravity, cardiac rhythm, and pH; with chronic hypercalcemia, assessment of activity tolerance and developmental level becomes important.

Carefully calculate calcium in total parenteral nutrition and other solutions, administer these solutions with caution, and use cardiac monitoring to prevent hypercalcemia in hospitalized children.

A generous fluid intake, appropriate to the child's age, is necessary to keep the urine dilute and to help reduce constipation (a common symptom of hypercalcemia).

Thiazide diuretics, which decrease calcium excretion, should not be given to the hypercalcemic child.

Provide a high-fiber diet to help reduce constipation.

Increasing mobility through assisted weight bearing helps to decrease the withdrawal of calcium from bones that is caused by immobility; if the hypercalcemia is caused by withdrawal of calcium from bones, the child is at risk for fractures with minor trauma and must be handled with special care.

Teach parents to avoid giving calcium-rich foods and calcium antacids (e.g., TUMS) to children with hypercalcemia; suggest juices and frozen fruit desserts as an alternative to milk and ice cream; vitamin D supplements should be avoided, as they increase calcium absorption from the gastrointestinal tract.

Hypocalcemia

Description and Etiology

Hypocalcemia is a serum deficit of calcium [less than 4.4 mEq/L (2.2 mmol/L) in children, 4 mEq/L (2 mmol/L) in newborns, or 3.4 mEq/L (1.7 mmol/L) in premature infants] (Umpaichitra, Bastian, & Castells, 2001); serum calcium levels may not reflect body stores of this mineral, as most of the body's calcium is stored in bone.

Hypocalcemia is caused by conditions that involve decreased calcium intake or absorption, shift of calcium to a physiologically unavailable form, increased calcium excretion, and loss of calcium by an abnormal route.

Decreased calcium intake or absorption causes hypocalcemia in children with chronic generalized malnutrition or with a diet that is low in vitamin D and calcium.

Female adolescents trying to lose or maintain a low weight often decrease foods that contain calcium and may develop chronic hypocalcemia; in these cases, premature bone loss and inadequate bone formation occur.

If a child does not ingest enough vitamin D, calcium is not absorbed efficiently from the duodenum.

Sunlight speeds formation of vitamin D in the skin, so children who are institutionalized without access to sunlight (e.g., severely developmentally delayed children), those with very dark skin, or children kept well covered when outside may become hypocalcemic due to lack of vitamin D.

Uremic syndrome is another cause of vitamin D deficiency because it interferes with the kidney's ability to activate vitamin D.

High phosphate intake can cause hypocalcemia.

Chronic diarrhea and steatorrhea (fatty stools) also reduce calcium absorption from the gastrointestinal tract.

Alkalosis causes more calcium to bind to plasma proteins and become physiologically inactive.

Citrate, found in transfused blood, can bind to body calcium.

Hypomagnesemia impairs parathyroid hormone function and may cause hypocalcemia.

Some types of neonatal hypocalcemia are associated with delayed parathyroid hormone function or hypomagnesemia.

A genetic abnormality can result in calcium-sensing receptor defect.

Infants of diabetic mothers may have hypocalcemia in response to glycosuria that leads to hypomagnesemia.

Very-low-birth-weight babies and newborns with respiratory impairment are prone to develop hypocalcemia.

Calcium shifts rapidly into bone when rickets is treated.

A high plasma phosphate concentration causes plasma calcium to decrease.

Children who receive liver transplants are hypocalcemic for several days due to impaired citrate metabolism.

Increased calcium excretion occurs in steatorrhea, when calcium secreted into the gastrointestinal fluid binds to the fecal fat in addition to the dietary calcium that is bound in the feces; a similar situation occurs in acute pancreatitis.

Loss of calcium by an abnormal route may contribute to hypocalcemia, as calcium is lost from the body through burn or wound drainage or sequestered in acute pancreatitis.

Many different medications can cause hypocalcemia, including antacids, laxatives, oil-based bowel lubricants, anticonvulsants, phosphate-containing preparations, protein-type plasma expanders during rapid infusion, and antineoplastics.

Clinical Manifestations

The signs and symptoms of hypocalcemia are manifestations of increased muscular excitability (tetany).

In children, symptoms include twitching and cramping, tingling around the mouth or in the fingers, carpal spasm, and pedal spasm.

Infants may demonstrate tremors, muscle twitches, and brief tonic-clonic seizures.

Laryngospasm, seizures, and cardiac arrhythmias are more severe manifestations of hypocalcemia and may be fatal.

Hypocalcemia may cause congestive heart failure, especially in neonates.

A chronic state of hypocalcemia may be manifested by spontaneous fractures in infants and in adolescents who exercise excessively.

Diagnostic Tests and Clinical Therapy

Laboratory assessment of serum calcium level may be performed.

Hypocalcemia is treated by oral or intravenous administration of calcium.

The original cause of the imbalance is treated; if hypocalcemia is due to hypomagnesemia, the magnesium must be replenished before the calcium replacement can be successful.

When the cause is chronic low dietary intake, counseling is needed about high-calcium foods and perhaps the necessity for vitamin D intake or supplements.

Nursing Management

Carefully assess growth in the female or male who is trying to diet; when an adolescent female is very thin, be sure to ask about excessive sports and other activities and about regularity of menstrual periods; if periods are irregular or not occurring, collect additional dietary information to help determine whether the girl is lacking in intake of calcium, calories, and other nutrients.

Assess for signs of inadequate nutrition such as fat and muscle wasting, dry hair, and cold hands and feet.

In those who may have acute hypocalcemia, assess for muscle cramps, stiffness, and clumsiness; grimacing caused by spasms of facial muscles and twitching of arm muscles; and laryngospasm.

Increased neuromuscular excitability may be detected by testing for Trousseau's sign or Chvostek's sign.

Monitor serum calcium levels and perform continuous cardiac monitoring to observe for cardiac arrhythmias in acute hypocalcemia.

To correct calcium deficiency in the hospitalized child, give oral or intravenous calcium as ordered; a 10% intravenous calcium gluconate solution should be readily available for emergency use in severe hypocalcemia. Calcium is never given intramuscularly because it causes tissue necrosis.

Take measures to ensure safety for the child who is hospitalized with hypocalcemia; seizure precautions may be necessary.

Explain the cause of muscle cramps to parents and older children.

Counsel the family about dairy products and nondairy foods rich in calcium; these include milk, cheese, yogurt, pudding, egg yolks, legumes, nuts, figs, chicken, salmon (canned with bones), grains (Cream of Wheat, farina, bran muffins), sardines (canned), tofu, and fruit drinks with added calcium.

ACID–BASE IMBALANCES
Respiratory Acidosis
Description and Etiology

Respiratory acidosis is caused by the accumulation of carbon dioxide in the blood. Because carbon dioxide and water can be combined into carbonic acid, respiratory acidosis is sometimes called *carbonic acid excess*; the condition can be acute or chronic and is controlled by the lungs.

Any factor that interferes with the ability of the lungs to excrete carbon dioxide can cause respiratory acidosis. These factors may interfere with the gaseous exchange within the lungs, may impair the neuromuscular pump that moves air in and out of the lungs, or may depress the respiratory rate.

As the carbon dioxide partial pressure (Pco_2) begins to increase, the pH of the blood begins to decrease. Compensatory mechanisms begin to act in the form of nonbicarbonate buffers, additional hydrogen ion excretion by the kidneys, and decreased bicarbonate excretion by the kidneys. These compensatory mechanisms may take several days to become clinically evident in most situations, depending on the underlying cause and the amount of compensation occurring.

Clinical Manifestations

Acidosis in the brain cells causes central nervous system depression, manifested by confusion, lethargy, headache, increased intracranial pressure, and even coma.

Acute respiratory acidosis can lead to tachycardia and cardiac arrhythmias.

The child's arterial blood gases always show an increased PCO_2, the laboratory sign of increased carbonic acid.

Serum pH can be decreased or normal.

Diagnostic Tests and Clinical Therapy

Laboratory tests involve arterial blood gases (see Table 14–4 for normal values).

Treatment of respiratory acidosis requires correction of the underlying cause—for example, treatment may include bronchodilators for bronchospasm, mechanical ventilation for neuromuscular defects, decreasing sedative use, or surgery for kyphoscoliosis.

Table 14–4 Normal Blood pH and Gases

	Infants	Children	Adolescents
Arterial blood pH	7.18–7.50	7.27–7.49	7.35–7.41
Arterial blood oxygen partial pressure	60–70 mm Hg (8.0–9.3 pKa)	80–108 mm Hg (10.7–14.4 pKa)	80–100 mm Hg (10.7–13.3 pKa)
Arterial blood carbon dioxide partial pressure	27–41 mm Hg (3.6–5.5 pKa)	32–48 mm Hg (4.3–6.4 pKa)	32–48 mm Hg (4.3–6.4 pKa)
Arterial blood bicarbonate	19–24 mmol/L	18–25 mmol/L	20–29 mmol/L

Nursing Management

Assessment

Assess respiratory rate, rhythm, and depth carefully.

Take the apical pulse and be alert for tachycardia or arrhythmia.

A cardiac monitor may be used.

Obtain serial arterial blood gas measurements in acute conditions to evaluate changing status.

Assess the level of consciousness and energy.

Observe for chronic fatigue, headache, or decreased level of consciousness.

Intervention

Ensure safety of the hospitalized child in respiratory acidosis; keep side rails raised, and turn and position the child frequently.

Evaluate mental status and document and report any changes in alertness.

When laboratory values of blood pH and PCO_2 are available, evaluate them promptly and report any changes or abnormalities.

Administer medications as ordered.

Carefully watch the doses of sedatives to avoid further respiratory depression.

Provide suctioning as needed and encourage deep breathing using age-appropriate techniques.

Patient and Family Education

Teach children at risk for respiratory acidosis and their parents preventive measures to use at home.

For the child with a chronic condition such as cystic fibrosis, muscular dystrophy, or kyphoscoliosis, demonstrate deep breathing and encourage its use several times each day.

Teach the family signs of infection—including fever, increased respiratory secretions, and discomfort with breathing—so the problems can be treated promptly to prevent further respiratory involvement.

Demonstrate techniques to position the child to facilitate chest expansion.

Teach parents about proper administration of any necessary medications.

Teach parents and older children about home respirator use when indicated.

Respiratory Alkalosis
Description and Etiology
Respiratory alkalosis occurs when the blood contains too little carbon dioxide; it is sometimes called *carbonic acid deficit.*

Excess carbon dioxide loss is caused by hyperventilation, in which more air than normal is moved into and out of the lungs.

Common causes of hyperventilation include the following:
- Hypoxemia
- Anxiety
- Pain
- Fever
- Salicylate poisoning
- Meningitis
- Encephalitis
- Septicemia caused by gram-negative bacteria
- Mechanical overventilation
- Hypoxia from severe asthma
  (Foster, Vaziri, & Sassoon, 2001)

Clinical Manifestations
The lack of carbon dioxide causes neuromuscular irritability and paresthesias in the extremities and around the mouth.

Muscle cramping and carpal or pedal spasms can occur.

The child may be dizzy or confused.

Diagnostic Tests
Arterial blood gas measurements show a decreased P_{CO_2} in respiratory alkalosis.

Blood pH is generally elevated (see Table 14–4).

Clinical Therapy
Clinical therapy focuses on correcting the condition that caused the hyperventilation, sepsis, hypoxia, or other condition so that the body's compensatory mechanisms can return carbon dioxide levels to normal.

Oxygen therapy may be helpful in some cases of hypoxia; salicylates are removed from the body.

Drugs that have interfered with breathing are stopped, and sepsis is treated with effective medications.

Anxiolytic medications may also be prescribed in certain situations.

Nursing Management

Assess the child's level of consciousness, and ask if the child feels light headed or has tingling sensations or numbness in the fingers, toes, or around the mouth.

Assess the rate and depth of respirations.

Monitor the hospitalized child's oxygen partial pressure with serial arterial blood gas measurements to evaluate changes in status.

A careful assessment is needed regarding the cause of hyperventilation.

When anxiety is the cause of respiratory alkalosis, instruct the child to breathe slowly, in rhythm with your own breathing; teach stress control techniques such as relaxation or imagery, and use other developmentally appropriate interventions for situations that cause anxiety in children and adolescents.

Use medications, imagery, distraction, positioning, massage, and other techniques to decrease pain and maintain pain management.

Have the child cough, or suction as needed; be certain that mechanical ventilation systems are working properly.

Provide a safe environment for the child who has a decreased level of consciousness.

Renal compensation to manage ongoing respiratory alkalosis requires adequate urinary output; regulate fluid intake to ensure urine output unless fluids are restricted due to medical condition.

Metabolic Acidosis

Description and Etiology

Metabolic acidosis is a condition in which there is an excess of any acid other than carbonic acid; it is sometimes called *noncarbonic acid excess.*

Metabolic acidosis is caused by an imbalance in production and excretion of acid or by excess loss of bicarbonate.

Excess accumulation occurs by one of two mechanisms: First, a child can eat or drink acids or substances that are converted to acid in the body (e.g., aspirin, boric acid, antifreeze); second, cells can make abnormally high amounts of acid that cannot be excreted [e.g., ketoacidosis of untreated diabetes mellitus, untreated growth hormone deficiency (Glaser, Shirali, Styne, & Jones, 1998), bladder construction that uses part of the bowel (Mundy, 1999), the starvation that can occur in anorexia or bulimia].

A disorder of excretion occurs in conditions such as oliguric renal failure.

Bicarbonate can be lost from the body through the urine or through excessive loss of intestinal fluid (e.g., diarrhea, fistulas, and ileal drainage are all possible causes).

Carbonic anhydrase inhibitors can cause loss of excess bicarbonate in the urine.

Clinical Manifestations

When the pH of the blood decreases below normal, the chemoreceptors in the brain and arteries are stimulated, and respiratory compensation begins; increased rate and depth of respirations (hyperventilation), or Kussmaul respirations, are observed.

Severe acidosis can cause decreased peripheral vascular resistance and resultant cardiac arrhythmias, hypotension, pulmonary edema, and tissue hypoxia.

Confusion or drowsiness may result, as well as headache or abdominal pain.

Diagnostic Tests

Laboratory tests include measurement of blood pH and blood gases; values show decreased blood pH and decreased bicarbonate and P_{CO_2}; the degree of alteration depends on the underlying cause and the body's attempt at compensation (see Table 14–4).

Clinical Therapy

Treatment of metabolic acidosis depends on identification and treatment of the underlying cause.

In severe metabolic acidosis, intravenous sodium bicarbonate may be used to increase the pH and to prevent cardiac arrhythmias.

Nursing Management

Assess the rate and depth of respirations.

Evaluate the child's level of consciousness frequently.

Be alert for signs or complaints of headache and abdominal pain.

Serial arterial blood gas measurements are usually obtained to evaluate changes in status.

Ensure safety, taking into account the child's level of consciousness and alertness.

Turn the child, and change his or her position to prevent pressure on the skin.

Limit the child's activities to decrease cardiac workload.

Position the child to facilitate chest expansion.

Provide oral care during rapid respirations because the mouth may become dry.

Monitor intravenous solutions and laboratory values indicating acid–base balance; report changes promptly.

Once the child is stabilized, provide teaching to compensate for knowledge deficits; teach parents of young children to keep medications and acids locked in a secure place and out of reach to prevent poisoning; teach about home management of diabetes and about early identification and treatment to avoid diabetic ketoacidosis.

Metabolic Alkalosis
Description and Etiology
Metabolic alkalosis occurs when there are too few metabolic acids; it is sometimes called *noncarbonic acid deficit.*

A gain in bicarbonate or a loss of metabolic acid can cause metabolic alkalosis.

Bicarbonate is gained through excessive intake of bicarbonate antacids or baking soda or through metabolism of bicarbonate precursors such as the citrate contained in blood transfusions.

Increased renal absorption of bicarbonate can occur with diuretic use, profound hypokalemia, primary hyperaldosteronism, or extreme deficit in extracellular fluid volume.

Acid can be lost through severe vomiting, such as that seen in infants with pyloric stenosis and in continued removal of gastric contents through suction.

Clinical Manifestations
Hypokalemia often occurs simultaneously (see description in Hypokalemia).

Respiratory rate and depth usually decrease.

Increased neuromuscular irritability, cramping, paresthesia, tetany, seizures, and excitation can occur.

Metabolic alkalosis can progress to weakness, confusion, lethargy, and coma.

Diagnostic Tests

Laboratory tests include blood pH and blood gases; blood pH, bicarbonate, and P_{CO_2} are usually elevated in metabolic alkalosis (see Table 14–4).

Clinical Therapy

Clinical therapy is directed at treating the underlying cause of the condition.

Increasing the extracellular fluid volume with intravenous normal saline is used to facilitate renal excretion of bicarbonate.

Medications such as acetazolamide may be used to increase renal excretion of bicarbonate.

Nursing Management

Assess the child's level of consciousness frequently; alertness may decrease after an initial period of excitement, so regular assessments are needed.

Monitor neuromuscular irritability.

Observe for nausea and vomiting.

Assess the rate and depth of respirations carefully.

Obtain serial arterial blood gas measurements as ordered.

Facilitate ease of respirations.

Ensure safety by keeping bed rails elevated and by turning the child frequently.

Position the child on the side to avoid aspiration of vomitus.

Administer intravenous infusions and medications as ordered.

If antacids are the cause of the alkalosis, teach the child and parents about correct use of these medications.

15. ALTERATIONS IN EYE, EAR, NOSE, AND THROAT FUNCTION

DISORDERS OF THE EYE
Infectious Conjunctivitis

Conjunctivitis is an inflammation of the conjunctiva, the clear membrane that lines the inside of the lid and sclera. There are several types of conjunctivitis, depending on the cause of inflammation. Bacteria, viruses, allergies, trauma, or irritants cause the conjunctiva to become swollen and red, with a clear, yellow, or white discharge.

Clinical Manifestations

Symptoms depend on the type of conjunctivitis and provide clues to diagnosis.

Bacterial conjunctivitis in an infant younger than 30 days of age is called *ophthalmia neonatorum*. These infections are usually acquired from the mother during vaginal delivery as a result of contact with infected vaginal discharge containing organisms such as *Chlamydia trachomatis* and *Neisseria gonorrhoeae*. Redness, swelling, and exudate are characteristic.

Bacterial conjunctivitis can occur in older children as well. It is characterized by edema of the eyelid, red conjunctiva, and enlarged preauricular lymph glands. There is usually mucopurulent exudate that causes matting, making the eyes difficult to open on awakening. Older children with conjunctivitis complain of itching or burning, mild photophobia, and a feeling of scratching under the lids.

Viral conjunctivitis may cause redness, swelling, and tearing of the eyes. Adenoviruses are common causes. Herpesviruses may be accompanied by herpes lesions on the face and are serious viral infections.

In allergic conjunctivitis, the child complains of intense itching. Eyes are red and swollen, with watery discharge; the conjunctivae have a "cobblestone" appearance. This condition is not infectious and is simply related to allergy.

Diagnostic Tests

Diagnosis is based on the history and symptoms.

Cultures may be taken, especially in infants or in cases suspected of being unusual bacterial illness or herpesviruses.

A Gram stain of discharge and conjunctival scraping for potential *Chlamydia* infection or herpes are performed.

Clinical Therapy

Clinical therapy includes routine prophylaxis of all infants to prevent ophthalmia neonatorum; 1% silver nitrate, 1% tetracycline, or 0.5% erythromycin may be used.

Antibiotic eye medication in droplet or ointment form for bacterial infection can be used; fluoroquinolones are frequently used.

For gonococcal conjunctivitis in newborns, ceftriaxone is recommended; the disease is resistant to penicillin; a single intramuscular (IM) or intravenous (IV) dose may be used if the infection is localized in the eye, or 7 days of IV therapy with cefotaxime is used for disseminated infection.

Chlamydial infections are treated with oral erythromycin or tetracycline (latter drug may be used only for those older than age 8 years).

Viral conjunctivitis may be treated with comfort measures such as cleaning drainage away with a warm clean cloth, avoiding bright lights, and avoiding reading.

Herpes simplex virus infections of the eye are treated promptly by an ophthalmologist, neonatologist, or others trained in treating this serious disease. Topical drugs are used and often are combined with a systemic antiviral agent such as acyclovir (Alcorn, 2001; Gross, 2002). Neonatal herpes simplex virus is treated vigorously with parenteral acyclovir for 14 days (or longer if central nervous system involvement is found on lumbar puncture) and with topical ophthalmic medication (trifluridine, iododeoxyuridine, or vidarabine). Recurrent lesions may necessitate suppressive or prophylactic treatment with oral acyclovir (American Academy of Pediatrics, 2003).

If an allergen is diagnosed as the cause of conjunctivitis, systemic or topical antihistamines may be prescribed. Decongestants can be combined with systemic antihistamines for short-term therapy. More current treatment involves use of mast cell stabilizers to decrease the activation of mast cells that accompanies allergic reactions. Most mast cell stabilizers have been tested and found to be safe in children 3 years of age and older (Alexander, 2003).

Nursing Management

Assess eyes of infants and children for any signs of conjunctivitis.

Refer the child to an ophthalmologist or other care provider for diagnosis and treatment.

Administer eye medications as prescribed.

Isolate children infected with bacterial or viral agents from others in the hospital; they should be kept home from school for bacterial conjunctivitis until treated with antibiotics for 24 hours.

Be alert for infections in childcare and school settings so that spread to other children can be minimized.

Teach parents correct administration of medications, comfort measures, and proper hygiene to prevent spread of infection to others.

Visual Disorders
Clinical Manifestations

In hyperopia (farsightedness), light rays focus posterior to the retina, resulting in an inability to focus on nearby objects.

In myopia (nearsightedness), light rays focus anterior to the retina, resulting in an inability to focus on far objects.

In astigmatism, light rays are refracted differently depending on their place of entry to the eye because the curvature of the cornea or lens is not uniformly spherical, causing blurred images.

Strabismus is an abnormal deviation or misalignment of the eye, usually inward or outward; the eyes are misaligned so that symmetric vision, or binocularity, is not possible.

In amblyopia, or reduced vision of the eye, generally one eye has much poorer vision than the other, resulting in loss of binocularity.

A cataract is opacity of the lens that is present at birth or develops during childhood.

Glaucoma is increased intraocular pressure that changes the structure of the eye and can lead to visual impairment and blindness if untreated.

Depending on the disorder and severity, the child may have asymmetric eye movements, have asymmetric light reflex, hold the head to one side, squint, have watering eyes or headaches, and/or show developmental delays.

See CM 15–1 for further detail on clinical manifestations of visual disorders.

Diagnostic Tests

Diagnostic tests include those for visual acuity and developmental testing, as well as ophthalmologic examination.

Clinical Therapy

Clinical therapy includes compensatory lenses, patching, and eye exercises.

Surgery for some conditions.

Medications for glaucoma or some cancers.

Nursing Management

Assessment

Observe for

- Visual acuity.
- Symmetry of eye movement.
- Ability to follow objects in all planes.
- Symmetry of light reflex.
- Developmental progression.

Obtain a complete and thorough history.

Examine for risk factors such as prematurity and low birth weight.

See Table 15–1 for assessment of visual disorders.

Implementation

Refer all abnormalities to eye specialist.

Teach importance of prescribed treatments.

Teach correct care for compensatory lenses, postsurgical care, and medication instillation.

Encourage interactions and skills that promote development.

Retinopathy of Prematurity

Clinical Manifestations

Retinopathy of prematurity occurs when immature blood vessels in the retina constrict and become necrotic. This condition, most common in infants of low birth weight or of short gestation, can heal completely or lead to mild myopia or retinal detachment and blindness.

Arteriole constriction, followed by vascular proliferation of abnormal vessels, occurs. In most cases, the abnormal vessels gradually

CM 15–1 Clinical Manifestations of Visual Disorders

Etiology	Clinical Manifestations	Clinical Therapy
Strabismus Can be congenital or acquired. Seen in 5% of all children. Most common types: Esotropia: inward deviation of eyes ("crossed eyes"). Exotropia: outward deviation of eyes ("wall eyes").	Eyes appear misaligned to observer. May occur only when child is tired. Symptoms include squinting and frowning when reading; closing one eye to see; having trouble picking up objects; dizziness and headache. Corneal light reflex and cover-uncover tests confirm diagnosis. Child may have no other abnormalities, but certain conditions such as cerebral palsy, hydrocephalus, Down syndrome, and seizure disorder are more commonly accompanied by strabismus. If treatment is begun before 24 months of age, amblyopia (reduced vision in one or both eyes) may be prevented.	Occlusion therapy (patching the fixating or good eye to force use of the weak eye). Compensatory lenses. Surgery of the rectus muscles to correct muscle imbalance. Eye drops to cause blurring of the good eye. Prisms. Vision therapy (eye exercises).

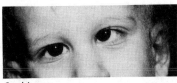

Reprinted from Paediatrics, 2nd ed., Thomas & Harvey, p. 130, 1997, by permission of the publisher Churchill Livingstone.

Strabismus

| **Amblyopia ("lazy eye")**
Reduced vision in one or both eyes; affects 7% of children.
Can result from anything that causes | Symptoms are the same as for strabismus.
Vision testing can be used to diagnose condition. | Compensatory lenses.
Occlusion therapy for 2–6 hr daily.
Occasionally vision therapy (eye exercises) is used in an attempt |

(continued)

Etiology	Clinical Manifestations	Clinical Therapy
Amblyopia (*continued*) visual deprivation to one eye. The most common causes are untreated strabismus, with the child "tuning out" the image in deviating eye, congenital cataract, or visual differences between eyes.		to improve the weaker eye. Atropine 1% 1 gtt/day in unaffected eye. Treatment is discontinued when visual faculty no longer improves; 20/20 acuity rarely attained. Treatment is most successful if received by 5–6 years of age.
Cataracts Occur when all or part of lens of eye becomes opaque, which prevents refraction of light rays onto retina. Seen in 1 of every 250 newborns.	Can affect one or both eyes and may be congenital or acquired. Clouding of lens indicates presence of cataract; however, cataracts are not always visible to naked eye. Symptoms include distorted red reflex, symptoms of vision loss (see Strabismus), white pupil. May be present alone but sometimes associated with fetal alcohol syndrome and Down syndrome.	Must be diagnosed at a young age for successful treatment; many cases are missed. Specific treatment depends on whether one or both eyes are affected, extent of clouding and presence of other ocular abnormalities. Surgical removal of lens and corrective lenses; contact lenses frequently used; results of surgery are good; surgery before the age of 2 months is associated with the best results; visual acuity in 55% of children is 20/40 or better. Lens implant may be used. Eye protectors and restraints are used postoperatively to prevent injury; antibiotic or steroid drops may be used for several weeks; treatment for amblyopia may be necessary.

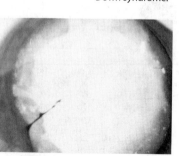

Congenital cataract

From Vaughan, D., Asbury, T., & Riordan-Eva, P. (1992). *General ophthalmology* (13th ed., p. 172). New York: McGraw-Hill Companies, with permission.

(*continued*)

CM 15-1 Clinical Manifestations of Visual Disorders (Continued)

Etiology	Clinical Manifestations	Clinical Therapy
Glaucoma		
Increased intraocular pressure damages eye and impairs visual function; ciliary body of eye produces aqueous fluid that flows between iris and lens into anterior chamber; if enough fluid accumulates, blindness results; affects 1 in 100,000 newborns. May be congenital (primary) or acquired (secondary) and affect one or both eyes.	Symptoms of congenital glaucoma include tearing, blinking, corneal clouding, eyelid spasms, and progressive enlargement of eye; photophobia (extreme sensitivity to light). Symptoms of acquired glaucoma include constant bumping into objects in child's periphery (painless visual field loss); seeing halos around objects. Diagnosis is made using tonometer, which measures intraocular pressure.	Surgery to reduce intraocular pressure is treatment of choice because medications used to combat glaucoma in adults are not as effective in children. Compensatory lenses used after surgery. Treatment is not always successful, especially if the child has congenital glaucoma, so parents' feelings regarding care of a visually handicapped child should be explored.

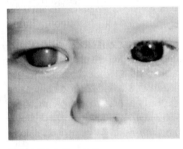

From Vaughan, D., Asbury, T. & Riordan-Eva, P. (1992). General ophthalmology. (13th ed., p. 172). New York: McGraw-Hill Companies, with permission.

Congenital glaucoma

Note: Data from Alterneier, W. A. (2000). Preschool vision screening: The importance of the two-line difference. Pediatric Annals, 29,264–267; Bacal, D. A., & Wilson, M. C. (2000). Strabismus: Getting it straight. Contemporary Pediatrics, 17,49–60; Starr, N. B. (2000). Vision therapy for learning disabilities and dyslexia. Journal of Pediatric Health Care, 14,32–33.

Table 15–1   Assessment Questions for Identifying Visual Disturbances in Children

Infant	Young Child	School-Age Child
Ask the parents the following:	Ask the parents the following:	Ask the parents the following:
Does your baby follow an object from one side to the other?	Does your child follow you with his or her eyes as you come into a room?	Does your child like to look at pictures and read?
What is your baby's reaction when you are directly in front and close?	Are other objects followed with ease?	Does your child hold toys or books close or sit very close to the television?
Does the baby seem to notice an object to the right and left sides?	Do both eyes work together or does one seem to wander off?	Does your child squint or rub the eyes?
Do your baby's eyes ever appear to move asymmetrically?	At what age did your baby sit, stand, and walk?	Is he or she performing at grade level in all subjects?
What is your baby learning to do right now?	Does your child have any difficulty picking up objects?	Has your child demonstrated any learning difficulties?
		Does he or she use a computer, watch television, or play computer games?
		Does your child play sports and games at the same level of ability as peers?

regress and normal vascularization occurs. Sometimes, however, the abnormal vascularization continues into the vitreous cavity, causing abnormalities of the retina, optic disk, and macula.

When visual impairment is present, the child usually manifests myopia. Total loss of vision can occur in the child who experiences a retinal detachment.

Diagnostic Tests
Ophthalmologic examination.

Infants at risk, particularly those under 2,000 g (4 lb, 3 oz) at birth or born before 33 weeks' gestation, are assessed frequently by an experienced ophthalmologist.

The disease does not manifest itself before 4–6 weeks after birth, so regular eye examinations are needed until the risk is discounted.

For infants with signs of disease, eye examinations continue every 1–2 weeks.

Clinical Therapy

Cryotherapy or laser therapy

Surgical procedures such as a scleral buckle procedure and vitrectomy for retinal detachments

Treatment of associated visual problems such as strabismus, amblyopia, and myopia to promote maximal development

See Table 15–2

Nursing Management
Assessment

Assess for risk factors such as prematurity, low birth weight, and oxygen therapy.

Monitor respiratory status.

Monitor ventilatory equipment for performance and proper settings.

Intervention

Refer to ophthalmologist as needed.

Table 15–2   Assessment and Treatment for Retinopathy of Prematurity (ROP)

Initial Assessment	Follow-Up Assessment	Treatment
Who? All infants less than 1,500 g or less than 28 weeks' gestation; babies 1,500–2,000 g who have other risk factors	Every 2–3 weeks if vasculature is immature and extends to zone II but no retinopathy is present; continue until normal vascularization is seen in zone III	Ablative therapy with laser or cryotherapy for infants reaching threshold disease; treatment needed within 72 hr of diagnosis to minimize chance of retinal detachment
When? 4–6 weeks postnatal age or 31–33 weeks of postconceptual age	Every 2 weeks if ROP is in zone II but not severe	
What? At least 2 funduscopic examinations with pupil dilation using binocular indirect ophthalmoscopy by an ophthalmologist; one examination is satisfactory if full retinal vascularization is seen bilaterally	Every 1–2 weeks if no ROP but having incomplete vasculature in zone I	
	Every week for infants with ROP in zone II, stage 3 ROP without plus disease or stage 2 ROP with plus disease or stage 3 ROP with plus disease not severe enough for surgery	

Note: Adapted from American Academy of Pediatrics Section on Ophthalmology (2001). Screening examination of premature infants for retinopathy of prematurity. Pediatrics, 108,809–811.

Provide kinesthetic, tactile, and auditory stimulation during play and in daily care.

Evaluate the environment for potential safety hazards based on age of child and degree of visual impairment.

Evaluate growth and development during all regular examinations as the child grows.

Patient and Family Education

Encourage parents of newborns at risk to return for scheduled appointments with ophthalmologist and developmental monitoring.

Help parents plan early, regular social activities with other children.

Refer parents to organizations, early intervention programs, and other parents of children with visual impairment.

Partner with parents during ongoing interventions to meet developmental, educational, and safety needs of the child with visual impairment.

See further suggestions for working with the child with visual impairment in Visual Impairment.

Visual Impairment
Clinical Manifestations

Legal blindness is defined as visual acuity of 20/200 or worse in the corrected eye or significantly reduced visual fields and occurs in 1 per 35,000 children; many more children have visual impairment.

Eyes may appear crossed or watery, and the lids may be crusty.

Verbal children may complain of itching; dizziness; headache; or blurred, double, or poor vision.

See Table 15–3 for further signs of visual impairment in children.

Table 15–3   Signs of Visual Impairment

Infants	Toddlers and Older Children
May be unable to follow lights or objects	May rub, shut, or cover eyes
Do not make eye contact	Tilt or thrust head forward
Have a dull, vacant stare	Blink frequently
Do not imitate facial expressions	Hold objects close
	Bump into objects
	Squint

Diagnostic Tests

Vision screening, followed by referral to an eye specialist for full examination for any abnormalities.

Responses to visual stimuli, symmetry of eye movements, location of corneal light reflex, cover-uncover testing, visual field testing, and funduscopic examination of retina.

Clinical Therapy

Surgery

Medication

Supportive aids such as glasses or contact lenses

Management by an interdisciplinary team of specialists to treat condition and maximize development

Nursing Management

Visual screening appropriate for age at each health promotion examination.

Visual acuity programs in schools.

Developmental screening; abnormalities may indicate visual impairment.

Teach safety, and encourage protective eyewear in activities such as sports (e.g., hockey, handball, football).

Work with school personnel to establish guidelines for protective eyewear for chemistry and other science or industrial education courses.

Keep laser pointers away from children because they can cause retinal damage, especially when stared at for 10 seconds.

For the child with visual impairment, nursing care focuses on encouraging the child's use of all senses, promoting socialization, helping parents to meet the child's developmental and educational needs, and providing emotional support to parents.

Announce another person's presence to the child when approaching.

When walking with a blind child, walk slightly ahead of the child so he or she can sense your movements.

Let the child hold the seeing person's arm rather than the reverse.

Identify the contents of meals and encourage the child to feed himself or herself.

Orient the child to new settings by explaining and allowing the child to feel objects.

Patient and Family Education

Stroke, rock, and hug infants and children who are visually impaired. Sing and talk to them. Infants with visual impairment appreciate and use touch and verbal interactions more, both in interactions with others, and when exploring new objects. These infants do not make eye contact and have rather blank expressions. Encourage parents to plan for interactions between the child and a variety of other children.

Teach parents to read body language and vocalization as expressions of emotion. Facial expressions give a great deal of information, but infants and children with poor vision do not have the ability to learn by visual imitation. Show parents how to use tactile means to teach appropriate facial expressions. For example, a touch on the arm can be soft and stroking to indicate a smile, but firmer to indicate dismay or frown.

Explain to parents that discipline and rewards for children with poor vision should be the same as those for other children in the family. The child should be given age-appropriate tasks.

Encourage contact with peers as the child grows older. Teach the child to look directly at persons who are talking to him or her. Play, sports, and other activities can be modified to give the visually impaired child the same social experiences as a sighted child.

Foster physical activity for visually impaired children by encouraging involvement in early intervention programs; recommending programs that increase cardiovascular strength, endurance, upper body strength, and flexibility; and facilitating participation in and reward for sports and athletics (Lieberman & McHugh, 2001). Ensure safety to prevent injury around the home, at school, and in other settings.

Provide parents with information about educational options before their child reaches school age. Education should take place in a setting that allows the child to have contact with other children and to participate in social activities. As the child enters middle and high school, it may be challenging to move to new schools or communities unfamiliar to the child. Help the parents to plan activities that will enable the youth to meet new friends.

The child may be mainstreamed with a tutor, be partially mainstreamed in a resource room, attend special classes, or be tutored at home. If the child is to attend public school, suggest to parents that they contact the school well before enrollment to ensure that school staff understands the child's disability.

Make sure that items such as large-print books, Braille materials, audio equipment, or a visual reading device is available. Ensure that frequent eye examinations are performed, and assist with proper use and care of prescribed glasses or contact lenses, as necessary.

Injuries of the Eye

Sports, darts, fireworks, air-powered BB guns, paint balls, blunt and sharp objects, chemical and thermal burns, physical irritants, and abuse are common causes of eye trauma in children (Behrman, Kliegman, & Jenson, 2004).

Teach about protective eyewear for sports and other hazardous activities.

Inquire about tetanus immunization history for all eye injuries; if a booster has not been administered in 5 years or more or if basic tetanus series is not completed, administer tetanus-diphtheria booster (form and dose appropriate for age of child).

See CM 15–2 for further information on clinical manifestations and treatment of eye injuries.

DISORDERS OF THE EAR
Otitis Media
Clinical Manifestations

Otitis media is common, with approximately 70% of infants having at least one case in the first year of life, and 93% affected by age 7 years. The short, horizontal eustachian tube of young children puts them at risk for this infection.

Risk factors include young age (6–12 months), males, attendance at childcare centers, having allergies, exposure to tobacco smoke, and pacifier use; winter months and conditions such as cleft lip and palate or Down syndrome also predispose children; breastfeeding is protective against otitis media.

Acute otitis media (AOM) is diagnosed when the child has acute onset of ear pain, marked redness of the tympanic membrane on otoscopy, and middle ear effusion; recurrent AOM is characterized by repeated episodes of AOM, such as three in 6 months, or four in 12 months.

Otitis media with effusion (OME) is evidence of fluid in the middle ear without inflammation.

CM 15–2 Clinical Manifestations and Emergency Treatment of Eye Injuries

Condition and Etiology	Clinical Manifestations	Clinical Therapy
Subconjunctival hemorrhage (caused by coughing, mild trauma, or increased physical activity)	Reddened area in conjunctiva	Usually heals spontaneously; child should see ophthalmologist if most of sclera is covered or if condition does not clear up in 1–2 weeks.
Periorbital ecchymosis	"Black eye," or bruising of the skin around the eye	Apply ice to eye area (both eyes) for 5–15 min every hour for the first 1–2 days after injury (even if only one eye is affected, both eyes may discolor), and then apply warm compresses beginning the second day after injury.
Foreign body on conjunctiva	Intense pain or feeling of something in the eye	Do not let child rub eye; remove material on surface of eye by closing upper lid over lower lid, irrigating or everting upper lid, visualizing material, and removing it with a slightly damp sterile gauze pad; patch eye and transport child to emergency department if foreign body cannot be removed.
Corneal abrasion	Intense pain and redness	Superficial corneal abrasions are diagnosed by touching a sterile fluorescein strip to lower conjunctiva; dye remains where corneal epithelial cells are disrupted; most corneal abrasions heal spontaneously, or antibiotic ointment may be prescribed and eyes patched in some children.
Burns (alkaline burns readily penetrate cornea and are more serious than acid burns)	Pain and/or complaints of "blindness" or vision loss	For child with chemical burn, irrigate eye for 15–30 min; transport child to emergency department, where irrigation should continue; pupils are dilated to reduce pain and prevent adhesions; after irrigation is complete, eyes are patched, and antibiotics are prescribed.

(continued)

Condition and Etiology	Clinical Manifestations	Clinical Therapy
Penetrating and perforating injuries	Pain	Obtain medical assistance immediately; never try to remove an object that has penetrated the child's eye; such objects should be removed by an ophthalmologist; prevent the child from rubbing injured eye; cover both eyes with shield before transportation to emergency department.
Eye injuries caused by severe blows to head and eye (blunt trauma can seriously injure all eye structures, including orbit, which can be fractured)	Pain and redness	Transport immediately to ophthalmologist's office or emergency department for evaluation and treatment. Personnel should be aware that retinal hemorrhage is a common presentation of the type of child abuse called *shaken child syndrome.*

Pulling at the ear is a sign of ear pain.

Diarrhea, vomiting, and fever are typical of otitis media.

Irritability with night awakenings and crying is common due to increased pressure when prone or supine.

Diagnostic Tests
Diagnosis of otitis media is based on otoscopic examination, often accompanied by pneumatic otoscopy and/or tympanography.

AOM is diagnosed by a history of acute onset, presence of middle ear effusion (bulging or decreased mobility of the tympanic membrane, air fluid behind the membrane or otorrhea or discharge), and signs and symptoms of inflammation (erythema of tympanic membrane or discomfort that makes sleep and other activities difficult for the child) (Subcommittee on Management of Acute Otitis Media, 2004).

OME is diagnosed by pneumatic otoscopy and tympanography; audiologic examination may be abnormal if hearing is affected.

Clinical Therapy
AOM treatment is delayed 48–72 hours in children aged 6 months to 2 years with nonsevere illness at presentation **and** uncertain diagnosis or in children 2 years and older without severe symptoms **or** with uncertain diagnosis; many children improve without specific treatment.

Section III: Body Systems

When needed, AOM is treated with antibiotic therapy for 10 days in children younger than age 6 years and 5–7 days for children 6 years and older.

Ibuprofen, acetaminophen, topical anesthetic eardrops, or herbal eardrops (a naturopathic herbal extract of *Allium sativum*, *Verbascum thapsus*, *Calendula flores*, and *Hypericum perforatum*) may be used for pain relief.

OME is not treated with antibiotics but is evaluated periodically to be sure there is not an additional AOM that needs treatment; improvement usually occurs within 3 months.

Because OME is more commonly associated with hearing loss and cochlear damage, follow-up with audiology is essential; if hearing is abnormal, speech testing should be performed (Otitis Media with Effusion, 2004).

If infections recur despite antibiotic treatment for AOM or if OME continues 4 months or more with persistent hearing loss present, myringotomy (surgical incision of the tympanic membrane) may be performed, and tympanostomy tubes (pressure-equalizing tubes) may be inserted to drain fluid from the middle ear.

Nursing Management
Assessment
The tympanic membrane is assessed by otoscopy at each health promotion visit and during examinations for illness; examine the color, transparency, mobility, presence of landmarks, and light reflex.

Ask parents if the child has had a fever, been fussy, or been pulling at the ears.

Observe for signs of impaired hearing, observing for the child's ability to hear whispered or soft sounds.

Intervention
Emphasize preventive measures to decrease risk factors for otitis media; prevention includes avoiding exposure to secondhand smoke, not placing babies to sleep with a pacifier, encouraging breastfeeding, and keeping immunizations up to date.

Explain treatment goals and plans; many parents may not understand why antibiotics are not used for every infection.

Prepare for day surgery if myringotomy and tubes are treatment choice.

Table 15–4   Severity of Hearing Loss

Type of Loss	Decibel Level (dB)	Hearing Ability
Slight/mild	26–40	Some speech sounds are difficult to perceive, particularly unvoiced consonant sounds.
Moderate	41–60	Most normal conversational speech sounds are missed.
Severe	61–80	Speech sounds cannot be heard at a normal conversational level.
Profound	81–90	No speech sounds can be heard.
Deaf	>90	No sound at all can be heard.

Continue to monitor hearing, speech, and developmental milestones.

Hearing Impairment
Clinical Manifestations

Conductive hearing loss occurs when conditions in the external auditory canal or tympanic membrane prevent sound from reaching the middle ear; it usually develops over time and can be treated. *Sensorineural hearing loss* occurs when the hair cells in the cochlea or along the auditory nerve (cranial nerve VIII) are damaged. This leads to permanent hearing loss. A *mixed hearing loss* indicates a hearing loss having a combination of conductive and sensorineural causes.

Lack of normal speech or language, developmental delays occur; findings are related to degree of hearing impairment (Table 15–4).

See Table 15–5 for behavioral signs typical of hearing impairment.

Diagnostic Tests
Audiologic testing should be conducted for all infants and regularly through childhood.

Otoscopic examination and tympanogram should be performed during health promotion visits.

Clinical Therapy
Removal of impediments in conductive loss.

Hearing aid, bone conduction hearing aid, surgical placement of cochlear implants.

Speech therapy and instructions in lipreading, signing, cueing, and fingerspelling.

See Table 15–6 for communication techniques.

Table 15–5 Behaviors Suggestive of Hearing Impairment

Age	Behavior
Infant	Has a diminished or absent startle reflex to loud sound
	Does not awaken when environment is very noisy
	Awakens only to touch
	Does not turn head to sound at 3–4 months
	Does not localize sound at 6–10 months
	Babbles little or not at all
Toddler and preschooler	Speaks unintelligibly, in a monotone, or not at all
	Communicates needs through gestures
	Appears developmentally delayed
	Appears emotionally immature, yells inappropriately
	Does not respond to doorbell or telephone
	Appears more interested in objects than people and prefers to play alone
	Focuses on facial expressions rather than verbal communications
School-age child and adolescent	Asks to have statements repeated
	Answers questions inappropriately, except when able to view speaker's face
	Daydreams and is inattentive
	Performs poorly at school or is truant
	Has speech abnormalities or speaks in a monotone
	Sits close to or turns television or radio up loudly
	Prefers to play alone

Nursing Management
Assessment

Conduct newborn hearing tests soon after birth; make observations of the infant's responses to sound.

Assess hearing at every well-child visit by observations of development, audiography, and tympanography.

Ask parents if they have concerns about their child's hearing; they are often the first to diagnose a hearing impairment.

Language milestones should be evaluated in the older infant and child with hearing impairment.

Evaluate hearing by audiography during screening programs in schools, and refer children who do not pass the screening test.

Monitor developmental milestones frequently in children with hearing impairment.

Table 15-6   Communication Techniques for Children Who Are Hearing Impaired

Technique	Description
Cued speech	Supplement to lipreading; eight hand shapes represent groups of consonant sounds, and four positions about the face represent groups of vowel sounds; based on the sounds the letters make, not the letters themselves; child can "see-hear" every spoken syllable a hearing person hears.
Oral approach	Uses only spoken language for face-to-face communication; avoids use of formal signs; uses hearing aids and residual hearing.
Total communication	Uses speech and sign, fingerspelling, lipreading, and residual hearing simultaneously; child selects communication technique depending on the situation.
Sign language	A language that allows the user to communicate quickly and accurately with others who understand signs. The signs, or hand movements, represent words or concepts. When a sign is not available, the word can be spelled out using signs. American Sign Language is most often used; British Sign Language is common in Europe.

Implementation

Encourage prevention of hearing loss due to exposure to loud noises such as from music and power and farm equipment; music should be turned down and ear protection worn for other activities.

Parents often need help to decide on the best method for hearing and language enhancement for the child.

Refer the parents to an early-intervention program as soon as the diagnosis of hearing impairment is made so as to foster the child's development.

Facilitate the child's ability to receive spoken language and to send information, help parents to meet the child's schooling needs, and provide emotional support to parents.

If a cochlear implant is planned, the child needs surgical care and follow-up to monitor results and integrate sound gradually into the child's life.

Patient and Family Education

Provide parents with information about adjustments that may have to be made for the hearing-impaired child who attends public school. By sitting at the front of the classroom, the child can hear and see more clearly. The teacher should always face the child when speaking, and background noise should be reduced.

Tell parents that children who are hearing impaired have the same intelligence quotient distribution as children without hearing impairment. However, communication and learning can be difficult, and extra support is needed.

Children with hearing impairment should reach their intellectual potential, although development in certain areas may take place more slowly than it does in children with no hearing impairment.

Teach care of hearing aids or other adaptive devices.

Teach the family about the community services available for medical, nursing, psychologic, and financial assistance. Link the family with the deaf or hearing-impaired community and resources.

Injuries of the Ear
Clinical Manifestations
Lacerations, infections, and hematomas may occur in the external ear structures, especially the pinna; children may place foreign objects in the ear, and insects may enter the ear canal. Rupture of the tympanic membrane may result from head injuries, blows to the ear, or insertion of objects into the ear canal. Serous drainage from the ear can indicate a basilar skull fracture due to accidents or child abuse (shaken child syndrome).

Earache, decreased hearing, imbalance problems, persistent bleeding, or other discharge (see Table 15–7 for emergency treatment of ear injuries).

Foreign bodies may need to be removed from the ears of young children. Ear is visualized with otoscope; objects may be removed with forceps, suction tip, hook, or irrigation (irrigation is avoided for materials that can absorb water because the object will swell, making removal even more difficult).

DISORDERS OF THE NOSE, MOUTH, AND THROAT
Epistaxis
Clinical Manifestations
Bleeding from the nose, unilateral or bilateral

Vomiting from swallowing large amounts of blood

Low hematocrit resulting from extended bleeding

Clinical Therapy
For anterior bleeding, child should sit upright quietly; the head should be tilted forward to prevent blood from trickling down the throat, which can lead to vomiting.

Table 15-7 Emergency Treatment of Ear Injuries

Injury	Treatment
Pinna	
Minor cuts or abrasions	Wash thoroughly with soap and water and rinse well; leave exposed to air if possible or apply adhesive bandage; monitor for infection.
Hematomas	Needle aspiration should be performed and pressure dressing applied; undrained hematomas may become fibrotic; "cauliflower ear" deformity may develop.
Cellulitis or abscesses	Apply moist heat intermittently; make sure that prescribed antibiotic is taken; minor surgery may be performed for an abscess.
Deep lacerations	Apply pressure to stop bleeding; transport to physician's office or emergency department for suturing.
Ear canal	
Foreign bodies	Have child lie on back and turn head over edge of bed, with affected side down; wiggle earlobe, and have child shake head; foreign object may fall out as result of gravity; if object remains in ear, call physician; do not try to remove foreign body with tweezers because this may push the object further into the ear.
Insects	Shine flashlight into ear to try to attract insect; instilling a few drops of mineral oil, olive oil, or alcohol kills insect, and irrigating ear canal gently may remove dead insect.
Tympanic membrane	
Ruptures	Call physician if child has persistent ear pain after blow, blast injury, or insertion of foreign object; cover external ear loosely with piece of sterile cotton or gauze; if tympanic membrane has been ruptured, systemic antibiotics are prescribed.

The nares should be squeezed just below the nasal bone and held for 10–15 minutes while the child breathes through the mouth; an ice bag can be applied to the nose or back of the neck.

If the bleeding does not stop, a cotton ball or swab soaked with phenylephrine (Neo-Synephrine), epinephrine, thrombin, or lidocaine may be inserted into the affected nostril to promote topical vasoconstriction or anesthesia.

Once the bleeding has stopped, the nostril may have to be cauterized with silver nitrate or electrocautery; if the bleeding cannot be stopped, absorbable packing may be used.

Alterations in Eye, Ear, Nose, and Throat Function 221

Posterior bleeding must also be stopped by packing, and the child must be monitored carefully; arterial ligation is occasionally needed.

Repeated or severe nosebleeds need further evaluation.

Nursing Management

Assess the child's hematocrit or hemoglobin if significant bleeding has occurred.

Children with frequent epistaxis should have a complete history taken and physical examination performed to rule out systemic disease.

Have the child avoid bending over, stooping, strenuous exercise, hot drinks, and hot baths or showers for 3–4 days after epistaxis.

Have the child sleep with the head elevated on two or three pillows; humidify the air with a vaporizer to prevent recurrence.

Nasopharyngitis

Known as the common cold or upper respiratory infection.

Infection and inflammation of the nose and throat by one of more than 200 viruses or bacteria.

Red nasal mucosa with clear nasal discharge and an infected throat with enlarged tonsils may be apparent; vesicles may be present on the soft palate and in the pharynx.

Lethargy, irritability, poor feeding, fever, muscle aches are common.

For infants who cannot breathe through the mouth, normal saline nose drops can be administered every 3–4 hours, especially before feeding.

For infants older than 9 months of age, nasal stuffiness can be treated with either normal saline nose drops or a decongestant such as phenylephrine (0.125–0.25%, depending on the child's age); older children can use nasal sprays.

Decongestant nose drops and sprays should not be used for more than 4 or 5 days or more often than recommended.

Room humidification may help prevent drying of nasal secretions.

Antipyretics such as acetaminophen or ibuprofen reduce fever and make the child more comfortable; aspirin is not recommended because of its association with Reye syndrome.

Ensure adequate intake of fluid to liquefy secretions.

Proper handwashing and disposal of tissues help to decrease the spread of the infection.

Sinusitis

Sinusitis is inflammation of one or more of the paranasal sinuses characterized by purulent nasal drainage or other symptoms; there is often accompanying facial pain, headache, and fever.

A history of recent upper respiratory infection is common, persistent cough from postnasal drip can occur, and nasal discharge or swelling can be apparent. Malodorous breath, fever, mouth breathing, hyponasal speech, and cervical lymphadenopathy may be present (Duchene, 2000; Hayes, 2001; Leung & Kellner, 2004).

Young children may be anorexic or have difficulty feeding; older children may complain of headache.

Most sinusitis is treated with antibiotics, and recurrent cases are referred for further care by an otolaryngologist and allergy specialist.

Pharyngitis

Acute pharyngitis is an infection that primarily affects the pharynx, including the tonsils, and is caused by a virus or bacteria (see CM 15–3 for common symptoms of viral and bacterial pharyngitis).

Diagnosis is made by assessment; throat cultures are taken in cases of suspected bacterial infection and with history of exposure to strep throat.

CM 15–3 Clinical Manifestations of Viral Pharyngitis and Strep Throat (Group A Beta-Hemolytic Streptococcus)[a]

Viral Pharyngitis	Strep Throat
Nasal congestion	Abrupt onset
Mild sore throat	Tonsillar exudate[b]
Conjunctivitis	Painful cervical lymphadenopathy[b]
Cough	Anorexia, nausea, vomiting, abdominal pain
Hoarseness	Severe sore throat
Mild pharyngeal redness	Headache, malaise
Minimal tonsillar exudate	Fever >38.3°C (101°F)
Mildly tender anterior cervical lymphadenopathy	Petechial mottling of soft palate
Fever ≤38.3°C (101°F)	

[a]Children 6 months to 3 years of age may have streptococcus with symptoms that resemble those of viral pharyngitis. Children with scarlet fever have the symptoms of strep throat plus a sandpaper-textured erythematous generalized rash and pallor around the lips.
[b]Classic signs of strep throat.

Strep throat should be treated with oral penicillin for 10 days or by long-acting penicillin given in one injection; erythromycin, azithromycin, doxycycline, ceftriaxone, cefixime, or ciprofloxacin is given if the child is allergic to penicillin.

Teach parents the importance of completing the entire course of antibiotics if prescribed for bacterial pharyngitis. After the child is on the medication for approximately 2 days, have the parents replace the child's toothbrush with a new one to avoid reinfection by bacteria that can survive on the moist brush.

Viral pharyngitis is treated symptomatically with acetaminophen, cool, nonacidic fluids and soft foods, ice chips, or frozen juice pops. Humidification, chewing gum, and gargling with warm salt water (5 g to 250 mL water; 0.25 teaspoon to 8 oz water) soothe an irritated throat.

Tonsillitis

Tonsillitis is an infection or inflammation (hypertrophy) of the palatine tonsils caused by virus or bacteria.

Symptoms and signs include frequent throat infections with breathing and swallowing difficulties, persistent redness of the anterior pillars, enlargement of the cervical lymph nodes, and dry and irritated mucous membranes.

Diagnosis is made on the basis of visual inspection and clinical manifestations; tonsils appear large and inflamed.

Symptomatic treatment for tonsillitis is the same as for pharyngitis.

Surgical removal of tonsils (tonsillectomy) is often recommended when children have recurrent throat infections (approximately three per year for 3 years), chronic tonsillitis, obstructive sleep apnea, or malformations causing nasal speech or a facial growth abnormality.

Care after tonsillectomy includes the following:
- Have the child drink adequate cool fluids or chew gum, as this reduces spasms in the muscles surrounding the throat.
- Give acetaminophen elixir as ordered (avoid aspirin and ibuprofen to decrease chance of bleeding).
- Apply an ice collar around the child's neck.
- Have the child gargle with a solution of 2.5 g (0.5 teaspoon) each of baking soda and salt in 8 oz of water.
- Have the child rinse the mouth well with viscous lidocaine and then swallow the solution.

Teach parents signs of complications such as hemorrhage or infection and how to seek emergency care for such conditions.

Mouth Ulcers

Mouth ulcers occur in a number of disease states and because of trauma.

Nurses examine mouth ulcers for size, location, drainage, and pain; for those at risk, such as children on chemotherapy, regular careful examinations of the oral mucosa are an important part of care.

Ensure that children have good oral care, including brushing teeth with a soft bristle brush or by use of mouth sponges.

Rinse the mouth after all meals and snacks.

Teach the family correct administration of oral medications and topical preparations designed to treat infection or provide comfort.

When oral mucosa ulcers are predicted, such as with chemotherapy or in acquired immunodeficiency syndrome, begin oral protocols before lesions occur to decrease their appearance and severity (Cheng, Molassiotis, Chang, Wai, & Cheung, 2001; Gibson & Nelson, 2000).

Encourage a diet that has only mild foods, avoiding spices and very sweet, sour, and acidic items; cold foods may be better accepted.

Monitor hydration status to ensure adequate fluid intake.

Teach parents the correct administration of acetaminophen or other analgesic treatment.

Use standard precautions to protect the child from infections and prevent their flora from being transferred to other children or family members.

Encourage parents to keep children with herpes gingivostomatitis out of contact with other children if active lesions or drooling is present (Blevins, 2003).

Mouth and Dental Emergencies

Teach the child and family to use mouth guards to protect from injury in sports.

When a tooth is removed during an injury, prompt treatment may influence the chance that it can be reimplanted. If the child's condition is stable, try to reimplant the tooth and then transfer the child to an emergency dental facility.

- Handle the tooth only by the crown (its top).

- Gently rinse the tooth in a bowl of tap water. Do not place it under running water.
- Insert into the socket.
- Have the child provide gentle pressure by biting a piece of gauze or a tea bag.
- If child is unstable or has other injuries, enlist emergency medical transportation (call 911); transport the tooth with the child.
- If the tooth cannot be inserted into the child's mouth, place it in milk, saline, saliva, or water; if a dental aid kit is available, it may contain a transport liquid called *Hank's Balanced Salt Solution*.

(Rudy, 2001)

16. ALTERATIONS IN RESPIRATORY FUNCTION

URGENT RESPIRATORY THREATS: RESPIRATORY DISTRESS AND RESPIRATORY FAILURE

Recognition of the child's respiratory signs and symptoms is critical, so care is provided to prevent the respiratory distress from progressing to respiratory failure. Assess the following:

Respiratory rate (see Chapter 2) and respiratory effort

Heart rate and quality of the pulse

Color

Cough

Behavior change

Signs of dehydration

Respiratory failure occurs when the body can no longer maintain effective gas exchange. As the child attempts to compensate for oxygen deficit and airway blockage, behavior and vital signs reflect beginning hypoxia. As respiratory distress progresses, the accessory muscles are used to assist oxygen intake. Hypoxia persists, and respiratory efforts waste more oxygen than is obtained. Without intervention, the oxygen deficit becomes overwhelming, and central nervous system changes are seen.

Clinical Manifestations

Signs of respiratory distress include tachypnea, retractions, nasal flaring, inspiratory stridor, and expiratory grunting.

Signs of respiratory failure include the following:

Early signs: restlessness, tachypnea, tachycardia, and diaphoresis

Early decompensation: nasal flaring, retractions, grunting, wheezing, anxiety and irritability, mood changes, headache, hypertension, and confusion

Signs of imminent respiratory arrest: dyspnea, bradycardia, cyanosis, stupor, and coma

With a chronic respiratory condition, development of respiratory failure may be gradual. Signs are subtle. Be alert to behavior changes in addition to respiratory signs.

Section III: Body Systems

227

Diagnostic Tests

Pulse oximetry and arterial blood gases assess respiratory distress and respiratory failure. Hypoxemia even with supplemental oxygen is a sign of respiratory failure.

Clinical Therapy

Reversal of severe hypoxemia is managed with oxygen, mechanical ventilation, and continuous positive end-expiratory pressure to increase functional residual capacity. Medical management is focused on treating the cause of respiratory failure. An endotracheal tube is used to stabilize the airway as necessary.

Nursing Management

Assessment

Perform the respiratory assessment. Attach a cardiorespiratory monitor and pulse oximeter. Monitor the child for changes in vital signs, respiratory status, and level of responsiveness.

If the child has an endotracheal tube or tracheostomy tube, assess for secretions, which may further obstruct the airway.

Implementation

Elevate the head of the bed, and keep the head in midline to help maintain the airway. Administer oxygen as ordered. Keep emergency equipment readily available.

Suction airway secretions as needed, and provide tracheostomy care if present. Provide good skin care around the endotracheal tube or tracheostomy to prevent breakdown over pressure points.

Provide support to parents and children, who will be stressed because of the life-threatening nature of the disorder.

RESPIRATORY CONDITIONS
Apparent Life-Threatening Event

An episode of central or obstructive apnea occurring in a term infant who is younger than age 4 months. Potential causes include infection, gastroesophageal reflux, seizures or breath-holding spells, cardiac arrhythmias, respiratory center dysfunction, obstructive sleep apnea, and metabolic and endocrine problems.

Clinical Manifestations

Apnea (central or obstructive) accompanied by a color change (cyanosis, pallor, or occasionally ruddiness), limp muscle tone, choking, or gagging.

Episodes may occur during sleep, wakefulness, or feeding.

Diagnostic Tests
A full diagnostic workup may include cardiorespiratory monitoring, cultures, complete blood counts, blood gas measurement, serum electrolyte measurement, electrocardiogram, echocardiogram, sleep study, barium swallow, and pH probe.

Clinical Therapy
The underlying cause is treated if one is found. Physical stimulation or emergency resuscitation is usually required to revive the infant.

Nursing Management

Assessment
Collect information about the characteristics and duration of the episode; relationship between the event and feeding; and any past episodes, recent infections, medications, seizure activity, birth history or perinatal insults, family history of infant deaths, apnea, or cardiac problems.

Assess respiratory function. Attach a cardiorespiratory monitor and pulse oximeter to monitor for sudden changes in respiratory status.

Implementation
Attempt to reduce parents' fear and anxiety. Explain tests and treatment to increase their understanding of the situation.

Encourage parents to hold infant and to participate in care. Encourage the mother to continue breastfeeding. Keep emergency resuscitation equipment and drugs accessible.

Teach parents how to use an apnea monitor if prescribed, to respond to an apneic episode, and techniques for choking intervention. Encourage parents to attend a cardiopulmonary resuscitation class.

Asthma
A chronic inflammatory disorder of the airway with acute exacerbations or persistent symptoms. The airway has increased airway responsiveness to stimuli, and the obstruction can be partially or completely reversed (Kieckhefer & Ratcliffe, 2004). Most children experience their first symptoms before 5 years of age.

The inflammation during an asthmatic episode causes bronchial constriction, airway swelling, and mucus production. Mucus clogs small airways, trapping air below the plugs. Decreased perfusion of the alveolar capillaries leads to hypoxemia. The child breathes faster to overcome the increased airway resistance.

Repeated episodes of bronchospasm, mucosal edema, and mucous plugging cause chronic inflammatory changes. Decreased airway elasticity and decreased lung function result.

Clinical Manifestations

Productive cough, expiratory wheeze, shortness of breath, respiratory fatigue, rapid and labored respirations, nasal flaring, intercostal retractions, decreased air movement, and respiratory fatigue, chest tightness.

Head bobbing when accessory muscles (sternocleidomastoids) are used to breathe.

In severe obstruction, wheezing may not be heard because of the lack of airflow.

Agitation to lethargic irritability due to hypoxia and side effects of medications.

Diagnostic Tests

A spirometer tests the volume of air the child can expel from the lungs after a maximal inspiration to assess the severity of airway obstruction.

A chest radiograph if other causes of the respiratory difficulty are suspected, such as a foreign body.

Skin testing may be used to identify allergens (asthma triggers).

Clinical Therapy

Pharmacologic therapies are matched to the severity of asthma for long-term control and management of acute episodes. Control of asthma symptoms is the goal, and the regimen should correspond to the asthma severity. See Table 16–1 for the national standard treatment of children older than age 5 years. See medications used in Meds 16–1.

Markers of good asthma control include the following:
- Minimal or no chronic symptoms day or night
- Minimal or no exacerbations
- No activity limitations, no school missed, and no missed work by parents
- Minimal use of short-acting beta$_2$-agonists (less than one time a day or less than one canister a month)
- Minimal or no adverse effects from medications
  (National Asthma Education and Prevention Program, 2002)

Table 16–1 Asthma Severity Classification and Preferred Clinical Therapy for Children Older than 5 Years of Age

Classification (Steps)	Description	Medications for Long-Term Control
Step 1: mild intermittent	Brief exacerbations with symptoms no more often than twice a week. Nighttime symptoms no more than twice a week. Asymptomatic and normal PEFR between exacerbations. No emergent visits and no asthma-related absences from school. PEFR = 80% of predicted, with variability less than 20%.	No daily medications needed. Severe exacerbation may occur, separated by long periods of normal lung function and no symptoms. A course of systemic corticosteroids is recommended.
Step 2: mild persistent	Exacerbations more than twice a week, but less than once a day. Nighttime symptoms more than twice a month. Exacerbations may affect activity and cause absences from school. PEFR = 80% of predicted, with variability of 20–30%.	Preferred treatment • Low-dose inhaled steroid • Alternate treatment • Cromolyn, leukotriene modifier, or nedocromil OR • Sustained release theophylline to serum concentration of 5–15 mcg/mL
Step 3: moderate persistent	Daily symptoms of coughing and wheezing. Exacerbations at least twice a week that may last for days. Nighttime symptoms more than once per week. Exacerbations affect activity and several school absences occur. PEF or FEV_1 greater than 60% but less than 80% of predicted, with variability greater than 30%.	Preferred treatment • Low- to medium-dose inhaled corticosteroid PLUS • Long-acting beta$_2$-agonists Alternate treatment • Increase inhaled corticosteroids to within medium-dose range OR • Low-dose inhaled steroid and either leukotriene modifier or theophylline • If needed (particularly in children and adolescents with recurring severe exacerbations)

(continued)

Table 16–1 Asthma Severity Classification and Preferred Clinical Therapy for Children Older than 5 Years of Age (Continued)

Classification (Steps)	Description	Medications for Long-Term Control
Step 3 (continued)		Preferred treatment • Increase inhaled corticosteroids within medium-dose range and add long-acting inhaled beta$_2$-agonists Alternative treatment • Increase inhaled corticosteroids within medium-dose range, and add either leukotriene modifier or theophylline
Step 4: severe persistent	Continuous daytime symptoms, limited physical activity. Frequent exacerbations. Frequent nighttime symptoms. Limited physical activity Hospitalizations frequent, with pediatric intensive care unit admissions for severe exacerbations. PEF or FEV$_1$ = 60% of predicted, with variability greater than 30%.	Preferred treatment • High-dose inhaled corticosteroids PLUS • Long-acting inhaled beta$_2$-agonists And if needed, • Oral corticosteroids at 2 mg/kg/day (not to exceed 60 mg/day). Repeated efforts should be made to reduce systemic corticosteroids and maintain control with high-dose inhaled corticosteroids.
Quick relief	Bronchodilator as needed for symptoms. Intensity of treatment depends on severity of exacerbation. Preferred treatment: short-acting inhaled beta$_2$-agonists by nebulizer, face mask, and space/holding chamber. Alternative treatment: oral beta$_2$-agonist. With viral respiratory infection Bronchodilator every 4–6 hr up to 24 hr (longer with physician counsel); in general, repeat no more than once every 6 weeks. Consider systemic corticosteroids if exacerbation is severe or patient has a history of previous severe exacerbations. Use of short-acting beta$_2$-agonists greater than 2 times a week in intermittent asthma (daily or increasing use in persistent asthma) may indicate the need to initiate (increase) long-term control therapy.	

FEV$_1$, forced expiratory volume in 1 second; PEF, peak expiratory flow; PEFR, peak expiratory flow rate.

Note: Adapted from National Asthma Education and Prevention Program. (2002). Expert Panel Report II: Guidelines for the diagnosis and management of asthma. Update on selected topics 2002. (NIH Publication No 02-5075). Bethesda, MD: National Heart Lung and Blood Institute, National Institutes of Health.

Meds 16–1　Medications Used to Treat Asthma

Medication	Action/Indication	Nursing Considerations
Rescue medication		
Beta$_2$-agonists (short-acting)—albuterol; metaproterenol; terbutaline; levalbuterol (inhalation, oral)	Relax smooth muscle in airway, increase water content in bronchial mucus to promote mucociliary clearance, resulting in rapid bronchodilation within 5–10 min	Use this rescue medication before inhaled steroid, wait 1–2 min between puffs; wait 15 min to give inhaled steroid. Child should hold breath 10 sec after inspiring. Then rinse mouth and avoid swallowing medication. Use spacer.
	Drug of choice for acute therapy (metered-dose inhaler or nebulizer)	Some side effects (tachycardia, nervousness, nausea and vomiting, headaches), but these are usually dose-related.
		Repetitive or excessive use can mask increasing airway inflammation and hyperresponsiveness and increase need for higher dosage to get same effect.
		Use of more than one canister a month indicates inadequate control.
Corticosteroids—Methylprednisolone (intravenous); prednisone; prednisolone (oral)	Diminish airway inflammation and obstruction, enhance bronchodilating effect of beta$_2$-agonists	Not used as primary treatment. Onset of action is 4–6 hr.
		Short-term therapy for 3–10 days until symptoms resolve or child achieves 80% peak expiratory flow personal best.
	Used for moderate to severe acute exacerbations when single beta$_2$-agonist dose given in emergency department does not resolve symptoms	Give with food.
		Give daily oral dose in early morning to mimic normal peak corticosteroid blood level.
		Assess for potential adverse effects of long-term therapy: decreased growth, unstable blood sugar, immunosuppression.
Anticholinergic—ipratropium (inhalation)	Inhibits bronchoconstriction and decreases mucus production	Not for primary treatment
		Side effects include increased wheezing, cough, nervousness, dry mouth, tachycardia, dizziness, headache, palpitations.
	Provides additive effects to short-acting beta$_2$-agonists during acute exacerbation	Avoid contact with eyes.

(continued)

Medication	Action/Indication	Nursing Considerations
Controller medication		
Beta$_2$-agonists (long-acting)—salmeterol; formoterol (inhalation)	Relax smooth muscle in airway, used for nocturnal symptoms and prevention of exercise-induced bronchospasm	Should not be used for acute asthma attack. Should not be used in place of inhaled corticosteroids. Caution against overdosage, as side effects such as tachycardia, tremor, irritability, insomnia last 8–12 hr. Report use of more than four puffs a day, as this may indicate need for stepped-up therapy.
Methylxanthines—theophylline (oral); aminophylline (intravenous)	Relax muscle bundles that constrict airways; dilate airway; provide continuous airway relaxation; sustained release for prevention of nocturnal symptoms Aminophylline may be used for emergency adjunct therapy in intensive care unit, but use is controversial	Tablet should not be crushed or chewed. Used for long-term control, so continuous administration needed; works best when a specific amount is maintained in the bloodstream (therapeutic serum level, 10–20 mcg/L). Requires serum level checks and dose adjustment. Side effects include tachycardia, dysrhythmias, restlessness, tremors, seizures, insomnia, hypotension, severe headaches, vomiting, and diarrhea.
Mast cell inhibitors—cromolyn sodium; nedocromil (aerosol)	Anti-inflammatory, inhibit early and late phase asthma response to allergens and exercise-induced bronchospasm; may be used for unavoidable allergen exposure	Not used at time of symptom development or acute exacerbation. Must be used up to four times a day to be effective. Therapeutic response seen in 2 weeks; maximum benefit may not be seen for 4–6 weeks. Adverse reactions include wheezing, bronchospasm, throat irritation, nasal congestion, and anaphylaxis.

Nursing Management
Assessment

Assess the ABCs—airway, breathing, and circulation—to make sure that the child's condition is not life-threatening.

Assess the respiratory system for rate, retractions, quality of breath sounds, presence or absence of wheezing, cough or stridor, color, and heart rate.

Attach a pulse oximeter to monitor oxygen saturation. Assess peak expiratory flow rate, skin turgor, intake and output, and urine specific gravity. Then complete the assessment to identify other associated problems.

Assess the child's anxiety.

Implementation
Maintain the airway; provide supplemental humidified oxygen by cannula or face mask.

Position child in semi-Fowler or upright position.

Restore and maintain fluid balance to help thin and break up mucous plugs. Give room-temperature beverages, as iced beverages may precipitate bronchospasms. IV hydration may be needed in some children. Prevent overhydration.

Provide aerosol medications, which rapidly deliver medications to the lungs for prompt onset of action. Monitor for side effects of medications.

Group tasks to promote rest, as the child is exhausted from labored breathing and hypoxia.

Reduce stress. Keep the parent and child informed about procedures.

Patient and Family Education
Identify knowledge of the condition:
- Review why asthma occurs. Assess parents' understanding of the physiologic process and its chronic and progressive nature, not an episodic illness.
- Help parents explore and understand how asthma affects their child.
- Identify asthma triggers and assess parents' understanding of how to prevent, avoid, or minimize their effect in a timely manner.
- The use of a peak expiratory flow meter can help to identify when obstruction occurs.
- Make sure the parents understand the need for daily management and how that enables the family and child to have control over asthma.
- Ensure that the family knows when and where to seek emergency medical help. Describe actions the family can take before seeking medical assistance.

Review medication therapy:

- Provide information about medications: Make sure the parents know the difference between controller medications and rescue medications.
- Regularly evaluate the child's technique for the use of an inhaler and nebulizer.
- Suggest diversions to help the child cooperate during the 8- to 10-minute nebulizer treatment.
- Provide a written action plan with daily management and steps for an asthma episode.

Review other care issues:

- Review plans for treatment at school or childcare. Supply medications for school or childcare and for home. Teach teachers to recognize respiratory distress and reduce the child's fear of going to the nurse for rescue medications.
- Medical identification bracelet or medallion is worn by child.
- Reduce triggers in the home, such as pets, smoking in home, wood smoke, controlling dust mites in child's bedroom, and control of cockroaches.
- Encourage regular health promotion and maintenance care and routine immunizations, including influenza. Promote exercise and physical fitness.

Bacterial Tracheitis

A secondary infection of the upper trachea following viral laryngotracheitis, caused by *Staphylococcus aureus*, alpha-hemolytic streptococcus, group A streptococcus, *Moraxella catarrhalis*, or *Haemophilus influenzae*. The subglottis becomes edematous and ulcerated. Thick mucopurulent exudate may obstruct the trachea and main bronchi.

Clinical Manifestations

Viral upper respiratory infection, croupy cough, and stridor.

Progression to high fever of more than 39°C (102.2°F), respiratory distress, and a toxic appearance; no drooling is present.

Diagnostic Tests

Blood cultures are performed after the child is found unresponsive to usual laryngotracheobronchitis (LTB) management. Endoscopic examination of the subglottic area may be performed to obtain culture and sensitivities.

Clinical Therapy

Bacterial tracheitis misdiagnosed as LTB worsens instead of improving with nebulized epinephrine. Antibiotics are given for 10–14 days. Most children are intubated for 3–11 days.

Nursing Management

Until intubated, the child is never left unattended or transported away from equipment or personnel who can perform emergency airway interventions. Postpone anxiety-provoking procedures, such as venipuncture, until the airway is secure.

The intubated child is cared for in the intensive care unit. Assess airway patency frequently. Suction the endotracheal tube as needed, and provide humidified air or oxygen. Children often prefer to lie flat to conserve energy. Administer prescribed antibiotics to treat the infection and IV fluids to provide hydration.

Support parents as they cope with the sudden onset of a life-threatening illness. Keep parents informed about the child's status, and permit them to stay with the child to help keep the child calm.

Bronchiolitis

An inflammation and obstruction of the bronchioles caused by respiratory syncytial virus (RSV), bacteria, mycoplasmas, and other viruses. RSV is the most common cause of lower respiratory tract infections in infants and children. Infection is most severe in infants younger than age 6 months and in children with lung or heart disease.

Clinical Manifestations

Upper respiratory symptoms such as nasal stuffiness, cough (not usually noted in infants), and fever [less than 39°C (102.2°F)] for a few days.

Progression to include the lower respiratory tract, rhinitis, low-grade fever, inspiratory and expiratory wheezing; a deeper, more frequent cough; tachypnea, retractions; and more labored breathing.

In severe cases, rapid, shallow respirations; nasal flaring and marked retractions; crackles; cyanosis; and decreased breath sounds occur.

Dehydration, abdominal distention may occur due to air swallowing, loss of appetite.

Diagnostic Tests

Laboratory tests include enzyme-linked immunosorbent assay or direct fluorescent assay that is performed on nasal wash specimens placed in viral transport medium. Chest radiographs show hyperinflation, patchy atelectasis, and other signs of inflammation.

Clinical Therapy

Cardiorespiratory monitor and pulse oximeter; children with apnea or respiratory failure are cared for in the intensive care unit.

Humidified oxygen therapy by hood or face tent, mask or nasal cannula.

Intubation and mechanical ventilation (positive end-expiratory pressure/continuous positive airway pressure).

Hydration with IV or oral fluids.

Postural drainage and chest physiotherapy.

Medications include acetaminophen or ibuprofen; bronchodilators, nebulized epinephrine, and corticosteroids are occasionally used. Antibiotics only for secondary bacterial infection. Ribavirin for life-threatening cases, such as infants with complicated congenital heart disease, bronchopulmonary dysplasia (BPD), cystic fibrosis, or other chronic lung disease (Wright, Pomerantz, & Luria, 2002).

To prevent RSV infection, give RespiGam (RSV immunoglobulin) IV or palivizumab (Synagis) intramuscularly to high-risk infants and children. Prematurity (younger than 32 weeks' gestation), chronic lung disease, complicated congenital heart disease, and immunocompromised status place infants and young children at higher risk (American Academy of Pediatrics Committee on Infectious Diseases and Committee on Fetus and Newborn, 2003). Monthly treatment for 5 months begins in October or November.

Nursing Management
Assessment
Assess airway and respiratory function carefully to identify worsening respiratory symptoms. A decreased oxygen saturation level below 90% is an indicator of severe disease.

Signs of life-threatening illness in the infant include central cyanosis, respiratory rate of more than 70 breaths per minute, listlessness, and apneic spells. Breath sounds may be very diminished on auscultation.

Implementation
Administer oxygen and pulmonary care therapies.

Clear the nasal passages. Elevate the head of the bed.

Provide small frequent feedings. Thickened formula may improve swallowing and prevent aspiration in infants with RSV bronchiolitis (Gadomski, 2002). An IV is used to rehydrate and maintain fluid balance until sufficient oral intake.

Decrease stress and anxiety to promote rest. Administer medications to control fever and promote comfort as needed. Partner with parents to comfort the child and provide care.

Patient and Family Education

When the child with less serious bronchiolitis is cared for at home, advise parents to call the healthcare provider if any of the following occur:

- Respiratory symptoms interfere with sleep or eating.
- Breathing is rapid or difficult.
- Symptoms persist in a child who is younger than 1 year old, has heart or lung disease, or was premature and had lung disease after birth.
- The child acts sicker—appears tired, less playful, and less interested in food, or the parents feel the child is not improving.

Bronchitis

An inflammation of the trachea and bronchi caused most often by a virus. May result from bacterial invasion or in response to an allergen or irritant. It can occur in any age child.

The classic symptom is a coarse, hacking cough that increases in severity at night. Coughing causes the chest and ribs to be painful. Breathing has a deep, rattling quality or audible wheezing. Treatment is supportive unless bacterial infection occurs.

Nursing Management

Support respiratory function through rest, humidification, hydration, and symptomatic treatment. Encourage parents who smoke to quit or refrain from smoking in the child's presence.

Bronchopulmonary Dysplasia (BPD) (Chronic Lung Disease)

A chronic lung disease caused by positive pressure ventilation and oxygen treatment for respiratory distress syndrome, inflammatory changes in the airways, and persistent hypoxia during the neonatal period. Occurs in an estimated 10–35% of very-low-birth-weight infants. Risk factors include prematurity, lung immaturity, patent ductus arteriosus, and vitamin A deficiency (Froh, 2002). Neonatal pneumonia, meconium aspiration syndrome, fluid overload, and lung hypoplasia also contribute to BPD (Capper-Michel, 2004).

Clinical Manifestations

Persistent signs of respiratory distress: tachypnea, wheezing, crackles, irritability, nasal flaring, grunting, retractions, pulmonary edema, and failure to thrive.

Intermittent bronchospasms and mucous plugging lead to persistent air trapping. Persistence over time results in a barrel-shaped chest.

Episodes of sudden respiratory deterioration with cyanosis or dusky color, agitation, and limited expiratory air flow.

Diagnostic Tests

A chest radiograph often shows hyperexpansion, atelectasis, and interstitial thickening (Capper-Michel, 2004).

Clinical Therapy

Treatment to support respiratory function and maturation of the lungs. Chest physiotherapy to help clear the airways.

Increased calories to support growth. Gastrostomy or nasogastric feeding to supplement calories. Restrict fluids to prevent pulmonary edema.

Supplemental oxygen with humidity to keep the SaO_2 at more than 90–92%, even during sleep and feeding. A tracheostomy for long-term airway management. Cautiously wean infants with severe BPD off of mechanical ventilation.

Medications used include diuretics, bronchodilators, anti-inflammatories, and inhaled corticosteroids. See Meds 16–2.

Oxygen and medications are gradually reduced as the child improves. Electrolytes may be monitored monthly.

Meds 16–2   Medications Used to Treat Bronchopulmonary Dysplasia

Medication	Action/Indication
Bronchodilators (beta$_2$-adrenergics, anticholinergics, theophylline, albuterol nebulizer)	Decrease airway resistance, increase expiratory flow in small airways, stimulate mucus clearance; different drugs work together for best response.
Anti-inflammatory agents (corticosteroids, inhaled cromolyn, beclomethasone)	Reduce pulmonary edema and inflammation in small airways; enhance effect of bronchodilators; help decrease the need for other drugs and oxygen; for moderate disease only.
Diuretics (furosemide, chlorothiazide, spironolactone)	Help remove excess fluid from lungs; decrease pulmonary resistance and increase pulmonary compliance; may cause electrolyte imbalances.
Potassium chloride	Prevents electrolyte imbalances associated with diuretics.
Antibiotics	Specific treatment for identified organisms.
Vitamin A	Plays a role in normal lung development.
Palivizumab (Synagis)	Protects infant from respiratory syncytial virus.

Long-term sequelae include asthma and respiratory infections, frequent rehospitalization. Potential complications include developmental delays, growth retardation, continuing airway obstruction, and persistent airway hypersensitivity.

Nursing Management

Assessment

Assess airway and respiratory function, vital signs, color, and behavior changes to identify signs of worsening respiratory symptoms even when oxygen is provided. Attach a cardiorespiratory monitor and pulse oximeter.

Observe for tracheostomy obstruction, and suction as needed.

Observe for signs of infection.

Monitor growth and development, as poor weight gain and developmental delays occur. Coordinate periodic hearing and vision testing.

Implementation

When the infant is hospitalized, eliminate unnecessary physical stimulation. Position the infant to facilitate breathing. Provide tracheostomy care. Provide humidified oxygen if ordered.

Manage fluids, as excess fluids can lead to pulmonary edema. Supplement calories as needed. Administer medications. Manage fever to help reduce energy needs.

For home care, make referrals for needed oxygen, respiratory supplies, medications, an early-intervention program, home health nursing, and follow-up care. Help families plan a schedule for needed care and to identify other family members to learn how to care for the infant.

A formula supplemented with carbohydrates and medium-chain triglycerides may be given to promote weight gain.

Patient and Family Education

Teach family members to identify signs of respiratory compromise indicating a need for rapid intervention. Infants can become very ill rapidly and need rehospitalization. Assist parents to develop an emergency care plan.

Educate parents on balancing fluid restrictions with nutritional requirements so that growth is supported and pulmonary edema is prevented. Teach procedures for nasogastric or gastrostomy feedings.

Promote the infant's normal development through rest, nutrition, stimulation, and family support.

Emphasize the need for frequent health promotion visits and immunizations. Encourage RSV prophylaxis.

Cystic Fibrosis

A common inherited autosomal recessive disorder of the exocrine glands that results in physiologic alterations in the respiratory, gastrointestinal, and reproductive systems. A defective cystic fibrosis transmembrane conductance regulator results in decreased chloride secretion and increased sodium absorption. Decreased water flows across cell membranes, and mucus becomes viscous and dehydrated. Mucous plugs damage the respiratory, gastrointestinal, and reproductive systems.

Natural enzymes necessary to digest fats and proteins are not secreted, resulting in poor digestion, malabsorption, and failure to thrive. Damage to the pancreas may interfere with insulin secretion, leading to cystic fibrosis–related diabetes mellitus. Excessive electrolyte loss through perspiration, saliva, and mucus secretion place children at risk for dehydration. The lungs are filled with thick mucus, leading to air trapping, hyperinflation, atelectasis, and secondary respiratory infections.

Clinical Manifestations

Up to 10% of newborns with cystic fibrosis present with a meconium ileus in the first 48 hours (McMullen & Bryson, 2004).

Steatorrhea and frothy, foul-smelling, and floating stools. Constipation is common, and intestinal obstruction may occur in older children.

Skin has salty taste.

Chronic moist, productive cough and frequent infections occur. Nasal polyps are often present.

Frontal headaches, facial tenderness, purulent nasal discharge, and postnasal discharge occur with chronic sinus infections.

Voracious appetite, difficulty maintaining and gaining weight occur because of food malabsorption and an increased metabolic rate due to frequent infections.

Clubbing of the distal extremities.

Children with mild disease may be adolescents or young adults before symptoms appear.

Diagnostic Tests

Newborn meconium ileus, malabsorption or failure to thrive, chronic recurrent respiratory infections, fecal impaction, and intussusception often trigger diagnostic testing.

Genetic testing is available, but rare CF gene alterations are not always detected (Cystic Fibrosis Foundation, 2004).

Newborn screening to detect immunoreactive trypsinogen is performed in some states, and when positive, genetic testing of the child's DNA is performed to verify the finding.

A sweat chloride test by pilocarpine iontophoresis.

Respiratory function tests every 6 months during cystic fibrosis center visits.

Sputum for culture and sensitivity when infections are suspected.

Clinical Therapy

The goal is to prevent or slow the progression of airway damage. Treatment is focused on controlling infection and inflammation and on reducing mucus accumulation. Numerous medications are used. See Meds 16–3. Bronchial hygiene therapy is performed by chest physiotherapy, positive expiratory pressure, flutter valve, or high-frequency chest wall oscillation.

A well-balanced diet with up to 1.5 times the daily caloric requirements to support growth and meet energy needs. Supplemental nasogastric or gastrostomy feedings help the child gain and maintain weight when oral intake is inadequate. Children with adequate nutrition have a longer life expectancy. Cystic fibrosis–related diabetes is challenging to manage because the large caloric intake must be balanced by insulin dosage.

The disease is ultimately terminal. Double-lung transplantation may temporarily halt the disease progression, and approximately 50% of cases survive for the first 5 years (McMullen & Bryson, 2004).

Nursing Management

Assessment

Auscultate the chest for breath sounds, crackles, and wheezes. Note any cyanosis or clubbing. Ask about the cough character and frequency and sputum characteristics. Compare to baseline data, as changes in the cough may be related to a new infection. Obtain oxygen saturation and spirometry readings if changes in respiratory status are suspected.

Evaluate the child's growth pattern, plotting the weight and height on a growth curve. Inquire about the child's appetite, food intake, and use of nutritional supplements, pancreatic enzymes, and vitamins. Growth delay and delayed appearance of secondary sex characteristics are often due to nutrition status.

Meds 16–3   Medications Used to Treat Cystic Fibrosis

Medications	Actions
Aerosol bronchodilators	Open large and small airways; used before chest physiotherapy and with symptoms; few studies exist to demonstrate their effectiveness.
Aerosol DNase	Loosens, liquefies, and thins pulmonary secretions; decreases risk of developing pulmonary infections requiring parenteral treatment in some patients (McMullen & Bryson, 2000).
Corticosteroids and high-dose ibuprofen on alternate days	Anti-inflammatory agents: reduce inflammatory response to infection; alternate-day use to decrease side effects of steroids; decrease progression of lung damage in preadolescents with mild disease.
Antibiotics (oral, intravenous, and inhalation)	Treat infections. Higher doses than normal and prolonged courses may be needed. Antibiotic selection should be based on culture sensitivities. Intermittent administration of tobramycin by inhalation improves pulmonary function.
Pancreatic enzyme supplements (Cotazym-S, Pancrease, Viokase)	Assist in digestion of nutrients decreasing fat and bulk; given before food ingestion, taken with meals and snacks.
Multivitamins and vitamin E in water-soluble form; vitamins A, D, and K given when deficient; iron supplementation	Cystic fibrosis interferes with vitamin production; supplements are required in water-soluble form for better absorption (vitamins A, D, E, and K are naturally fat soluble); iron deficiency results from malabsorption syndrome.
Ursodeoxycholate	May slow progression of hepatic lesion in cystic fibrosis. Given when patient has elevated liver enzymes or evidence of portal hypertension.
Lactulose	May abort early distal intestinal obstruction syndrome and prevent recurrences.

Assess the child's stooling pattern. Identify any problems with abdominal pain or bloating and if these problems are related to eating, stooling, or other activities. Palpate the abdomen for liver size, fecal masses, and evidence of pain.

Assess hearing periodically, as tobramycin is associated with hearing loss.

Identify how the child's illness affects day-to-day functioning, conflicts with family activities, and how the family has adapted to the child's need for care. Ask how the child or adolescent feels about the daily care routine.

Implementation

Periodic hospitalization for a severe infection or for a pulmonary and nutritional "tune-up." Place the child in a single room with standard precautions to reduce risk for transfer of *Pseudomonas* and *Burkholderia cepacia*. Respect and support the parents who need to take advantage of the respite from daily care.

Chest physiotherapy is performed one to three times per day before meals to facilitate removal of secretions from the lungs. DNase is given by nebulizer to help thin respiratory secretions. Identify the chest physiotherapy regimen most acceptable to the child and family.

Antibiotics for an acute exacerbation by oral, inhalation, and IV routes. With an increased clearance of nearly all antibiotics, higher dosages and up to 14 days of treatment are needed. Monitor renal function, and test antibiotic serum drug levels to ensure therapeutic dosing.

Give pancreatic enzymes with all meals and snacks to promote absorption of dietary nutrients and water-soluble vitamin supplements. Fats and extra salt are needed in the diet. Increase calorie intake with snacks between meals and before bed. The goal is to achieve near-normal, well-formed stools and adequate weight gain. Make a referral to a nutritionist before discharge.

Assist the child and parents with issues relating to discipline; body image (stooling and odor, clubbing, barrel chest); frequent rehospitalization; the potential fatal nature of the illness; the child's feeling of being different from friends; and overall financial, social, and family concerns. Refer families to psychosocial counseling as needed.

Assist families with a newly diagnosed child to obtain necessary equipment. Make referrals to social services as needed for financial assistance.

Help adolescents establish appropriate educational and occupational goals for their future and to transition to adult healthcare services.

Initiate palliative care planning with adolescents and young adults as the disease progresses to respiratory failure.

Patient and Family Education

During hospitalization, review basic and new information about the disorder, respiratory care, medications, and nutrition.

Review the child's use of bronchodilators and airway clearance techniques.

Encourage a regular, vigorous exercise regimen and aerobic fitness.

During periods of exercise and increased sweating, encourage the child to drink more fluids and increase salt intake. Teach parents to recognize early symptoms of salt depletion (fatigue, weakness, abdominal pain, and vomiting) and to contact the child's healthcare provider if these symptoms occur.

Review dietary needs and methods to provide extra calories needed for growth and increased energy expenditures.

Teach adolescents to assume responsibility for daily disease management. Discuss ways to perform the daily care regimen and interact with peers at school. Provide information about potential infertility and guidelines for safe sexual practices. Discuss the need for contraception with adolescent females. Refer to genetic counseling.

Laryngotracheobronchitis, or Croup

A viral invasion of the upper airway that extends throughout the larynx, trachea, and bronchi common in children 3 months to 4 years of age. Viruses causing LTB include parainfluenza virus type I, II, or III; influenza A and B; adenovirus; RSV; and measles (Perkin & Swift, 2002). Inflammation and edema narrow the subglottic area of the airway and cause obstruction.

Clinical Manifestations

Upper respiratory symptoms that progress to a cough and hoarseness.

Low-grade fever, runny nose, tachypnea, inspiratory stridor, and a seal-like barking cough.

Expiratory stridor, severe tachypnea, retractions.

Physical exhaustion can diminish the intensity of retractions, and stridor and breath sounds may actually diminish. Responsiveness decreases as hypoxemia increases.

Diagnostic Tests

Diagnosis by history and clinical signs. Pulse oximetry is used to detect hypoxemia. A radiograph of the upper airway may show a tapered, symmetric subglottic narrowing and rule out a foreign body.

No throat cultures or visual inspection of the inner mouth and throat are performed, as these procedures can cause laryngospasms and further compromise the airway.

Clinical Therapy

Management involves humidification, medications, and supplemental oxygen when the saturated oxygen level is less than 92%. See Meds 16–4 for medications used to treat LTB. Airway obstruction is a potential complication. Intubation and transfer to the pediatric intensive care unit if total obstruction is imminent.

Nursing Management

Assessment

Assess the child's respiratory status, and continuously monitor for development of airway obstruction (absence of voice sounds, increasing degree of respiratory distress, inability to swallow, and acute onset of drooling). If any of these signs occur, get medical assistance immediately. The quieter the child, the greater the cause for concern.

Monitor the level of consciousness—for anxiety, lethargy, or stupor as hypoxia increases.

Implementation

Provide supplemental oxygen with humidity if hypoxemia is present.

Meds 16–4 Medications Used for Laryngotracheobronchitis Treatment

Medication	Action/Indication	Nursing Considerations
Beta-agonists and beta-adrenergics (e.g., albuterol, racemic epinephrine): aerosolized through face mask	Rapid-acting bronchodilator, decreases bronchial and tracheal secretions and mucosal edema, used to decrease symptoms of moderate to severe respiratory distress and constriction of subglottic mucosa and submucosal capillaries. Used until dexamethasone begins working.	Provides only temporary relief; improvement in 30 min that lasts approximately 2 hrs, it gives time for the steroid to work; the child may experience tachycardia (160–200 beats/min) and hypertension; dizziness, headache, and nausea may necessitate stopping medication; reduces the need for artificial airway.
Corticosteroids (e.g., dexamethasone): intramuscular, oral, nebulized budesonide	Anti-inflammatory, used to decrease edema; has a long half-life of 36–54 hr.	The child may experience cardiovascular symptoms (hypertension); requires close observation for individual response; children less frequently need emergency airways; stridor resolves faster.

Allow the child to assume a position of comfort to help maintain the airway, usually sitting or lying with the head elevated. Administer medications.

Be immediately available to attend to the child's respiratory needs, as the child will have difficulty communicating about worsening respiratory symptoms.

Encourage the child to drink cool, noncarbonated, nonacidic beverages to liquify secretions and provide calories for energy and metabolism.

Teach parents about actions to take if symptoms recur.

Pneumonia

An inflammation or infection of the bronchioles and alveolar spaces of the lungs. Risk factors for developing pneumonia include chronic lung disease, anatomic problems, gastroesophageal reflux with aspiration, neurologic disorders that compromise the airway, and altered immune status (Sectish & Prober, 2004). Viral, bacterial, mycoplasmal, and fungal organisms cause pneumonia.

Clinical Manifestations

Mycoplasma pneumoniae: insidious onset, malaise, muscle aches, headache, fever, sore throat, rhinorrhea, dry hacking cough that becomes productive, fine crackles, and anorexia.

Viral pneumonia: sudden or insidious onset, rhinitis, slight cough that may become productive, fever and chills, crackles, and wheezes.

Streptococcus pneumoniae: sudden onset, high fever, cough, shaking, chills, chest pain, nasal flaring, retractions, fine crackles, dullness on percussion, and fremitus.

Staphylococcus aureus: upper respiratory infection and abrupt change in condition, high fever, cough, shaking, chills, lethargy, chest pain, nasal flaring, retractions, fine crackles, dullness on percussion, and fremitus.

Chlamydia pneumoniae: insidious onset, minimal or absent fever, tachypnea, malaise, persistent cough, and pharyngitis.

Newborns and infants may have grunting, nasal flaring, irritability, lethargy, and a diminished appetite. Diminished breath sounds may be noted.

Diagnostic Tests

History, physical signs and symptoms, and chest radiography help distinguish the type of pneumonia present. Children with recurrent pneumonia need to be evaluated for immunodeficiency syndromes, foreign-body aspiration, obstruction or compression of the airway, structural abnormality, cystic fibrosis, and asthma.

Clinical Therapy

Airway management, fluids, fever management, pain management, and rest; some children need oxygen and IV fluids to maintain hydration.

Hospitalization is required when respiratory symptoms increase in severity.

Antibiotics are prescribed for mycoplasma and bacterial pneumonias or for secondary bacterial infection of viral pneumonia.

Nursing Management

Assessment

Assess the respiratory rate, heart rate, and temperature, and observe color for pallor or cyanosis. Attach a pulse oximeter to monitor the SpO_2 level. Assess hydration status. Assess for the presence of pain with coughing.

Implementation

Promote deep breathing to fully aerate the lungs and to promote coughing to clear secretions and cellular debris. Teach the child and parent how to splint the chest.

Provide pain medication (acetaminophen or ibuprofen), which can provide the added benefits of temperature control and may aid in sleep. Give medications as prescribed.

Maintain hydration with clear fluids. IV fluids are used when oral fluids are inadequate. Encourage soft foods when tolerated.

Patient and Family Education

Educate family members about proper administration of medications and any side effects.

Teach family members to recognize signs indicating a worsening condition and needing immediate care, such as increased difficulty breathing and refusal to take fluids.

Encourage pneumococcal conjugate vaccine immunization. For children older than age 2 years who are immunosuppressed or have chronic diseases, encourage immunization with the 23-valent pneumococcal vaccine.

Tuberculosis

Tuberculosis (TB) is caused by the organism *Mycobacterium tuberculosis*, which is transmitted through the air by droplets when a person with active infection coughs, sneezes, speaks, or sings. Inhaled bacilli are small enough to travel directly to the alveoli and replicate. The risk of transitioning from latent TB to an active infection is greatest during the first 2 years of life and during adolescence. Foreign-born children have accounted for more than one-third of newly diagnosed cases in children 14 years of age or younger in recent years (American Academy of Pediatrics, 2003). Children have a greater risk for developing extrapulmonary TB, such as TB meningitis and miliary (disseminated) TB (Maltezou, Spyridis, & Kafetzis, 2000).

Clinical Manifestations

Latent TB is asymptomatic. Signs and symptoms may develop 1–6 months after becoming infected.

Infants have a persistent cough, weight loss or failure to gain weight, and fever. Wheezing, crackles, and decreased breath sounds may be present.

Children have fatigue, cough, anorexia, weight loss or growth delay, night sweats, chills, and a low-grade fever.

Diagnostic Tests

Intradermal purified protein derivative (PPD); only those children at high risk of exposure or at high risk for acquiring the infection because of immune status are routinely tested.

Confirmation of the diagnosis with cultures and acid-fast stains of blood, gastric aspirate or sputum, and a chest radiograph. A pleural biopsy may also be performed for culture and tissue examination.

Clinical Therapy

Combinations of medications are used for treatment of active and latent TB for 6 months (Meds 16–5). For infants, children, and adolescents with latent TB, a single daily dose of isoniazid is given for 9 months. Direct observed drug therapy is recommended to reduce treatment failure and development of drug-resistant organisms. Active TB cases are reported to the public health department.

Nursing Management

Assessment

Identify children at higher risk for exposure to TB (recent contact with a case of TB, family history of TB, positive PPD in household member, exposure to individuals with HIV infection, foreign birth, or prolonged travel to a country with high TB rates) (American Academy of Pediatrics, 2003).

Monitor the health of infants and young children who have a PPD conversion. Assess for weight loss, fever, fatigue, coughing, and respiratory status.

Meds 16–5   Medications Used to Treat Latent and Active Tuberculosis in Infants, Children, and Adolescents

Medication	Nursing Considerations
Isoniazid (bactericidal)	Obtain baseline bilirubin and liver function studies, as hepatotoxicity can occur. Obtain a baseline weight. Assess ophthalmologic and hematopoietic status studies. Give 1 hr before or 2 hr after meals unless gastrointestinal irritation occurs; then give with food. Tablets can be crushed. Interferes with hepatic metabolism of phenytoin and may cause toxicity. Monitor for symptoms of hypersensitivity, signs of hepatotoxicity (anorexia, fever, malaise, nausea, vomiting, diarrhea, weight loss), dark urine, jaundice. Adolescents should avoid alcohol. Pyridoxine supplementation (vitamin B_6) is recommended for children and adolescents with meat- and milk-deficient diets, those with nutritional deficiencies, and those who are pregnant or human immunodeficiency virus–infected to prevent peripheral neuritis and seizures.
Rifampin (bactericidal)	Obtain baseline bilirubin and liver function studies, as this drug can alter the pharmacokinetics and serum concentrations of other drugs. Assess renal and hematopoietic status studies. Give 1 hr before or 2 hr after meals unless gastrointestinal irritation occurs; then give with food. Capsule contents can be sprinkled on applesauce or suspended in flavored syrup. Monitor for symptoms of jaundice and other side effects. Assess medications taken for interaction with rifampin (e.g., diazepam, beta-adrenergics, barbiturates, analgesics, corticosteroids, oral contraceptives, digitalis). Inform parents and child about orange-colored body fluids. Contact lenses become permanently discolored if used. Sexually active adolescent females should not use oral contraceptives, as rifampin makes them ineffective.
Pyrazinamide	Obtain baseline liver function studies and renal and hematopoietic status studies. Monitor for symptoms of hepatotoxicity. Monitor blood glucose level in children with diabetes, as glycemic control may be affected. When used in combination with isoniazid and rifampin, a 6-month course of therapy is possible.

(continued)

Medication	Nursing Considerations
Ethambutol (bacteriostatic or bactericidal, depending on dosage used)	Obtain baseline liver function studies and renal and hematopoietic status studies. Perform a baseline and monthly ophthalmologic test of visual acuity, visual fields, and color discrimination, as the drug may cause reversible or irreversible optic neuritis, particularly in children with impaired renal function. Give with meals if gastrointestinal irritation occurs. Inform parents and child to report any vision changes.
Streptomycin (may occasionally be used for initial 4–8 weeks of treatment for active tuberculosis)	Intramuscular injections are painful, so provide guidance for pain management. Monitor for ototoxicity; assess hearing acuity regularly. Monitor intake and output, looking for signs of reduced kidney function. Educate parents to immediately report these symptoms: nausea, vomiting, incoordination, dizziness, impaired hearing, fullness in ears.

Implementation

Implement standard precautions until the infection status is known. Provide supportive care if hospitalized.

Assist with the collection of blood, sputum, and gastric aspirate cultures.

Patient and Family Education

Emphasize the importance of keeping appointments for "directly observed drug therapy" and of subsequent daily home administration of medications. Drugs are given on an empty stomach. Emphasize the importance of completing the full course of medications.

Encourage proper nutrition and rest to promote recovery.

The child can return to school or childcare when effective therapy is instituted, adherence to therapy is documented, and clinical symptoms have diminished (American Academy of Pediatrics, 2003).

Facilitate PPD testing of family members and close contacts.

INJURIES OF THE RESPIRATORY SYSTEM
Foreign-Body Aspiration

Inhalation of any object (solid or liquid, food or nonfood) into the respiratory tract, causing partial or complete obstruction. Infants and young toddlers are at high risk because of increasing mobility and tendency to mouth objects, but aspiration occurs at all ages. Common aspirated items include the following:

- Foods such as nuts, popcorn, hard candy, or small pieces of raw vegetables or hot dog
- Small, loose toy parts such as small wheels and bells
- Household objects and substances such as beads, safety pins, coins, buttons, balloon pieces, and colorful liquids (mouthwash, perfume) in enticing packages (small screw bottle tops)

Most aspirated foreign bodies cause bronchial obstruction, often in the right lung. An object lodged in the trachea is life-threatening.

Clinical Manifestations

Clutching the neck is universal sign of choking, seen in older children.

Spasmodic coughing, gagging, dysphonia, wheezing without fever or other symptoms of illness; may be brief or last of hours.

Signs of increased respiratory effort such as dyspnea, tachypnea, nasal flaring, and retractions.

Concentrated focus on breathing, an anxious expression, and sitting in a forward position with the neck extended, as if to straighten out the airway.

Behavior changes such as irritability and decreased responsiveness as the child becomes hypoxic.

Diagnostic Tests

A chest radiograph or a forced expiratory film.

Clinical Therapy

Perform back blows and chest thrusts for an infant and abdominal thrusts for older children.

Administer oxygen.

Fluoroscopy and fiberoptic bronchoscopy performed in the operating room to locate and extract the foreign body; removal of visible foreign body with a laryngoscope and Magill forceps.

Treatment for pneumonia if present.

Nursing Management

Assessment

Continuously assess the child, as a complete obstruction may occur.

Monitor for increasing respiratory distress. Breath sound changes from noisy to decreasing to absent on the affected side can indicate that the object is moving and blocking a mainstem bronchus.

Attach a cardiorespiratory monitor and pulse oximeter to assess increasing hypoxia.

Assess the family's level of distress and coping ability.

Implementation

Keep emergency resuscitation equipment immediately accessible.

Allow the child to select the position of comfort, such as sitting upright or a semi-Fowler position.

Avoid any procedure that increases the child's anxiety.

Provide a quiet environment and keep parents close to help reduce the child's anxiety.

Provide education about potential safety hazards in the home. Encourage the parents to learn CPR.

Pneumothorax

Air enters the pleural space because of tears in the tracheobronchial tree, the esophagus, or the chest wall, resulting in lung collapse. Causes of pneumothorax include the following:

- Complication of mechanical ventilation or high peak inspiratory or end-expiratory pressure
- Gas trapping and alveolar hyperinflation in chronic lung conditions such as neonatal respiratory distress syndrome, status asthmaticus, and cystic fibrosis
- Blunt trauma to the chest

An open pneumothorax results from any penetrating injury that exposes the pleural space to atmospheric pressure.

A tension pneumothorax is a life-threatening emergency that results when the air leaked in the chest on inhalation cannot be vented to escape during exhalation. Internal pressure builds, compressing the chest contents and collapsing the lung. As the pressure continues to build, a mediastinal shift impairs venous blood return to the heart and causes decreased cardiac output.

Clinical Manifestations

Open pneumothorax: a sucking sound may be heard as the air moves through the opening on the chest wall; restlessness, cyanosis, or air leakage into the tissue.

Closed pneumothorax: decreased or absent breath sounds on the injured side; respiratory distress.

Tension pneumothorax: increasing respiratory distress, absent breath sounds, cardiovascular instability, and a tracheal shift to the unaffected side.

Diagnostic Procedures
Physical signs are used to make the diagnosis. A chest radiograph reveals the lung collapse.

Clinical Therapy
Immediate treatment for an open pneumothorax is covering the wound with an airtight seal.

For a closed pneumothorax, a thoracostomy is performed and a chest tube inserted. A closed drainage system helps remove the air and reinflate the lung.

Immediate care for a tension pneumothorax is a needle thoracentesis to allow air to escape and relieve the tension. A chest tube is inserted and attached to a closed drainage system.

Nursing Management
Assess for respiratory distress or change in respiratory function and monitor vital signs. Nursing care focuses on chest tube and drainage system management. When the chest tube is removed, the site is covered with an occlusive dressing, and the child's respiratory status is carefully monitored for signs of respiratory distress.

Pulmonary Contusion
Bruising damage to the lung tissues after the energy from blunt trauma is transferred directly through the child's chest wall to the internal organs. The capillaries bleed into the alveoli, and capillary rupture in the air sacs may occur. As blood and fluid from damaged tissues accumulate in the lower airways, pulmonary edema develops. Lower airway obstruction and atelectasis may result in impaired gas exchange, acute respiratory distress, and respiratory failure (Hazinski, 1999).

Clinical Manifestations
Initially, the child may appear asymptomatic.

Signs of respiratory distress often develop over several hours and include wheezing, hemoptysis, fever, and crackles. Agitation and lethargy can signal increasing hypoxia.

Diagnostic Tests
Careful observation is required during the first 12 hours after the injury to detect decreased perfusion related to ventilatory impairment. A chest radiograph may reveal lower airway obstruction and atelectasis.

Clinical Therapy

Intubation and mechanical ventilation as the lung tissues heal; humidified oxygen; diuretics to decrease edema in the interstitial pulmonary tissue. The child is carefully monitored for acute respiratory distress syndrome.

Nursing Management

Monitor respiratory function to detect signs of deterioration using level of consciousness as a key indicator. Inspect the thorax for symmetric chest wall movement. Observe for hemoptysis (fresh blood in the sputum), dyspnea, decreased breath sounds, wheezes, crackles, and a transient temperature elevation. Cyanosis in children is often a late indicator of respiratory distress.

Provide physiologic support, such as oxygen therapy, pulmonary management, positioning, ventilatory support to provide positive end-expiratory pressure, and comfort measures. Carefully manage fluids to prevent large increases in pulmonary edema.

Smoke-Inhalation Injury

Exposure of the child's face and airway to fire or high heat leads to airway obstruction from thermal injury and edema. Exposure to noxious chemicals and irritants results in mucosal airway damage, bronchospasm, depletion of alveolar surfactant, and mucous plugging from soot and sloughed airway mucosa.

When the child is trapped in a closed space, carbon monoxide exposure rapidly produces hypoxia. Confusion, myocardial depression, and ventricular arrhythmias result as the vital organs are deprived of oxygen.

Soot carried deep into the lungs combines with moisture in the lungs to produce acid chemicals that burn and cause loss of cilia, loss of surfactant, and edema. Gas exchange is disrupted, and sloughing lung tissue obstructs the airways. Microorganisms grow in damaged tissue, and pneumonia often results.

Clinical Manifestations

Burns of the face and neck, singed nasal hairs, soot around the mouth or nose, and hoarseness with stridor or voice change.

Respiratory distress may develop over a few hours, when tachypnea, stridor, coughing, and wheezing may be seen. Respiratory distress may progress to respiratory failure.

If carbon monoxide poisoning is present, the child is confused or unconscious and has cardiac arrhythmias.

Diagnostic Tests

Diagnosis is based on history of the child being exposed to smoke in a closed area and signs of soot around the nose and mouth.

Clinical Therapy

Hospitalization and monitoring for progression of respiratory distress.

Initial treatment is 100% humidified oxygen administered through a nonrebreather mask.

If respiratory distress develops, an endotracheal tube, mechanical ventilation, and monitoring are provided in the intensive care unit.

Aerosol bronchodilators may be prescribed. Pulmonary physiotherapy.

All other fire-related injuries are treated.

Nursing Management

Monitor for development of respiratory distress, and check vital signs frequently. Attach a pulse oximeter. Auscultate the lungs for crackles, wheezes, and decreased breath sounds. Assess for level of consciousness and behavior changes that could indicate increasing hypoxia.

Provide oxygen as ordered. Position the child to promote respiratory function. If the child's condition deteriorates, assist with procedures to secure the child's airway and prepare the child for transfer to the intensive care unit. Assess the family's response to the life-threatening crisis and offer support with information about the child's condition.

17. ALTERATIONS IN CARDIOVASCULAR FUNCTION

CONGESTIVE HEART FAILURE (CHF)

Cardiac output is inadequate to support the body's circulatory and metabolic needs, and it may result from one of the following:

- A congenital heart defect that causes increased pulmonary blood flow or obstruction to the systemic outflow tract (the most common cause)
- Problems with heart contractility
- Conditions that require high cardiac output: severe anemia, acidosis, or respiratory disease
- Acquired heart disease: cardiomyopathy, rheumatic heart disease, or Kawasaki syndrome

Clinical Manifestations

Pulmonary venous congestion leads to tachypnea, wheezing, crackles, retractions, cough, dyspnea on exertion, grunting, nasal flaring, skin color changes (mottling, pallor, or cyanosis), feeding difficulties, irritability, tiring with play, and exercise intolerance.

Systemic venous congestion leads to hepatomegaly, ascites, periorbital edema, peripheral edema, weight gain, and neck vein distention in children.

Impaired cardiac output leads to tachycardia, weak, thready pulses, hypotension, S_3 gallop rhythm, capillary refill time of more than 2 seconds, pallor, cool extremities, oliguria, fatigue, restlessness, and enlarged heart.

High metabolic rate leads to weight loss, failure to thrive or slow weight gain, and diaphoresis.

Diagnostic Tests

Chest radiograph, echocardiography, an electrocardiogram (ECG)

Clinical Therapy

Medications include diuretics, inotropic medications and afterload-reducing agents, digoxin, and beta-blockers (Meds 17–1).

Meds 17–1   Medications Used in Treatment of Congestive Heart Failure

Drug	Action
Digoxin	Increases myocardial contractility, improving systemic circulation
Furosemide	Rapid diuresis, blocks reabsorption of sodium and water in renal tubules
Thiazides: chlorothiazide (suspension), hydrochlorothiazide (tablets)	Maintains diuresis, decreases absorption of sodium, water, potassium, chloride, and bicarbonate in renal tubules
Spironolactone	Maintenance diuresis (potassium sparing)
Angiotensin-converting enzyme inhibitor	Promotes vascular relaxation and reduced peripheral vascular resistance, reduces afterload
Propranolol	Increases contractility
Carvedilol	Improves left ventricular function, promotes vasodilation of systemic circulation for chronic heart failure and dilated cardiomyopathy

Supportive medical therapy includes airway management, ventilatory support, oxygen, rest, and fluid and dietary management.

Surgery or interventional catheterization to correct a congenital heart defect; cardiac transplantation for end-stage cardiomyopathy or complex congenital heart defects such as hypoplastic left heart syndrome.

Nursing Management
Assessment
Obtain a detailed history of the onset of symptoms.

Assess vital signs: quality of pulses and respirations and color. Assess for signs of fluid overload; intake and output; serial abdominal measurements; signs of exercise intolerance; feeding difficulty; irritability, behavior changes; growth status; diaphoresis; and skin redness and breakdown. Inspect, palpate, and auscultate the heart.

Conduct a family assessment for knowledge of the child's condition; correct medication dosing, and identify changes in child's condition needing care; ability to provide needed care; anxiety level and coping strategies; support system and respite care; and financial status.

Perform a developmental assessment.

Observe for changes in feeding habits (decreased intake, vomiting, sleeping through feedings, and increased perspiration with feedings) that may indicate deteriorating cardiac status.

Implementation

Administer and monitor prescribed medications. Read labels carefully and double-check doses.

- Give digoxin at the same times daily.
- Check the apical heart rate for a full minute before giving any dose. If bradycardia is present, call for advice before giving the drug.
- Check the serum potassium level if diuretics are ordered, as a low potassium level increases the risk for digoxin overdose.
- Observe the child carefully for digoxin toxicity (tachycardia in young children or bradycardia in older children, nausea, vomiting, anorexia, dizziness, headache, weakness, fatigue, and arrhythmia). Certain antibiotics (macrolides, azithromycin, tetracyclines, and β-lactams) increase digoxin serum concentration.

Provide frequent skin care when edema is present.

Monitor the oxygen flow rate, ensure delivery device is working properly, and provide humidification. Position the child in semi-Fowler or a 45-degree angle.

Group assessments and interventions to provide uninterrupted rest each hour. Encourage quiet activities. Encourage development with appropriate toys, short periods of activity, singing, talking, and music.

Teach parents feeding techniques. Burp infants frequently to permit rest and prevent vomiting. Encourage breastfeeding if mother chooses. Some ways to decrease the work of feeding, either with breast or bottle, include the following (Cook & Higgins, 2004):

- Hold the infant at a 45-degree angle to help to decrease venous return to the heart and reduce metabolic demand. If the parent gets fatigued, the infant can be shifted to an infant seat at a 45-degree angle.
- Limit feeding time to 40 minutes, so the infant does not become overtired.
- Permit the infant to set his or her own rhythm for feeding and resting.
- Follow the infant's cues for hunger, satiety, and tiring.

Ensure adequate calories for the increased metabolic rate and growth, with a high-calorie formula. Supplement nutrition by nasogastric or gastrostomy tube as needed.

Provide emotional support to the family.

Teach family about medication administration and safety and toxic effects of digoxin and other medications, signs of worsening condition, and feeding techniques to maximize food intake.

CONGENITAL HEART DISEASE

A defect in the heart or great vessels or persistence of a fetal structure after birth. Congenital heart defects are categorized by the pathophysiology and hemodynamics.

Defects That Increase Pulmonary Blood Flow

A connection between the left and right side of the heart (septal defect) or between the great arteries (patent ductus arteriosus) allows blood to flow between two sides of the heart. The higher pressures on the left cause left-to-right shunting, and the volume of blood pumped to the lungs is increased. CHF, pulmonary vascular resistance, and right ventricular hypertrophy may develop.

Clinical Manifestations

Increased heart and respiratory rates and increased metabolic rate.

Diaphoresis with feeding; poor weight gain.

Signs of CHF (dyspnea, tachypnea, intercostal retractions, and periorbital edema); frequent respiratory infections.

See Box 17–1 for specific heart defects.

Box 17–1   Heart Defects That Increase Pulmonary Blood Flow, Their Clinical Manifestations and Clinical Therapy

Atrial Septal Defect (ASD)

An opening in the atrial septum permits left-to-right shunting of blood.
Asymptomatic if opening is small. A soft systolic ejection murmur in the pulmonic area with wide fixed splitting of S_2. CHF, easy tiring, and poor growth occur with a large ASD.
Surgery to close or patch the ASD or closure by a septal occluder during cardiac catheterization.

Atrioventricular (AV) Canal (Endocardial Cushion Defect)

A combination of defects in the atrial and ventricular septa and portions of tricuspid and mitral valves. The most complex malformation results in one AV valve and large septal defects between both atria and ventricles.
CHF, tachypnea, tachycardia, poor growth, recurrent respiratory infections, and repeated respiratory failure. A holosystolic murmur is loudest at left lower sternal border (mitral regurgitation). Accentuated S_1 and split S_2.
Palliative pulmonary artery banding reduces blood flow to the lungs and CHF before corrective surgery. Patches are placed over septal defects, and valve tissue is used to form functioning valves. Mitral valve may be replaced.

Patent Ductus Arteriosus (PDA)

Persistent fetal circulation. Blood is shunted from the aorta through the PDA to the pulmonary arteries, increasing circulation to the pulmonary system.

CHF, intercostal retractions, hepatomegaly, and growth failure. Infant is at risk for frequent respiratory infections, pneumonia, and infective endocarditis. Continuous "machinery" murmur during systole and diastole, a thrill in the pulmonic area.

Surgical ligation of PDA. IV indomethacin often stimulates PDA closure in premature infants.

Ventricular Septal Defect (VSD)

An opening in the ventricular septum allows blood to flow from the left ventricle directly across the open septum into the pulmonary artery.

Small VSDs are asymptomatic. Large VSDs cause tachypnea, dyspnea, poor growth, reduced fluid intake, CHF, increased number of pulmonary infections, and pulmonary hypertension. A systolic murmur at the third or fourth left intercostal space at the sternal border.

Small VSDs often close spontaneously by 6 months of age. Surgical patching of VSD or closure of VSD by transcatheter device during cardiac catheterization.

Diagnostic Procedures

Chest radiograph, ECG, echocardiogram, and cardiac catheterization.

A complete blood count, urinalysis, coagulation studies, platelet counts, and serum electrolytes before surgery.

Clinical Therapy

Surgery may be performed early in infancy to prevent irreversible pulmonary vascular disease, or surgery may be postponed until the child is symptomatic or older. Indomethacin may be given to preterm infants with a PDA when immediate ductus closure is needed. Therapeutic cardiac catheterization may be performed for some conditions. See Box 17–1.

Nursing Management of the Child Undergoing a Cardiac Catheterization

Assessment

Before the procedure, assess the vital signs, hematocrit and hemoglobin, capillary refill, skin temperature and color, and strength of the pedal and popliteal pulses for postcatheterization comparison.

After the procedure, assess vital signs (check for arrhythmia) and perfusion of leg below catheter site (pedal and popliteal pulses, skin temperature, color, capillary refill, and sensation). Monitor intake and output, as the contrast medium causes diuresis. Diuretic treatment increases risk for dehydration.

Assess the pressure dressing over the catheterization site every 15 minutes for 1 hour and then every 30 minutes for 1 hour. Monitor for bleeding (checking under buttocks for blood) and hematoma or thrombus formation at the catheterization site.

Implementation
Before the procedure
- Keep the child NPO for several hours, except for medications. Give the ordered sedative to older children. Infants and young children are given deeper sedation to keep them still during the procedure.
- Provide age-appropriate information to prepare the child for the procedure. Explain the sensations that will be experienced.

After the procedure
- Apply direct pressure over the catheterization site for 15 minutes after wires and catheters are removed. Place a pressure bandage for 6 hours.
- Keep the child on bed rest for 6 hours and avoid flexion of the hips. Then limit activity for 24 hours.
- Begin with clear liquids and progress to other fluids and food as tolerated. Maintain hydration.

Patient and Family Education
Check for signs of complications several times in the first 24 hours after catheterization—for example, fever, bleeding or a bruise increasing in size at the catheterization site, and loss of feeling in foot or cooler foot on side of catheterization.

If the child is treated with diuretics, observe for signs of dehydration (dry mucous membranes, no tears, sunken fontanel).

Notify physician immediately if any of these signs are noted within the first 24 hours after the catheterization.

Encourage fluids to help flush the dye out of the body and to prevent dehydration.

Permit quiet play such as crayons or markers, board games, puzzles, books, music, and videos for 24 hours.

Children whose heart defect is corrected by cardiac catheterization have the same risks for infective endocarditis as children with surgical correction.

Nursing Management before Surgery

Monitor the infant for poor growth and signs of CHF as described in Congestive Heart Failure.

Provide psychosocial support to the parents coping with the infant's diagnosis.

Provide nursing care as described for the infant with CHF.

Teach parents to care for the child at home until surgery, encouraging adequate nutrition, reducing exposure to infectious diseases, monthly prophylaxis for respiratory syncytial virus with palivizumab during the peak season, and other routine health promotion and maintenance visits.

Nursing Management at the Time of Surgery
Assessment

Assess child to detect an acute illness. Assess behavioral patterns, cardiac function, respiratory function, weight, and fluid status.

After surgery, assess vital signs, temperature, breath sounds, respiratory effort, and surgical incision site for erythema or wound drainage. Auscultate the apical pulse to detect arrhythmia. Use pulse oximetry to assess oxygen saturation. Monitor intake and output. Identify signs of surgical complications such as infection, arrhythmias, and impaired tissue perfusion.

Assess the child's pain.

Implementation

Provide pain management with intravenous (IV) opioids 24 hours a day until the child is taking fluids. Then provide oral analgesics around the clock. Carefully lift and move the child to avoid stress on the incision and pain. Do not lift the child under the arms.

Encourage deep breaths and coughing, or perform spirometry exercises regularly. Chest physiotherapy is used for children younger than 3 years old.

Encourage oral fluids and nutrition when permitted. Oral fluids are rarely limited.

Inspect incision for infection. Administer antibiotics as ordered.

Encourage a gradual increase in activity with longer periods out of bed every day. Ensure adequate rest periods to promote healing.

Patient and Family Teaching

Sponge bathe the infant or use a tub bath with low water level to bathe the child. Clean the incision daily with gentle baby or pH-balanced soap. Keep the incision clean and dry.

Demonstrate methods to lift and move the child to prevent pain and stress on the incision.

Encourage a nutritious diet and snacks so the infant or child has an opportunity to catch up for previous growth deficits.

Call the healthcare provider for signs of wound infection (redness, swelling, tenderness, or drainage around the incision), fever of more than 40.3°C (101°F), flu-like symptoms, a change in appetite or activity level, irritability, or an increased respiratory rate.

Give appropriate dose of acetaminophen or ibuprofen for pain control.

Place a small blanket over the incision for protection while in the care safety seat.

Allow the child to gradually increase activity. Report increased fatigue or decreased activity tolerance to the physician. No rough play, bike riding, or climbing for 6 weeks until the sternum incision has healed completely.

Prepare parents for the child's potential response to hospitalization stress (nightmares, separation anxiety, and overdependence on parents).

When a complete correction of the cardiac defect has been performed, encourage parents to allow the child to live a normal and active life.

Give prophylactic antibiotics for dental and surgical procedures according to American Heart Association guidelines.

Defects Causing Decreased Pulmonary Blood Flow and Mixed Defects

Defects causing decreased pulmonary blood flow often permit little or no blood to reach the lungs for oxygenation. When an atrial septal defect or ventricular septal defect exists, higher right-sided pressures result in right-to-left shunting. Polycythemia develops to increase the hemoglobin available to carry oxygen and places the child at higher risk for the following:

- Impaired clotting and risk of bleeding with surgery
- Thromboembolism (cerebral or pulmonary) due to sluggish blood flow through the small vessels
- Brain abscesses
- Mixed defects: Many complex congenital heart defects make the newborn dependent on the mixing of the pulmonary and systemic circulations for survival, resulting in a general desaturated systemic blood flow and cyanosis. Increased pulmonary

blood flow and obstruction of systemic flow causes pulmonary congestion.

Clinical Manifestations

Defects causing decreased pulmonary blood flow (see Box 17–2 for specific heart defects)

- Cyanosis when the ductus arteriosus closes, dyspnea, and a loud murmur.
- Fatigue, clubbing of the fingers and toes, exertional dyspnea, tiring and diaphoresis with feeding, poor weight gain, and delayed developmental milestones.
- Low oxygen saturation level because unoxygenated and oxygenated blood mixes; supplemental oxygen does not improve the oxygen saturation level or cyanosis.
- Hypercyanotic episodes (see Hypercyanotic Episodes).
- Exercise-induced dizziness and syncope in an older child.

Box 17–2   Defects with Decreased Pulmonary Blood Flow, Their Clinical Manifestations and Clinical Therapy

---

Pulmonic Stenosis

Narrowing of the pulmonic valve obstructs blood flow into the pulmonary artery. Increased preload and right ventricular hypertrophy results.

Dyspnea and fatigue on exertion. CHF and chest pain on exertion in severe cases. A loud systolic ejection murmur, widely split S_2, and thrill in the pulmonic area.

Dilation by balloon valvuloplasty during cardiac catheterization or surgical valvotomy when other defects are present.

Tetralogy of Fallot

A combination of pulmonic stenosis, right ventricular hypertrophy, ventricular septal defect, and overriding of aorta. An open foramen ovale or atrial septal defect in some cases.

Hypoxia and cyanosis occur as the ductus arteriosus closes. Polycythemia, hypoxic spells, metabolic acidosis, poor growth, clubbing, and exercise intolerance may develop. Systolic murmur in the pulmonic area transmitted to suprasternal notch. A thrill in the pulmonic area.

Hypercyanotic episodes managed with knee–chest positioning, calming, oxygen, IV morphine, and IV propranolol. A surgical total repair is performed at approximately 6 months of age.

Pulmonary Atresia/Tricuspid Atresia

Pulmonary atresia: no communication between the right ventricle and the pulmonary artery. The right ventricle pushes blood back through the tricuspid valve for passage through the foramen ovale. The ductus arteriosus provides the only flow of blood to the pulmonary arteries.

Tricuspid atresia: no communication between the right atrium and ventricle. Blood flows through the foramen ovale as in pulmonary atresia.

Cyanosis at birth. Tachypnea, CHF, pulmonary edema, hepatomegaly, acidosis, hypoxic spells, clubbing, polycythemia, and growth delays. A continuous murmur from the patent ductus arteriosus in pulmonic area. A single S_2 in aortic area, and a harsh systolic murmur in the tricuspid area.

Prostaglandin E_1 is given to maintain a patent ductus arteriosus. Digoxin and diuretics are used. The Rastelli balloon atrial septostomy is performed to increase the atrial opening. A Rastelli or modified Fontan procedure improves survival.

Mixed defects (see Box 17–3 for various defects)

- Varying degrees of cyanosis and CHF.
- When the pulmonary blood flow is decreased, cyanosis and polycythemia are more severe (Suddaby, 2001).

Box 17–3 Mixed Heart Defects Causing Cyanosis, Their Clinical Manifestations and Clinical Therapy

Transposition of the Great Arteries

The pulmonary artery is the outflow tract for left ventricle, and the aorta is the outflow tract for the right ventricle, creating parallel circulations.

Cyanosis at birth, does not improve with oxygen; progresses to hypoxia, acidosis, and CHF. Tachypnea (60 respirations/minute) without retractions or other signs of dyspnea. Growth failure. A systolic murmur if a ventricular septal defect (VSD) is present; otherwise no murmur, loud S_2.

Prostaglandin E_1 (PGE$_1$) to maintain a patent ductus arteriosus until surgery (arterial switch) before 1 week of age. Balloon atrial septostomy may be first stage during cardiac catheterization. Other defects repaired in stages as the infant grows.

Truncus Arteriosus

A single large vessel empties both ventricles and provides circulation for the pulmonary, systemic, and coronary circulations. A VSD may be present.

Cyanosis soon after birth, increased pulmonary blood flow with severe CHF, dyspnea, retractions, fatigue, poor feeding, poor growth, polycythemia, clubbing, bounding peripheral pulses, increased pulse pressure, frequent respiratory infections, and cardiomegaly. The VSD produces a harsh systolic murmur at lower sternal border. A systolic click at apex and pulmonic area.

Rastelli procedure to close the VSD and create a passage to pulmonary arteries. Repeated surgery to enlarge pulmonary artery conduit. Digoxin and diuretics.

Total Anomalous Pulmonary Venous Return

The pulmonary veins empty into right atrium or veins leading to the right atrium rather than into the left atrium. The foramen ovale must remain patent for blood to pass to the systemic circulation.

Mild cyanosis and frequent respiratory infections. Increased cyanosis if the pulmonary veins are obstructed and increased pulmonary blood flow, resulting in tachycardia, dyspnea, pulmonary edema, retractions, crackles, hepatomegaly, poor feedings, irritability, and failure to thrive. A palpable precordial bulge. Wide, fixed split S_2 with ejection murmur in the pulmonic area, gallop rhythm.

PGE_1 to maintain patent ductus arteriosus. Hypoxemia and CHF are treated. Balloon atrial septostomy initially, then surgery to reconnect or baffle the pulmonary veins to the left atrium.

Double-Outlet Right Ventricle

Both great arteries leave the right ventricle, increasing pulmonary blood flow and reducing systemic blood flow. The only outlet for the left ventricle is a large VSD.

Growth retardation, tachypnea, signs of CHF, cyanosis, clubbing. Loud S_2 and upper left sternal border systolic murmur, systolic thrill.

Digoxin and diuretics. Pulmonary artery banding or balloon atrial septostomy when symptomatic. An arterial switch or Senning procedure with an intraventricular tunnel between the VSD and the pulmonary artery.

Diagnostic Procedures

Chest radiograph, ECG, echocardiogram, cardiac catheterization, hematocrit and hemoglobin, and clotting time.

Clinical Therapy

A palliative procedure initially to preserve life, let the infant grow, and improve the success of corrective surgery.

Prostaglandin E_1 (PGE_1) is given to reopen the ductus arteriosus if its closure causes life-threatening cyanosis.

Hemoglobin and hematocrit values are monitored for polycythemia or anemia. Red blood cell pheresis is performed if the blood viscosity is too high.

Hypercyanotic episodes are treated aggressively (see Hypercyanotic Episodes).

Antibiotic prophylaxis to prevent infective endocarditis.

Nursing Management

Assessment

Before surgery

- Closely monitor the infant's cardiovascular status when on PGE$_1$ therapy. Assess vital signs, heart rhythm, skin color, peripheral pulses, capillary refill time, pulse oximetry, and blood gases.
- For infants at risk for CHF, assess for tachycardia, tachypnea, crackles, frothy secretions, low urine output, and edema.

Before or between stages of surgery at health visits
- Assess growth and plot on growth curve.
- Identify signs of progressive deterioration in cardiac status (increased cyanosis in the morning or at other high-risk times, note clubbing of the fingers and toes).
- Observe for headache, dizziness, excessive irritability, and paralysis associated with thromboembolitic complication.

After surgery
- Monitor the heart's functioning. Assess vital signs, pulse oximetry, skin color, perfusion of the skin by capillary refill, and distal pulses. Early signs of hemorrhage include a sudden, sustained increase in pulse and respirations and a decrease in peripheral perfusion.
- Monitor fluid intake and output.
- Note any signs of respiratory distress.
- Assess for pain.

Implementation
Home care of the child before surgery

Make referrals to community-based early-intervention programs to promote the child's development. Reduce parental anxiety about developmental delays with information about the long-term developmental outcomes of children with periods of cyanosis and subsequent surgery.

Children with mild cyanotic lesions do not need to adjust activity. The child with moderate to severe disease should be able to tolerate crying for a few minutes, but prevent prolonged crying. Do not let child travel to high-altitude locations without physician approval. Supplemental oxygen when traveling on an airplane may be necessary.

Teach parents to observe for signs of worsening cyanosis that could signal a hypercyanotic episode. Provide guidelines for the initial management of the hypercyanotic episode (see Hypercyanotic Episodes). Assist them to develop an emergency care plan.

Teach parents to seek early medical care for acute illnesses (e.g., fever, vomiting, or diarrhea). Educate parents about the signs of infective endocarditis and the need for antibiotic prophylaxis.

Care of the newborn

- Monitor and carefully maintain the central, umbilical, or peripheral IV lines in the newborn receiving continuous infusion of PGE_1. Observe for common side effects of prostaglandin treatment (cutaneous vasodilation, bradycardia, tachycardia, hypotension, seizure activity, fever, and apnea).
- Have emergency equipment for apnea and IV fluids for hypotension.

After surgery

- Monitor for postoperative bleeding (especially in the chest tube), as bleeding times are prolonged and platelet counts are low in children with polycythemia.
- Nursing care is the same as described for the child having surgery for increased pulmonary blood flow.

Defects Obstructing Systemic Blood Flow

Stenosis of a valve or in the great artery obstructs blood flow, increases pressure (afterload) on the ventricle, and decreases cardiac output to the pulmonic or systemic circulation.

Clinical Manifestations

Signs of low cardiac output: diminished pulses, poor color, delayed capillary refill time, and decreased urinary output.

CHF and pulmonary edema in severe obstructions; in mild obstructions, leg cramps, and cooler feet than hands.

Stronger pulses and higher BP in the arms than the legs.

See Box 17–4 for specific heart defects.

Box 17–4 Defects That Obstruct the Systemic Blood Flow, Their Clinical Manifestations and Clinical Therapy

Aortic Stenosis (AS)

Narrowing of the aortic valve obstructs blood flow to systemic circulation. Usually asymptomatic, but life-threatening AS and congestive heart failure (CHF) seen in some newborns. Normal blood pressure with a narrow pulse pressure; weak peripheral pulses; tolerates exercise; some have chest pain after exercise. Fainting and dizziness are serious signs. Systolic heart murmur and thrill in the aortic or pulmonic areas, transmission to neck, ejection click. Split S_2 with severe aortic stenosis.

Newborns with life-threatening aortic stenosis need prostaglandin E_1 (PGE$_1$) to maintain a patent ductus arteriosus until the aortic valve can be dilated by balloon valvuloplasty during cardiac catheterization. Surgical valvuloplasty or aortic valve replacement.

Coarctation of the Aorta

Narrowing, or constriction, in the descending aorta, often near the ductus arteriosus or left subclavian artery, obstructs the systemic blood outflow.

Asymptomatic initially, but constriction of aorta is progressive. Lower blood pressure in legs and higher blood pressure in arms, neck, and head. Bounding brachial and radial pulses and weak or absent femoral pulses. Loud, single S_2. Systolic ejection murmur at the upper right and middle or lower left sternal border. A thrill in the suprasternal notch.

Balloon dilation and surgical resection with the subclavian artery.

Hypoplastic Left Heart Syndrome

Absence or stenosis of mitral and aortic valves, abnormally small left ventricle, a small aorta, and aortic or mitral stenosis or atresia.

With closure of ductus arteriosus, progressive cyanosis, tachycardia, tachypnea, dyspnea, retractions and decreased peripheral pulses. Systolic murmur may be present. Poor peripheral perfusion, pulmonary edema, and CHF eventually lead to shock, acidosis, and death.

PGE$_1$ to maintain a patent ductus arteriosus. No supplemental oxygen. Treatment options are comfort or palliative care, the Norwood procedure, or heart transplantation (see Heart Transplantation).

Diagnostic Procedures

Chest radiograph, ECG, echocardiogram, cardiac catheterization, magnetic resonance imaging, and stress testing may all be used, depending on the type of defect.

Clinical Therapy

PGE$_1$ and inotrope medications may be required to support the systemic circulation until the obstruction is relieved or ventricular function improves. Balloon dilatation during cardiac catheterization or surgery may be performed, depending on the defect. See Box 17–4.

Nursing Management

Care for children with aortic stenosis and coarctation of the aorta is similar to those having defects that increase pulmonary blood flow.

Care for infants with hypoplastic left heart syndrome is similar to those having defects causing decreased pulmonary blood flow and mixed defects. There is no cure, and parents must make decisions very quickly about the best treatment while being faced with the potential death of their newborn. Share information about each treatment option and associated mortality, the intense care a surviving child needs, potential neurocognitive and neurodevelopmental outcomes, and unknown long-term survival. If parents choose comfort or palliative care, PGE_1 is discontinued, and the infant is given pain medication and comfort. Provide supportive care to the family.

Heart Transplantation

Heart transplant indications vary by age (Odim, Laks, Burch, et al., 2000):

- In infants, hypoplastic left heart syndrome and other complex defects
- In children and adolescents, cardiomyopathy and congenital heart disease (myopathy is acquired due to past reconstructive and palliative procedures)

Rejection and infection are the major causes of mortality and morbidity.

Clinical Manifestations

Signs of rejection include increasing resting heart rate, arrhythmias, or bradycardia; presence of a third heart sound; cool and mottled extremities; inspiratory crackles, diaphoresis, tachypnea, and pulmonary edema; hepatosplenomegaly; and oliguria (Duitsman, Suddaby, & Masterson, 1999).

Diagnostic Procedures

Diagnostic procedures include endomyocardial biopsy to detect rejection and echocardiograms to assess cardiac function.

Clinical Therapy

Tacrolimus or cyclosporine, azathioprine, and corticosteroids are given for immunosuppression. High-dose IV steroids for episodes of acute rejection.

Treatment for bacterial, fungal, and viral infections.

Lovastatin to reduce the serum cholesterol level.

Calcium channel blockers for hypertension.

Second heart transplant.

Nursing Management

Encourage return to school, activities, and exercise. Encourage a diet and exercise program to reduce the child's risk for obesity and osteoporosis.

Promote positive self-esteem when side effects of immunosuppression occur (hair growth, gum hyperplasia, weight gain, short stature, moon facies, acne, and rashes).

No live virus immunizations are given. If immunizations are not given before transplant, notify schools to report cases of measles, mumps, rubella, and chickenpox to family so child can receive preventive treatment if necessary. Encourage handwashing and other methods to reduce the spread of infection.

Educate the parents and child to follow the immunosuppression regimen, to recognize the signs of rejection, and to seek treatment promptly.

Hypercyanotic Episodes

A life-threatening condition occurring in infants with congenital heart defects that decreases pulmonary blood flow. Crying, feeding, exercise, warm bath, or straining with defecation triggers an abrupt decrease in systemic resistance and pulmonary blood flow combined with a sudden increase in cardiac output and venous return. Hypoxemia worsens as increased respiratory effort further increases the cardiac output.

Clinical Manifestations

Increased rate and depth of respirations; increased cyanosis, pallor, and poor tissue perfusion; increased heart rate; diaphoresis; irritability and crying; and loss of consciousness. The child may have a seizure or cerebrovascular accident and die.

Clinical Therapy

Aggressive treatment to decrease the pulmonary vascular resistance by calming the child, giving oxygen. Administer IV morphine, IV propranolol, and IV fluids. Give dopamine and phenylephrine (Neo-Synephrine). If the child is anemic, packed red blood cells are given to improve tissue oxygen delivery.

Knee–chest position to increase the systemic vascular resistance.

Immediate palliative or corrective surgery is often scheduled.

Nursing Management

Immediately place the infant in knee–chest position and administer oxygen. Attempt to calm the infant.

Administer morphine as ordered. Immediately notify the physician for further orders if the episode continues despite interventions.

Avoid any unpleasant or anxiety-provoking procedures.

Patient and Family Education

Initial management of the hypercyanotic episode—call for an ambulance and try to calm the infant.

Place in knee–chest position by holding the infant facing the chest, with one arm under the knees, and folding the legs upward toward the infant's chest. Use the other arm to support the infant's back.

Give oxygen if available without further upsetting the infant.

Pulmonary Artery Hypertension

A complication of congenital heart defects that increases pulmonary blood flow, pulmonary conditions, or congenital diaphragmatic hernia. The pulmonary vascular bed tries to reduce excessive pulmonary blood flow by vasoconstriction, leading to increased smooth muscle in the small pulmonary arteries. The pulmonary artery pressure increases to push blood across the vascular bed, resulting in inflammation, hypertrophy of pulmonary vessels, fibrosis, a right-to-left shunt, and impaired right heart function. Hypoxemia and acidosis result and help maintain the vasoconstriction.

Clinical Manifestations

Infants—tachypnea, cyanosis, retractions, fatigue, difficulty feeding, weight loss with fluid and electrolyte imbalance

Older children—exertional dyspnea, chest pain, and syncope

Clinical Therapy

Congenital heart defect—surgery to correct an obstructive lesion or close a defect.

Noncardiac condition—bronchodilators, antibiotics, corticosteroids, and low-flow oxygen.

Short-term nitric oxide therapy (Kinsella, Parker, Ivy, et al., 2003).

No cure. Life can be prolonged with above measures (Barst, 1999).

Nursing Management

Promote rest, monitor fluid intake and output, and administer medications and oxygen. Permit exercise that does not cause dyspnea. Give parents needed support and information.

Postpericardiotomy Syndrome

Pericardial and pleural inflammation may occur within a few weeks to a few months after surgery that required a pericardiotomy (incision through the pericardium).

Clinical Manifestations
High fever up to 40°C (104°F) and severe chest pain that worsens with deep inspiration and in supine position. The condition lasts 2–3 weeks.

Clinical Therapy
Mild cases are treated with bed rest and nonsteroidal anti-inflammatory drugs.

Severe cases may need hospitalization, pericardiocentesis, diuretics, and corticosteroids (Park, 2002).

ACQUIRED HEART DISORDERS
Cardiomyopathy
Dilated Cardiomyopathy
As the ventricles stretch or dilate to accommodate increased blood volume, the heart muscle does not contract and pump blood effectively. The blood flows more slowly through the heart, and clots may form, increasing risk for emboli. Neuromuscular disorders, such as muscular dystrophy, and viral myocarditis are the most common causes (Lipshultz, Sleeper, Towbin, et al., 2003). Other cases have an unknown cause and develop during the first year of life.

Clinical Manifestations
CHF, with tachypnea, wheezing, and poor cardiac output; arrhythmias may cause cardiac arrest.

Clinical Therapy
Anticoagulants, vasodilators, antiarrhythmics, diuretics and digoxin, and heart transplant. An implantable cardioverter-defibrillator is used for ventricular arrhythmias.

Nursing Management
Nursing management is the same as for CHF unless or until a heart transplant is performed (see Congestive Heart Failure).

Hypertrophic Cardiomyopathy
Hypertrophy of the ventricular muscles or ventricular septum makes the ventricular walls rigid, and reduces the size of the ventricular chamber, and obstructs blood flow. Up to 60% of cases are autosomal dominant trait transmission (Park, 2002).

Clinical Manifestations
Exertional dyspnea, fatigue, dizziness, fainting, palpitations, and chest pain.

Abnormal heart rhythms may cause sudden death.

Clinical Therapy

Digoxin is contraindicated, and diuretics may worsen symptoms (Park, 2002).

Surgery for subaortic stenosis may be performed if this is the cause of left ventricular outflow obstruction.

Antiarrhythmic medications or an implantable cardioverter-defibrillator.

Nursing Management

Monitor child's condition during health visits, and review progress with antiarrhythmic medications. See Cardiac Arrhythmias.

Dyslipidemia

A condition with an abnormal serum level of total cholesterol, low-density lipoproteins, triglycerides, and/or high-density lipoprotein that increases the risk for the presence of coronary artery calcium, obesity and increased body mass index, elevated BP in childhood, and dyslipidemia (Kavey, Daniels, Lauer, et al., 2003). Primary dyslipidemia is familial. Secondary dyslipidemia results from a diet rich in saturated fat and too little exercise, diseases such as diabetes, and drugs such as anabolic steroids (Kingsbury, 2003).

Clinical Manifestations

Children and adolescents rarely have signs or symptoms.

Diagnostic Tests

A fasting serum lipid panel is recommended for all children older than age 2 years who have the following risk factors (Kavey et al., 2003):

- Family history of cardiovascular disease before age 55 years (parents or grandparents), a parent who has an elevated total serum cholesterol (240 mg/dL or higher), or unknown family history
- BP of more than 90th percentile for age, sex, and height percentile
- Overweight, body mass index of more than 85th percentile
- Other risk factors such as smoking, diabetes

See laboratory values in Chapter 6 for recommended blood levels.

Clinical Therapy

Dietary changes are made to reduce total fat to no more than 30% of calories, polyunsaturated fat up to 10% of calories, monounsaturated fats at 10–15% of calories, and cholesterol to less than 300 mg/day. Exercise and other lifestyle changes are made.

Cholestyramine or colestipol, niacin, and lovastatin may be prescribed for children older than age 10 years.

Nursing Management

Identify children who need to have serum lipids measured.

Assess the child's diet, and provide dietary teaching for the entire family to reduce risk. Promote exercise and limit sedentary activity.

Assess the child's history of exercise patterns and weight and body mass index percentiles. Obtain data on familial heart disease, hypertension, diabetes, and smoking to determine risk factors.

Discourage smoking by the child and family.

Hypertension

Secondary hypertension in infants and prepubescent children is often associated with kidney disease or heart defects. Other causes include coarctation of the aorta, endocrinopathies, increased intracranial pressure, and ingestion of cocaine or amphetamines. Primary or essential hypertension may be associated with a genetic or familial predisposition and obesity.

Clinical Manifestations

Children rarely have symptoms.

Diagnostic Procedures

Diagnosis is based on three separate readings of an elevated BP. Secondary causes are identified through blood urea nitrogen, creatinine, glucose, electrolytes, a complete blood count with differential and platelet count, urinalysis and culture, and a lipid panel.

If kidney disease is suspected, renal ultrasonography, a 24-hour urine creatinine clearance and protein excretion, and urine and serum catecholamines are performed.

Echocardiogram to assess for coarctation of the aorta.

Ambulatory BP monitoring.

Clinical Therapy

Nonpharmacologic therapy includes weight reduction, increased exercise, and dietary modification to reduce sodium; provision of three to five fruit servings daily; consuming less than 10% of calories from saturated fats, and adequate intake of calcium and dietary fiber.

Discourage smoking, alcohol, and drugs.

Medications for children with persistent, severe hypertension include angiotensin-converting enzyme inhibitors, angiotensin receptor blockers, calcium channel blockers, and beta-agonists (Flynn, 2003).

Nursing Management

Assessment

Take a complete history of the child with borderline hypertension, including family history, diet, sodium intake, and exercise routines.

Assess the BP with the correct size cuff, including at least one measurement in the leg, at different times of the day. Have the child sit quietly for 5 minutes before taking the BP. The systolic reading in the leg is normally at least 10–20 mm Hg higher than the arm reading (Flynn, 2003). Compare readings to normal BP for age, height percentile, and gender (see Chapter 2).

Implementation

Teach the importance of weight reduction and dietary changes. Provide suggestions about substitute seasonings for salt, lists of salty foods to avoid, and increased intake of low-fat dairy products and fruits.

Discuss ways to increase activity and reduce time watching television and playing computer games.

Provide suggestions for the management of stress and stressful situations.

Instruct the family on correct administration of prescribed medications when used.

Infective Endocarditis

An inflammation of the lining, valves, and arterial vessels of the heart caused by bacterial, enterococci, and fungal infections. The causal organism enters the bloodstream and lodges on damaged or abnormal endocardial tissue. Children at greater risk have complex congenital heart disease with implanted vascular grafts, patches, or prosthetic valves, or have indwelling venous catheters (Ferrieri, Gewitz, Gerber, et al., 2002). It is also associated with IV drug use.

Clinical Manifestations

A prolonged low-grade fever, fatigue, weakness, weight loss, joint and muscle aches, diaphoresis, a new or changing murmur, CHF, decreased oxygen saturation levels, dyspnea, hematuria, petechiae, and splenomegaly (Brook, 1999)

Indwelling catheters—pulmonary symptoms or signs of septic pulmonary embolism

Newborns—feeding difficulties, respiratory distress, and tachycardia

Diagnostic Procedures

Blood, urine, and cerebrospinal fluid cultures, erythrocyte sedimentation rate, C-reactive protein, complete blood cell count, ECG, two-dimensional echocardiography, color Doppler

Duke Criteria used for diagnosis

Clinical Therapy

IV antibiotics such as penicillin G, ampicillin, vancomycin, nafcillin, or gentamicin. IV administration for 2–8 weeks until the infective organism is eradicated. Serum levels of antibiotics are monitored to maintain a therapeutic range.

Surgery to replace a heart valve or because of the risk of embolism.

CHF treatment with bed rest and medications (digoxin and furosemide).

Nursing Management

Assessment

Monitor the vital signs, oxygen saturation, level of consciousness, intake and output, and level of comfort. Monitor for signs of CHF or embolism. Assess the parents' coping.

Intervention

Prevent infective endocarditis when possible; however, not all cases can be prevented.

- Educate parents of children and adolescents to ask for prophylaxis before professional teeth cleaning and other dental procedures; tonsillectomy or adenoidectomy; bronchoscopy; and surgery on the respiratory, gastrointestinal, and genitourinary systems.
- Discourage those at risk from body piercing and tattoos. There is an increased incidence of endocarditis with piercings of the nose, tongue, and nipple (Goldrick, 2003).

Care of the child who has infective endocarditis

- Take the vital signs and assess gastrointestinal discomfort.
- Administer IV medications as ordered, and monitor serum antibiotic levels. Monitor for side effects of antibiotics and for infiltration or extravasation at the infusion site.
- Keep invasive procedures to a minimum. Use careful aseptic technique in performing venipunctures, urinary catheterizations, and other procedures.

- Inform parents and the adolescent about nursing care and potential for complications. Plan appropriate activities, as the child is often lethargic and on bed rest.
- Arrange for home health nursing for home antibiotic infusion therapy, home schooling, encourage social interactions with peers, and emphasize need for future infective endocarditis prophylaxis.

Kawasaki Syndrome

An acute febrile, multisystem inflammatory illness of unknown cause that involves the small and medium-sized arteries. Coronary artery damage may result in aneurysms, ischemic heart disease, and infarcts. A leading cause of acquired heart disease in children.

Clinical Manifestations

Acute stage—irritability, fever, conjunctival hyperemia, red throat, swollen hands and feet, rash on the trunk and perineal area, unilateral enlargement of the anterior cervical lymph nodes, diarrhea, and hepatic dysfunction

Subacute stage—cracking lips and fissures, skin desquamation on the tips of the fingers and toes starting at approximately 10 days after the fever begins, joint pain, cardiac disease, and thrombocytosis

Convalescent stage—6–8 weeks after disease onset; child appears normal, but lingering signs of inflammation may be present

Diagnostic Procedures

Diagnosed when a fever higher than 39°C (102.2°F) is present for 5 days or longer, along other physical signs, such as
- Bilateral conjunctivitis without exudate
- Dry, swollen, cracked lips and a strawberry tongue
- Intense erythema and induration of the hands and feet, followed by desquamation
- An erythematous maculopapular rash on the trunk
- Acute cervical lymphadenopathy
  (Rowley & Shulman, 1999)

A two-dimensional echocardiogram is used to identify specific vascular changes in the heart and coronary arteries.

Clinical Therapy

IV immunoglobulin (2 g/kg given in a single infusion) and oral aspirin; if a second dose of immunoglobulin is ineffective, corticosteroids may be administered.

Careful monitoring for cardiac disease continues for several weeks or months. Coronary aneurysms and coronary artery stenosis are the most serious complications. Coronary artery angioplasty or coronary artery bypass grafts are needed by some children.

Nursing Management

Assessment

Take the temperature every 4 hours and before each dose of aspirin. Carefully assess heart sounds and rhythm.

Assess the extremities for edema, redness, and desquamation every 8 hours. Examine the eyes for conjunctivitis and the mucous membranes for inflammation.

Monitor dietary and fluid intake and weigh the child daily.

Implementation

Administer aspirin and monitor for side effects.

Administer IV immunoglobulin as a blood product, regulating the infusion rate to run slowly (not be over 1 mL/min). Stop the infusion immediately if reaction is noted.

Keep the child's skin clean and dry, and lubricate the lips. Use cool compresses and tepid sponges to make the feverish child more comfortable. Change the child's clothes and bed linens frequently.

Give frequent, small feedings of soft foods and liquids that are neither too hot nor too cold.

Use passive range-of-motion exercises to facilitate joint movement.

Plan rest periods and quiet, age-appropriate activities.

Patient and Family Education

Teach the parents to administer aspirin as ordered and to watch for side effects. Take the child's temperature daily and report any fever above 37.8°C (100°F) to the physician.

Limit strenuous activity if coronary aneurysms or stenosis. Emphasize the need for follow-up care to monitor for cardiac complications.

Postpone measles and varicella immunizations, if not already given, for 11 months after immunoglobulin administration, but other immunizations may be given on schedule, including influenza vaccine.

Rheumatic Fever

An inflammatory connective tissue disorder affecting the heart, joints, brain, and skin tissues that follows an initial infection by some strains of group A beta-hemolytic streptococci. One possible cause is an autoimmune response in a genetically predisposed child (Steeg, Walsh, & Glickstein, 2000).

Clinical Manifestations

Hallmark signs occur 1–3 weeks after an untreated streptococcal infection and include the following:

Carditis (Aschoff bodies, hemorrhagic bullous lesions) develops in the connective tissue of the heart and may involve the mitral and aortic valves, myocardium, and pericardium.

Arthritis—large joints are more commonly affected, with pain, swelling, tenderness, erythema, and heat. Signs may migrate from joint to joint (migratory polyarthritis).

Subcutaneous nodules.

Erythema marginatum—pink macules and blanching in the middle of the lesions on the trunk and proximal extremities but not on the face.

Sydenham's chorea (St. Vitus dance)—aimless movements of the extremities and facial grimacing.

Diagnostic Procedures

Diagnosis is based on conclusive evidence of a preceding streptococcal infection (positive throat culture or rapid streptococcal antigen test, or elevated or rising streptococcal antibody titer) and physical signs of carditis, joint pain, fever, erythema marginatum, subcutaneous nodules, and chorea.

Clinical Therapy

Antibiotics (penicillin, sulfadiazine, or erythromycin).

Aspirin for 3–4 weeks or longer if carditis is present; serum salicylate levels are monitored; steroids may be used for severe carditis with CHF.

Monitor for residual heart involvement by echocardiogram.

Long-term antibiotic prophylaxis to reduce the risk of recurrent attacks; children with cardiac valve damage also need infective endocarditis prophylaxis.

Nursing Management

Prevention of rheumatic fever

- Perform a throat culture for all sore throats, especially if family members or other contacts have had a streptococcal infection.

- Emphasize importance of giving the entire 10-day course of antibiotics when a culture is positive.

During the acute inflammatory phase while hospitalized
- Monitor vital signs and take temperature every 4 hours. Auscultate the heart for any new sounds. Observe for changes in skin, joints, or behavior.
- Keep child on bed rest while monitoring for carditis onset and for 4 weeks if carditis develops. Provide quiet activities.
- Perform throat cultures on family members.
- Administer antibiotic and aspirin as ordered. The child is usually lethargic and often has joint pain. Place the child's joints in neutral position and handle them carefully. Aspirin often relieves pain dramatically after a few doses.

During the recovery phase at home
- Limit activities, especially if heart damage is suspected. Help parents plan quiet activities. Arrange rest periods after the child returns to school.
- Emphasize the importance of taking a daily oral low-dose antibiotic or monthly long-acting antibiotic injection until adulthood. Emphasize the need for follow-up care. Educate about the need for infective endocarditis prophylaxis.
- Educate the child and parents that future sore throats may be streptococcal and need a throat culture even when the child is taking daily antibiotics. The child may need additional antibiotics for the infection.

CARDIAC ARRHYTHMIAS
Long QT Syndrome
A rhythm disturbance of autosomal dominant and autosomal recessive inheritance that increases the risk for ventricular fibrillation and sudden death. It may also result from electrolyte abnormalities, malnutrition associated with anorexia and bulimia, myocarditis, and central nervous system trauma (Berul, 2000).

Clinical Manifestations
The arrhythmia commonly occurs without warning and often results in death. Early signs include a heart rate too fast to count, irritability, lethargy, poor feeding, poor perfusion (cool, pale skin, increased capillary refill time), decreased responsiveness, and decreased BP.

Clinical Therapy
If the child is resuscitated, an ECG detects the arrhythmia.

Treated by beta-adrenergic blockade, antiarrhythmic agents, and often a pacemaker (Lewin, 2000).

Several medications may trigger episodes (e.g., antihistamines, macrolide antibiotics) and should not be prescribed (Erickson & Jones, 2000).

Nursing Management
Educate parents and children to avoid triggers that cause arrhythmia episodes such as competitive athletics, swimming, loud noises, and hypokalemia. Teach the parents and adolescents to remind the primary care provider about prescription medications to avoid. The list is available at http://www.longqt.com.

Supraventricular Tachycardia (SVT)
An extremely fast heart rate due to a congenital heart defect or Wolff-Parkinson-White syndrome. Prolonged episodes of SVT (more than 24 hours) are life-threatening and can progress to CHF or cardiogenic shock if untreated.

Clinical Manifestations
An abrupt onset of a rapid, regular heart rate that may be up to 260 beats per minute in infants or between 150 and 240 beats per minute in older children. Early signs in infants include poor feeding, irritability, and pallor. Older children may have palpitations, chest discomfort, dizziness, syncope, or cardiac arrest. Recurrent attacks are common.

Diagnostic Procedures
Perform ECG, and if symptoms are episodic, a 24-hour Holter monitor or an event monitor may be used to capture the arrhythmia.

Clinical Therapy

SVT episodes are initially treated with vagal maneuvers (ice to face, rectal stimulation with a thermometer, Valsalva maneuver, gag reflex, blowing forcefully on the thumb) to slow the heart rate when the infant or child is stable.

IV adenosine when the vagal maneuvers are unsuccessful.

Digoxin, amiodarone, or propranolol may also be used during acute episodes if more aggressive therapy is needed. Long-term digoxin and propranolol may be given to reduce the frequency of episodes (Starr & Freitas-Nichols, 2000).

In urgent or life-threatening situations the child is sedated and synchronized cardioversion is used to convert the tachycardia to sinus rhythm.

Radiofrequency ablation may be performed in the cardiac catheterization laboratory.

Nursing Management

Assessment

Monitor the vital signs and use a cardiorespiratory monitor and pulse oximetry to identify deterioration of the child's condition. Identify changes in level of consciousness, color, weakness, irritability, and feeding pattern, as hypoxia and life-threatening shock may develop.

Implementation

Assist with vagal maneuvers if ordered for SVT, and monitor for recurrence of the arrhythmia.

Administer medications as ordered and monitor for response.

Provide for rest and adequate nutrition.

Have emergency drugs and resuscitation equipment available at bedside.

Patient and Family Education

Educate about danger signs indicating a recurrence of the acute condition. Encourage parents to become trained in CPR and to have an emergency care plan.

Emphasize the need to avoid cardiac stimulant medications such as decongestants that could trigger another episode. Educate parents about medications that may be provided long term.

INJURIES OF THE CARDIOVASCULAR SYSTEM

Cardiogenic Shock

An abnormality of myocardial function in which the heart fails to maintain adequate cardiac output and tissue perfusion. Causes include CHF, cardiovascular surgery, severe obstructive congenital heart disease, cardiomyopathy, and arrhythmias. As the cardiac output falls, myocardial ischemia and progressive myocardial dysfunction develop. Multisystem organ failure occurs from persistent ischemia.

Clinical Manifestations

Low cardiac output—tachycardia, tachypnea, decreased oxygen saturation, hypotension, diminished peripheral pulses, and cool, pale extremities similar to hypovolemic shock. Disorientation and restlessness occur as the compensatory mechanisms fail. Respiratory distress occurs when CHF develops. The cardiac output and BP fall.

Clinical Therapy

An enlarged heart and pulmonary congestion are seen on chest radiograph. The goal of medical treatment is rapid restoration of myocardial function, with adequate ventilation, resolution of the initial metabolic insult, correction of arrhythmias, fluid management, and administration of diuretics and inotropic drugs.

Hypovolemic Shock

Inadequate tissue and organ perfusion resulting from the movement of blood or plasma out of the intravascular compartment, leading to inadequate intravascular volume. Impaired delivery of oxygen and nutrients to cells and accumulation of toxic waste in the capillaries result. Cellular hypoxia and acidosis develop simultaneously. Causes include hemorrhage, burns, nephrotic syndrome, sepsis, dehydration, diabetic ketoacidosis, and diabetes insipidus. The child's body attempts to compensate with adrenergic and renal mechanisms until 20–25% of volume loss occurs, and then life-threatening hypotension and hypoxemia occur.

Clinical Manifestations

Early shock—persistent tachycardia of more than 130 beats per minute, increased respiratory effort, capillary refill time of more than 2 seconds, weak distal pulses, pallor or mottled color, cold extremities, BP often normal for age, child irritable and anxious, decreased urine output (less than 1–2 mL/kg/hour in newborns and less than 0.5–1.0 mL/kg/hour in infants and children)

Uncompensated shock—tachycardia, absent distal pulses, decreasing systolic BP, capillary refill time of more than 3 seconds, cold extremities, cyanosis, confusion, lethargy, decreased level of consciousness, oliguria. Progresses to cardiopulmonary failure if untreated

Diagnostic Procedures

No laboratory values diagnose the volume deficit rapidly. Laboratory tests performed include hematocrit and hemoglobin, arterial blood gases, serum electrolytes, glucose, osmolality, blood urea nitrogen, and urinalysis.

Clinical Therapy

Establish and maintain a patent airway, give supplemental oxygen, and control bleeding.

Start an IV or intraosseous line to give large volumes of Ringer's lactate or normal saline. A fluid volume of 20 mL/kg is administered rapidly over 5 minutes and repeated in 5 minutes if the child's physiologic condition does not improve. Blood or albumin is usually ordered if there is no response after the second fluid bolus.

Inotropic medications provided in IV drips to sustain cardiac output and increase renal perfusion are used for some children.

Monitor the child's circulatory status, especially when the liver or spleen is injured, for signs of continued bleeding.

Nursing Management

Assessment

Assess the severity of acute illnesses to determine if dehydration is present. If external bleeding is apparent, determine the amount of blood lost. If no external bleeding is evident, assess for potential injury causing internal bleeding.

Frequently assess the child's vital signs, capillary refill time, level of consciousness, color, and skin temperature. Monitor urine output and specific gravity hourly. Signs of the child's improved status include the following:

- A decrease in heart rate, respiratory rate, and capillary refill time
- An increase in systolic BP and urine output
- Improved color, level of consciousness, and skin temperature
- Regaining of lost weight

Implementation

Assist with the child's assessment and IV access. Calculate and prepare the IV fluid boluses needed for the child's weight (20 mL/kg). Ensure rapid fluid administration by IV push or pressure bag. Monitor the child's physiologic response to the fluid bolus within 5 minutes.

Keep the child warm. Use warmed IV fluids for resuscitation.

When packed red blood cells are given, verify that the correct blood has been obtained. Change the IV fluid to normal saline. Assess the child carefully for a transfusion reaction.

Support to the child and family during the acute phase of treatment. When the parent is present during the resuscitation, assign a health-care provider to provide information and support. Explain the care being provided and how it helps the child. Listen to their concerns and correct any misconceptions.

Maldistributive Shock

An abnormal distribution of blood volume usually resulting from a decrease in systemic vascular resistance, allowing blood to accumulate in the extremities. Less blood returns to the heart, so preload and cardiac output fall. Common causes include sepsis, anaphylaxis, and spinal cord injury.

Clinical Manifestations

Septic shock has three phases: compensated, uncompensated, and refractory.

Compensated phase—tachycardia and tachypnea; fever (more than 38°C, or 100.4°F) or hypothermia (less than 36°C, or 96.8°F); warm, dry extremities; a bounding pulse and a brisk capillary refill time; normal urine output; diminished level of responsiveness.

Uncompensated phase—hypotension and inadequate oxygen and nutrient delivery to the tissues; poor tissue perfusion of the vital organs; multiple organ failure begins.

Refractory phase—shock becomes irreversible, cardiac output falls.

Clinical Therapy

Treatment of sepsis, with appropriate antibiotics effective for the organisms.

Aggressive fluid administration to stabilize the circulation and ensure adequate tissue perfusion. Hemodynamic monitoring and vasopressors to maintain the BP. Metabolic acidosis is treated.

Nursing Management

See Hypovolemic Shock.

18. ALTERATIONS IN IMMUNOLOGIC FUNCTION

To understand normal actions of the immune system, an overview of the types of cells and tissues in the immune system, as well as the classes of immunoglobulins, is necessary.

IMMUNODEFICIENCY DISORDERS

Immunodeficiency, a state of decreased responsiveness of the immune system, can occur in response to several congenital or acquired events and causes a deficiency in B cells or T cells, or both.

Congenital or **primary immunodeficiency**, when infants are born with a lack of humoral antibody formation (B-cell disorder), a deficient cellular immune system (T-cell disorder), or a combination of both defects

Acquired or **secondary immunodeficiency**, as in human immunodeficiency virus (HIV) infection

See Table 18–1.

Severe Combined Immunodeficiency Disease

Severe combined immunodeficiency disease (SCID) is a congenital condition characterized by absence of humoral and cellular immunity, which is manifested by lack of functioning T cells and B cells. SCID occurs in X-linked recessive, autosomal recessive, and sporadic forms. The disorder is more common in males than females (Cooper, Pommering, & Koranyi, 2003).

Clinical Manifestations

Susceptibility to infection by 3 months of age, after loss of maternal immunity.

Manifestations include oral candidiasis, failure to thrive, chronic diarrhea, sepsis, and chronic infections, such as otitis media or pneumonia (Box 18–1).

Diagnostic Tests

Complete blood count.

Erythrocyte sedimentation rate.

B- and T-cell lymphocyte counts (see Table 18–2).

Table 18–1 Selected Congenital Immunodeficiency Disorders

Disorders	Laboratory Findings
B cell	
X-linked hypogammaglobuline-mia	Reduced IgA, IgM, IgE, IgG (<100 mg/dL), absence of B cells in peripheral blood, normal T cells
Selective IgA deficiency	IgA <10 mg/dL
Common variable immunodeficiency	IgA, IgM reduced; IgG <250 mg/dL
T cell	
DiGeorge syndrome	Lymphopenia; absent T-cell functions, decreased T cells, normal B cells
Immunodeficiency with hyper-IgM	Reduced IgG, IgA; elevated IgM; mutations in T-cell surface proteins
Combined	
Severe combined immunodeficiency syndrome	Complete absence of T and B cells and NK immunity
Wiskott-Aldrich syndrome	Thrombocytopenia, low platelet volume, nonfunctional B cells, normal IgG, decreased IgM, increased IgA, increased IgE; inability to respond to polysaccharide antigens

IgA, immunoglobulin A; IgE, immunoglobulin E; IgG, immunoglobulin G; IgM, immunoglobulin; NK, natural killer.

Immunoglobulin levels are significantly reduced. See Table 18–1 for laboratory findings in SCID.

A chest radiograph is conducted to assess thymus size.

Clinical Therapy

Intravenous immune globulin is administered to provide protection until humoral immunity is established.

Hematopoietic stem cell transplantation can be curative for the child with SCID. However, the donor must be a histocompatible donor, such as a sibling.

Box 18–1 Warning Signs of Primary Immune Deficiency

Persistent, frequent, and unusual types of infections
Infections that are resistant to treatment
Failure to thrive
Delayed development
Family history of primary immunodeficiency

Table 18–2 Cells Evaluated in Laboratory Studies for Immune Conditions

Test and Type of Cell Evaluated	Action	Implication of Increased or Decreased Levels
White blood cell count (normal values in parentheses)		
Neutrophil (polys) (54–62%)	Phagocytic cell that defends against bacteria	Increased in bacterial infection, inflammatory processes, and some malignancies
Eosinophil (1–3%)	Associated with antigen–antibody reaction	Increased in allergic reaction; decreased in children receiving corticosteroids
Lymphocytes [T, B, and non-B/non-T (natural killer)] (25–33%)	Major components of immune system	Increased in many infections; decreased in children with immune deficiency
Immunoglobulins (Ig)		
IgM, IgG, IgA, IgD, IgE	Many roles in a number of immunologic reactions	Increased in presence of infection or allergic response; decreased in children with immune deficiency

Thymic hormones have been given to some children with limited success.

Enzyme-replacement therapy may be implemented in certain forms of autosomal recessive SCID.

Prevention of infection is essential. Antibiotic therapy targeting specific infectious agents should be aggressive (Koleilat, Williams, & Ryan, 2003).

Nursing Management

Assessment and Diagnosis

Obtain a thorough history of infections, including age of onset, type of causal organism, frequency, and severity.

Assess family history, and determine whether the child has had any unusual reactions to vaccines, medications, or foods.

Measure the child's height and weight accurately to identify failure to thrive.

Assess the child's nutritional intake and fluid and electrolyte balance.

Assess for any evidence of infections involving the skin, subcutaneous tissues, respiratory system, or mucous membranes.

Palpate the abdomen for hepatomegaly and the lymph nodes for lymphadenopathy.

Perform a developmental assessment, and assess for delays in achievement of developmental milestones.

Assess family support systems and coping mechanisms when the child is diagnosed with the disorder.

Intervention

Prevent Systemic Infection

Frequent and thorough handwashing is essential.

Implement sterile aseptic techniques when caring for all sites where needles, catheters, central lines, endotracheal tubes, pressure-monitoring lines, peripheral intravenous lines, or other invasive equipment enters the child's body.

Food and other items entering the hospital room may require special treatment.

Inform parents that, because of the risk of infection to the child, live vaccines may not be recommended.

Live vaccines, including measles-mumps-rubella and varicella, are permitted in household members (Champi, 2002; Centers for Disease Control and Prevention, 2005).

Administer immune serum globulin as prescribed.

Promote Skin Integrity

Provide good skin care, and closely observe all possible pressure areas for signs of breakdown or infection.

Implement measures to avoid skin trauma.

Reposition the child frequently, and encourage range-of-motion exercises.

Promote Nutritional Balance

Encourage adequate fluid and nutritional intake.

Provide foods that the child prefers.

For children with evidence of failure to thrive, offering small frequent feedings of high-calorie, protein-rich foods is advised.

Protein intake can be increased by adding dried milk powder to foods.

Energy intake can be increased by adding small amounts of cooking oil, margarine, or butter.

Foods that are soft and moist are easier to chew for children with mouth ulcers.

Yogurt can help reduce diarrhea, which often accompanies various drug regimes.

Wiskott-Aldrich Syndrome
A combined congenital immunodeficiency syndrome, Wiskott-Aldrich syndrome is an X-linked recessive disorder that occurs in males and causes mutation in the Wiskott-Aldrich syndrome gene and changes in the Wiskott-Aldrich syndrome protein (Elder, 2000).

Clinical Manifestations
Thrombocytopenia and bleeding

Eczema

Hemorrhagic tendencies

Recurrent infections (Champi, 2002)

Malignancy (leukemia or lymphoma) in some cases

Diagnostic Tests
Complete blood count

Platelet count

Stool for guaiac

Prothrombin time and partial thromboplastin time

Clinical Therapy
Antibiotic prophylaxis with platelet infusions, and monthly intravenous immune globulin infusions

Splenectomy, if hypersplenism is present

Stem cell transplantation to correct the inherent genetic defect

Nursing Management
Assessment
Assess for splenomegaly, cervical lymphadenopathy, and hepatomegaly.

Observe for bleeding, such as excessive bleeding after circumcision and bloody diarrhea.

Assess skin for infections and irritations.

Thorough assessments for signs of infection.

Intervention

Refer the parents for genetic counseling to help them understand the transmission of the disease and the probability of having another child with the same disorder.

Provide care during periods of infection.

Encourage activities that promote normal developmental milestones.

Arrange for psychologic support for those parents who may be overwhelmed with guilt from learning that the illness is inherited.

Human Immunodeficiency Virus and Acquired Immunodeficiency Syndrome
Clinical Manifestations
See Table 18–3 for HIV staging.

The neonate is asymptomatic at birth. The time period for the development of opportunistic infections varies; however, the interval from HIV infection to the onset of overt acquired immunodeficiency syndrome (AIDS) is shorter in children than in adults and shorter in children infected perinatally than in those infected through transfusion. See CM 18–1 for clinical manifestations of HIV in children.

Most children with AIDS have nonspecific findings, including
- Lymphadenopathy.

Table 18–3   Clinical Staging of Pediatric Human Immunodeficiency Virus (HIV) Infection

Diagnosis of HIV infection in children
  HIV infected (two or more positive tests for HIV or demonstrates acquired immunodeficiency syndrome)
  Perinatally exposed (born to a mother known to be infected with HIV)
  Seroconverter (born to a mother known to be infected with HIV, but has had two negative HIV tests)
When infected, the child with HIV is classified as
  Category N (not symptomatic)
  Category A (mildly symptomatic)
  Category B (moderately symptomatic)
  Category C (severely symptomatic; multiple, recurrent infection)

Note: From Centers for Disease Control and Prevention. (1998). Guidelines for the use of antiretroviral agents in pediatric HIV infection. Morbidity and Mortality Weekly Reports Recommendation Reports 47(RR-4), 1–43.

CM 18–1   Clinical Manifestations of Human Immunodeficiency Virus in Children

Etiology	Clinical Manifestation	Clinical Therapy
Frequent, chronic, or unusual infections due to poor immune response	Chronic bilateral otitis media Oral candidiasis *Pneumocystis carinii* pneumonia Skin disorders Fever	Vigorous antimicrobial therapy for treatment of infections Limit exposure to groups of people. Obtain recommended immunizations.
Poor nutritional intake owing to lack of appetite caused by disease and medications	Failure to thrive (eating disorder of childhood) Weight and body mass index below 10th percentile Chronic diarrhea Skin irritation	Monitor growth. Supplemental intake, such as enteral feedings at night and total parenteral nutrition if needed Meticulous skin care to prevent breakdown
Immune system overgrowth to compensate for lack of proper immune response	Hepatosplenomegaly and lymphadenopathy	Assess abdomen frequently. Teach about safe transport to avoid injury to liver and spleen.

Note: Be alert for the possibility of human immunodeficiency virus infection in infants with some combinations of the clinical manifestations, especially in infants known to be at risk.

- Hepatosplenomegaly.
- Nephropathy.
- Oral candidiasis.
- Failure to thrive and weight loss.
- Delayed development.
- Chronic diarrhea.
- Chronic eczema and dermatitis.
- Fever.
- Severe or persistent symptoms usually appear within 2 years in children born with HIV infection.
- Bacterial and opportunistic infections, such as *Streptococcus, Haemophilus influenzae, Salmonella*, and *Pneumocystis carinii* pneumonia, and malignancies, such as lymphomas, frequently occur as the disease progresses.
- Lymphocytic interstitial pneumonitis.
- Encephalopathy, resulting in developmental delay or a deterioration of motor skills and intellectual functioning.
- Adolescents with HIV infection often are also infected with hepatitis B virus (Rogers, 2000).

Diagnostic Tests

Serologic tests for detection of the virus are monitored in infants born to HIV-positive mothers. These tests are performed within 48 hours of birth (as many as 40% of infected infants can be identified at this time).

Infants with initially negative virologic tests should be retested at age 1–2 months. Those who had negative virologic assays at birth and age 1–2 months should have the test repeated at 3 and 6 months, then again between 15 and 18 months.

The preferred test is polymerase chain reaction; other tests include p24 antigen or HIV culture, which is not universally available. Any positive result is confirmed by retesting. HIV infection is confirmed by two positive assays (polymerase chain reaction or viral culture) on two separate specimens. A positive HIV antibody test at older than 18 months indicates HIV infection.

Clinical Therapy

Medical management begins with prevention of the spread of HIV from mother to newborn.

Early identification of infected infants is important to ensure the most effective treatment.

HIV-infected mothers should be identified during pregnancy, and their infants should undergo periodic laboratory testing, as described earlier.

Pregnant women infected with HIV who are treated with zidovudine and deliver their babies by cesarean section reduce the chance of transmission of the virus to the baby down to a rate of 1%. The neonate is also treated prophylactically with zidovudine.

Medication Therapy

Treatment with highly active antiretroviral therapy, a drug regimen aimed at maximizing the effect of viral load suppression, has had a dramatic impact on the health of HIV-infected children.

Combination therapy is recommended for all infants, children, and adolescents who are treated with antiretroviral agents, including nucleoside reverse transcriptase inhibitors, such as zidovudine, didanosine, zalcitabine, lamivudine, and stavudine (Edmunds & Mayhew, 2004).

The protease inhibitors ritonavir, nelfinavir, amprenavir, and lopinavir/ritonavir have now been approved for use in children older than

2 years and are used in combination with nucleoside reverse transcriptase inhibitors.

The antineoplastic drug, hydroxyurea, can be used in combination with nucleoside reverse transcriptase inhibitors (Kline, Calles, Simon, et al., 2000).

Nursing Management

Assessment and Diagnosis

For infants at risk of HIV infection, obtain the HIV test results of the mother, if available. When the results are positive, the infant should be screened for HIV infection according to the Centers for Disease Control and Prevention guidelines as previously described in Diagnostic Tests.

Facilitate the screening, and explain the necessity of the screening to the family.

Screen adolescents at risk of HIV infection (see Box 18–2).

Physiologic Assessment

Observe and evaluate potential sites of infection.

Assess breath sounds, respiratory status, arterial blood gases, level of consciousness, and mental status.

Assess the child's height and weight frequently. Observe for signs of failure to thrive, and assess for anemia.

Assess for *Candida* infections in the mouth and the diaper area.

Box 18–2   Questions to Screen the Adolescent at Risk for Human Immunodeficiency Virus (HIV)

1. Do you inject drugs and/or share needles, syringes, or other equipment?
2. Have you engaged in unprotected vaginal, anal, or oral sex with anyone who might be infected with HIV (e.g., someone with multiple or anonymous sexual partners, men who have had sex with other men, a partner who injects drugs, someone who has been treated for sexually transmitted infections)?
3. Have you engaged in unprotected sex with more than one partner?
4. Have you been diagnosed or treated for a sexually transmitted infection?
5. Have you ever experienced a fever or illness of unknown cause?

From Centers for Disease Control and Prevention. (2001). Revised guidelines for HIV counseling, testing, and referral and revised recommendations for HIV screening of pregnant women. Morbidity and Mortality Weekly Report, 50(RR 19), 1–58. http://www.cdc.gov/mmwr/preview/mmwrhtml/rr5019a1.htm, accessed 7/20/2005.

Note any developmental delays in motor skills or intellectual functioning (Pearson, McGrath, Nozyce, et al., 2000).

Psychosocial Assessment

Assess family support systems and coping mechanisms, as the stressors of caring for a child with HIV or AIDS may overwhelm parents.

Assess the family's ability to care for the child. If the mother is infected, inquire about the extended family's ability to provide daily care as well as emotional support.

Support the family when they decide to inform a school-age child or adolescent of the diagnosis.

When assessing an adolescent with AIDS, evaluate the teen's understanding of how AIDS is transmitted and the response to the diagnosis.

Implementation

Prevent disease by evaluating test results and instituting measures to interrupt perinatal transmission of HIV to the infants of infected mothers.

Testing, prophylaxis for HIV and *Pneumocystis carinii* pneumonia, and follow-up visits for evaluation of general health and development for all infants at risk of the disease are advised.

The American Academy of Pediatrics recommends that pediatricians offer HIV testing and counseling to adolescents who are sexually active or involved in substance abuse (Committee on Pediatric AIDS and Committee on Adolescence, 2001).

Intervention

Prevent infection with HIV, and prevent infections of various types in children with HIV infection:

- Educate sexually active adolescents on the importance of practicing safe sex and the ramifications of high-risk sexual behaviors and intravenous drug abuse.
- Protection of the neonate from HIV-infected maternal secretions is essential. Measures to implement include avoidance of the use of fetal scalp electrodes and other invasive devices during labor.
- Bathe the newborn as soon as possible after delivery, and wash the eyes and face before administration of prophylactic eye drops or ointment.
- Heel-sticks and newborn injections should be delayed until after the newborn has been bathed. To avoid transmission of HIV through breast milk, encourage the mother to formula-feed the baby instead.

- Proper disposal of needles and contaminated materials or equipment is essential to reduce the transmission of HIV.
- Frequent handwashing and prevention of exposure of the child to individuals with upper respiratory or other infections are the best interventions to protect the child with HIV from acquiring other infections.
- A modified immunization schedule is recommended (see Chapter 8).
- Tuberculosis is more common in children with AIDS; therefore, annual skin tests that are performed and read by health professionals are recommended (Cohen, Chen, Sunkle, et al., 2000).

Promote Medication Regimen Adherence
The treatment regimen with antiretroviral therapies for the child with HIV or AIDS may be complex and time consuming, presenting an overwhelming challenge to the child and their family.

Educate the child, when old enough to understand, and the parent and/or care provider regarding the purpose of the medication, the benefits of adhering to the regimen, and the potential consequences of not adhering to the regimen.

Use behavior modification techniques and positive reinforcement to promote the child's adherence.

Promote Respiratory Function
Encourage the child to cough and deep breathe every 2–4 hours to improve respiratory function.

Blowing cotton balls with a straw, blowing bubbles, or other games may engage the interest of a younger child.

Reposition infants frequently so that all areas of the lungs can fully expand.

Rest periods to conserve energy and lower the body's demand for oxygen should be included in the plan of care.

Promote Adequate Nutritional Intake
Because many children with AIDS have failure to thrive, nutrition is an important part of their care.

A nutritionist should be involved in planning an appropriate diet for the child that provides necessary calories, protein, and other nutrients.

Vitamins may be especially lacking in the diets of infected children.

Antioxidants (vitamin A, vitamin E, zinc, and selenium) are known to enhance general immune system function and should be consumed at recommended levels.

Adequate nutrition is sometimes provided by hyperalimentation, nasogastric feeding, or gavage feeding.

Antidiarrheal medications or alternative formulas may be prescribed.

Carefully monitor hydration status, skin turgor, and urine output. Provide careful perineal skin care to prevent infection.

The frequency of *Candida* infections leads to blisters, cracking, and discharge involving the oral mucous membranes.

Mouth care with a non–alcohol-based solution, such as normal saline or lemon–glycerin swabs, should be performed every 2–4 hours to keep the child's lips and mouth moist.

Precautions to guard against food-borne illness are particularly important for the HIV-infected child.

Provide Emotional Support
Spend time with the family to provide them with an opportunity to discuss their fears and feelings.

Clarify any misconceptions the older child with HIV or AIDS may have about the transmission of the disease. Routes of transmission and the need for safe sexual practices must be clearly discussed with adolescents.

Providing support for adolescents is particularly important because the dependence that this chronic and terminal disease brings can make it difficult to meet the developmental task of independence.

Adolescents may benefit from contact with other infected peers.

Discharge Planning and Community Care
Be honest and direct. Education is essential and begins at the time of admission or diagnosis.

Explain that there is no evidence that casual contact among family members can spread the infection.

Discuss the family's finances as well as health insurance coverage for the child's care.

Assess the family's ability to provide nutritious food, required medications, and a supportive environment.

Refer to services, as needed, to ensure provision of quality care for the child after discharge.

Support groups, home healthcare nursing services, financial assistance, and psychological counseling are usually needed at some point during the child's illness, and the family should be aware of the availability of such services.

Assist the family with coping mechanisms to deal with feelings of guilt about the child's condition.

AUTOIMMUNE DISORDERS

In an immune system damaged by pathologic changes, an immune response may occur to some of the body's own proteins, resulting in the production of autoantibodies. These pathologic conditions in which the body directs the immune response against itself—identifying *self* as *nonself*—are called *autoimmune disorders*.

Systemic Lupus Erythematosus

A generalized disorder mainly occurring in females is a chronic inflammatory, autoimmune disease of unknown origin that involves many organ systems.

The disease is characterized by remissions and exacerbations.

The disease is more common in blacks, Hispanics, and Asians than in whites. Females are affected more than males with a 9:1 ratio (Mulvihill, 2003).

The majority of cases are diagnosed during the teenage and early adult years.

The five classifications of systemic lupus erythematosus are as follows:

- Systemic lupus—involves one or more of the following systems: cardiovascular, central nervous system, hematologic, kidneys, lungs, and musculoskeletal.
- Drug-induced lupus—associated with some antineoplastic drugs, isoniazid, hydralazine (Apresoline), and others. The symptoms generally subside after the drugs are discontinued.
- Discoid/cutaneous lupus—involvement of the disorder is limited to the skin.
- Overlap—several autoimmune disorders overlap with lupus, including rheumatoid arthritis, scleroderma, and Sjögren's syndrome.
- Neonatal lupus—occurs when maternal autoantibodies are acquired by the infant during delivery. Symptoms affecting the skin, heart, and blood of the newborn may develop (Lupus Foundation of America, 2004).

Clinical Manifestations

See CM 18–2.

CM 18–2   Clinical Manifestations of Systemic Lupus Erythematosus

System	Clinical Manifestations
Integumentary	A butterfly rash on the face, consisting of a pink or red rash over the bridge of the nose extending to the cheeks, is a characteristic finding Photosensitivity Alopecia Mouth or nose ulcers
Hematologic	Hemolytic anemia Leukopenia (low white blood cells) Thrombocytopenia (low platelet count) Bleeding disorders
Musculoskeletal	Joint pain Raynaud's phenomenon (fingers turning white and/or blue in the cold) Arthritis Arthralgia
Neurologic	Chorea Dizziness Seizures Cerebral vascular accident and resultant quadriplegia
Pulmonary	Pleural effusions Pleuritis
Cardiac	Pericarditis Vasculitis
Renal	Glomerulonephritis Renal failure Lupus nephritis
Other	Hypergammaglobulinemia Extreme fatigue

Manifestations of systemic lupus erythematosus may be acute with onset of nephritis, arthritis, or vasculitis or may be noted as a gradual onset with nonspecific symptoms.

Symptoms vary and depend on the organ involved and the amount of tissue damage that has occurred.

Initial symptoms include fever, chills, fatigue, oral ulcers, malaise, and weight loss.

The most common symptom is joint pain, occurring in approximately 80–90% of patients with systemic lupus erythematosus (Mulvihill, 2003), and skin rash.

A butterfly rash on the face, consisting of a pink or red rash over the bridge of the nose extending to the cheeks, is a characteristic finding.

Diagnostic Tests

Serum measurement (CBC and anti-DNA antibody).

Radiologic examinations include chest radiographs and computed tomography scans, as well as magnetic resonance imaging of affected joints.

A 24-hour urine collection and imaging studies, as well as renal biopsies, may be performed to evaluate lupus nephritis.

Clinical Therapy

Several medications may be used.

Diet may be restricted if the child has excessive weight gain or fluid retention from steroids and renal damage.

Nursing Management
Assessment and Diagnosis

Because systemic lupus erythematosus generally consists of multiorgan involvement, careful assessment of each of the systems is essential to detect any complications as early as possible.

A thorough physiologic assessment as well as a thorough psychosocial assessment is essential.

Assess the child's nutritional status, including baseline weight and history of recent weight loss or weight gain.

The skin is assessed for rashes, ulcer photosensitivity, ecchymosis, petechiae, cyanosis, and hair loss.

Respiratory assessment includes breath sounds and respiratory rate and assessing for pleural effusion or pleuritis.

Cardiovascular assessment includes vital signs and heart tones and assessing for symptoms of pericarditis or friction rub.

Musculoskeletal assessment includes joint deformity or discomfort, general pain, weakness, and ability to perform activities of daily living.

Neurologic assessment includes changes in affect or cognitive abilities and seizure activity.

Gastrointestinal assessment includes splenomegaly, abdominal pain, and anorexia.

Renal assessment includes intake, output, and weight.

Assess family interactions, exploring stressful situations such as divorce or trauma.

Treatment-related restrictions associated with medications and changes in appearance, such as weight gain, cushingoid appearance, and skin rashes, can lead to withdrawal, depression, and suicidal tendencies.

Perform psychological assessments periodically as the child grows and adapts to the disorder or faces new developmental challenges with a chronic disease.

Implementation
Maintain Fluid Balance
Because most children with systemic lupus erythematosus have renal involvement, nursing care includes maintaining accurate intake and output measurements and frequent evaluation of the child's fluid and electrolyte status.

Renal dysfunction may be manifested by edema, muscle cramps, diarrhea, tetany, and seizures.

Promote Adequate Nutrition
The diet may be restricted according to renal involvement, weight gain, weight loss, or other complications.

The child is at risk for weight gain associated with treatment with steroids and a decreased activity level during exacerbations of this disease.

A well-balanced, nutritious diet as well as appropriate fluid intake for age should be encouraged.

Promote Skin Integrity
Presence of the rash on mucous membranes can cause weakening of the tissues, placing the child at increased risk for infection.

Encourage the use of good hygienic measures and a mild soap.

Recommend that adolescents limit their use of cosmetics.

Reinforce the importance of avoiding sunlight as much as possible and the use of sun protection factor of 15 or higher at all times when in the sun.

Encourage the child to wear protective clothing to limit exposure to sunlight.

Avoid unprotected fluorescent lighting (Mulvihill, 2003).

Encourage the adolescent to avoid the use of tanning beds.

Provide instructions on oral care to maintain intact oral mucosa.

Provide instructions on the care of the head if alopecia occurs.

Promote Rest and Comfort
Encourage frequent rest periods such as naps and time-outs.

Encourage a nutritious diet to maximize energy stores.

A physical therapist can plan a therapeutic exercise program to encourage mobility and increase muscle strength.

Implement measures such as application of heat to painful areas.

Avoid Triggers That Cause Disease Exacerbation
Many children and their parents can recognize the signs of an impending exacerbation and the triggers that precede them.

Partner with the parents and child to implement measures to avoid these triggers.

Discuss preventive behaviors such as avoiding sun exposure and stressors.

Adolescents should be warned that alcohol, smoking, and drugs also pose an increased risk due to the potential to stimulate flares.

Female adolescents who are sexually active should avoid birth control pills that contain the hormone estrogen because the extra estrogen may exacerbate symptoms. Alternate birth control methods should be discussed with the adolescent.

Prevent Infection
Infections are a leading cause of death for patients with systemic lupus erythematosus.

Prophylactic antibiotics may be required for dental work and surgical procedures.

Instruct the patient and family to inform all healthcare providers of the disease to plan for prophylactic measures.

Educate the patient and family on the importance of adhering to the immunization schedule and obtaining a yearly influenza vaccine to prevent infection.

Instruct the family on handwashing and infection control measures in the home.

Warn adolescents about the dangers of tattooing and body piercing because of the risk of infection.

Provide Emotional Support

Adolescents may have an altered body image as a result of rash, alopecia, arthritic changes in the joints, and chronic disease.

Referral to a lupus support group, social services, or counseling may be helpful.

Juvenile Rheumatoid Arthritis

Juvenile rheumatoid arthritis (JRA) is a chronic autoimmune inflammatory disease characterized by joint inflammation, resulting in decreased mobility, swelling, and pain and occurs slightly more often in girls than in boys. JRA is the most common type of arthritis in children and adolescents, and usually occurs in children between 2 and 5 or 9 and 12 years of age (Ilowite, 2002).

There are three major types of JRA: pauciarticular arthritis, systemic arthritis, and polyarticular arthritis.

Pauciarticular arthritis primarily affects the knees, ankles, and elbows and occurs more frequently in females. Approximately 50% of children with JRA have pauciarticular arthritis. It generally manifests between infancy and age 5 years. Four or fewer joints are affected in this type of JRA.

Systemic arthritis affects males and females equally and characteristically is manifested by high fever, polyarthritis, and rheumatoid rash. Systemic arthritis affects internal organs and joints. Approximately 15% of children with JRA have systemic arthritis.

Polyarticular arthritis involves many joints (five or more), particularly the small joints of the hands and fingers. It may also affect the hips, knees, feet, ankles, and neck. This type of arthritis affects approximately 35% of the children with JRA.

Clinical Manifestations

One of the most common complaints is morning joint stiffness accompanied by joint swelling. This commonly affects the knees and the joints in the hands and feet.

Fever and rash are common.

Symptoms may also include:

- Lymphadenopathy.
- Splenomegaly.
- Hepatomegaly.
- Older children may develop symmetric involvement of the small joints of the hand.

Diagnostic Tests

Rheumatoid factor (may or may not be elevated)

Human leukocyte antigen B27

Antinuclear antibody tests

Erythrocyte sedimentation rate (elevated)

Clinical Therapy

Relieve pain.

Suppress the inflammatory process.

Prevent contractures.

Preserve joint function.

Promote normal growth and development.

Physical and/or occupational therapy increases strength and mobility of joints while protecting them from injury.

Exercises such as swimming involve a majority of the muscles and joints with minimal impact and stress on joints.

Surgery is occasionally performed to relieve pain and maintain or improve joint function in children with joint contractures.

Children with polyarticular and systemic JRA should be examined by an ophthalmologist for eye inflammation every 6 months, and children with pauciarticular arthritis should be examined every 3 months.

Nursing Management

Assessment

A careful history is important because it is sometimes the primary mode of diagnosis.

Assess for joint swelling and deformities, pain, decreased mobility, morning stiffness, fever, nodules under the skin, delayed growth, and enlarged lymph nodes.

Implementation

Promote Improved Mobility

Physical therapy.

Range-of-motion exercises, stretching, hydrotherapy, and swimming.

Encourage the child to perform activities of daily living.

Exercise may be painful or even difficult for the child.

Emphasize the importance of establishing a regular exercise and activity routine.

Encourage periods of rest during exacerbations, as the child fatigues more easily.

Teach the child methods to reduce stress on joints, such as using wrist splints when lifting.

Encourage Adequate Nutrition

Promote general health by encouraging a well-balanced diet.

Encourage adequate hydration to reduce the risk of constipation associated with immobility.

Dietary consultation will help ensure that the child receives adequate calories and a well-balanced diet.

Monitor the child's food and liquid intake and output.

Manage Side Effects of Medication

Aspirin and corticosteroids may lead to gastric irritation. To decrease the risk of stomach irritation or pain, aspirin should be administered with food, milk, or a prescribed antacid.

Monitor for signs and symptoms of aspirin toxicity, including tinnitus, decreased hearing, nausea, vomiting, drowsiness, irritability, and rapid, shallow breathing.

Caution the family not to use products with aspirin or nonsteroidal anti-inflammatory agents; contact a health professional for treatment of childhood illnesses.

Community Care

The child will need assistance to facilitate performance in school. Walking in hallways, reaching a locker, writing, and other activities may produce pain; partner with family and school personnel to plan alternative approaches.

Assist the family to adjust to the periodic disruption of family life when the child has exacerbations. Provide support and referral to other families experienced with JRA.

ALLERGIC REACTIONS
Allergy

Allergy is an abnormal or altered reaction to an antigen. Antigens responsible for clinical manifestations of allergy are called *allergens*. Allergens can be ingested in food or drugs, injected, absorbed through contact with unbroken skin, or inhaled (Box 18–3). An allergic reaction is an antigen–antibody reaction and can manifest itself as

- Anaphylaxis
- Atopic disease
- Serum sickness
- Contact dermatitis

See CM 18–3 for a list of the various clinical manifestations common in allergic reactions.

The **hypersensitivity response**, an overreaction of the immune system, is responsible for allergic reactions. Hypersensitivity reactions have been classified into four types:

Type I hypersensitivity reactions, the most common allergic reactions, are immediate reactions that occur within seconds or minutes of exposure to the antigen. Symptoms can include a wheal and flare in the skin, edema, spasm of smooth muscle, wheezing, vomiting, diarrhea, or anaphylaxis. The release of chemical substances such as histamine is responsible for the signs and symptoms exhibited.

Type II hypersensitivity reaction is immediate, within 15–30 minutes after exposure to the antigen. Symptoms vary and may include fever and dyspnea.

Box 18–3	Common Childhood Allergens	
Common childhood allergens include		
Animal dander	Medications, such as penicillin	Seafood
Cockroaches	Mites	Shellfish
Cow's milk	Mold	Soy
Dust	Plant pollens	Tree nuts
Egg whites	Peanuts	Wheat

CM 18–3   Clinical Manifestations of Allergic Reactions in Children

System	Clinical Manifestations
Respiratory system	Asthma
	Rhinitis (seasonal and perennial)
	Serous otitis media
	Cough
	Pneumonia
	Croup
	Edema of glottis
	Nasal congestion or discharge
Gastrointestinal system	Abdominal pain and colic
	Stomatitis
	Constipation
	Diarrhea
	Bloody stools
	Geographic tongue
	Vomiting
Skin	Angioedema
	Urticaria
	Eczema
	Atopic dermatitis
	Erythema multiforme
	Purpura
	Drug and food rashes
	Contact dermatitis
Nervous system	Headache
	Tension
	Fatigue
	Seizures
	Ménière syndrome
	Tremors
	Irritability
	Sleep disorders
	Decreased concentration
Eyes	Conjunctivitis
	Cataract
	Ciliary spasm
	Iritis
	Itching eyes
	Tearing

(*continued*)

CM 18–3 Clinical Manifestations of Allergic Reactions in Children (Continued)

System	Clinical Manifestations
Hematologic	Thrombocytopenic purpura
	Hemolytic anemia
	Leukopenia
	Agranulocytosis
Musculoskeletal system	Arthralgia
	Myalgia
	Rheumatoid arthritis
	Torticollis
Genitourinary system	Dysuria
	Vulvovaginitis
	Enuresis
Miscellaneous	Anaphylactic shock
	Serum sickness
	Autoimmune diseases

Type III hypersensitivity reaction may be difficult to distinguish from type II reaction. Type III hypersensitivity reactions generally peak within 6 hours.

Type IV reactions are delayed responses that do not appear until several hours after exposure and require 24–72 hours to fully develop. Symptoms include contact dermatitis, itching, and blistering.

Nursing Management

Intervention

Educating the child and family on methods to minimize or avoid exposure to allergens is important.

Parents of children who have had severe reactions to bee or wasp stings should be taught how to take precautions and provide emergency treatment if the child is stung.

An EpiPen may be prescribed, and the parents and child will require instructions on its proper use.

Partner with the family to determine effective measures to allergy-proof their home. Pets, dust, carpets, fabrics, feather pillows and bedding, and cigarette smoke can all cause allergic reactions.

When the child has type I reactions to an environmental substance, avoidance of the allergen is most critical.

In addition, care providers, families, and school personnel must be able to treat anaphylaxis if exposure to the allergen occurs.

School nurses keep records regarding children's allergies and inform school personnel about the allergies and cautions that should be followed.

Be sure to label the child's chart and bed and apply a red armband to the child to alert others to allergies when the child is hospitalized.

Nurses must be aware of the resuscitation procedures and equipment in all facilities, such as hospital units, offices, childcare centers, and schools.

Anaphylaxis

Anaphylaxis, also called anaphylactic shock, is a potentially life-threatening systemic reaction to an allergen. Symptoms can occur within minutes or up to 2 hours after exposure to an allergy-causing substance.

Clinical Manifestations

See CM 18–4 for clinical manifestations of anaphylaxis.

Clinical Therapy

Essential to preservation of life is the immediate recognition and treatment of anaphylactic reaction.

Establish a stable airway and intravenous access. Epinephrine is the medication of choice for treating an anaphylactic reaction (Tang, 2003).

Epinephrine may be administered subcutaneously, intramuscularly, or via an endotracheal tube. Epinephrine reverses the symptoms of an anaphylactic reaction by causing vasoconstriction and reversing airway constriction.

Antihistamines, such as diphenhydramine (Benadryl), and steroids are often administered to the child experiencing an anaphylactic reaction.

Place the child in a supine position, and elevate the legs to increase venous return.

Obtain intravenous access for fluid resuscitation. Large volumes of fluids may be required to treat hypotension caused by increased vascular permeability and vasodilation.

Administer oxygen.

CM 18–4 Clinical Manifestations of Anaphylactic Shock

System	Clinical Manifestations	Clinical Therapy
Respiratory	Wheezes Stridor Dyspnea Laryngospasm Bronchospasm Pulmonary edema Cyanosis	Administer epinephrine, oxygen, and fluids (protocol for anaphylactic shock). Monitor respiratory status. Monitor breath sounds. Monitor arterial blood gases.
Cardiovascular	Profound hypotension Tachycardia Dysrhythmias Decreased central venous pressure	Monitor heart rate, blood pressure, and cardiac rhythm. Monitor peripheral pulses.
Neurologic	Anxiety Restlessness Lethargy Progression to coma	Conduct neurologic assessment at regular intervals. Assess for changes in level of consciousness. Assess for changes in anxiety level.
Gastrointestinal	Vomiting Diarrhea Abdominal pain	Assess for vomiting or diarrhea. Assess for abdominal pain. Assess bowel sounds.
Integumentary	Edematous face, lips, tongue, hands, feet Skin warm	Assess for edema and rashes. Assess skin temperature.
Renal	Oliguria progressing to anuria	Assess urine output hourly. Monitor intake hourly. Monitor serum blood urea nitrogen and creatinine.

The child may require endotracheal intubation and mechanical ventilation.

Monitor the child for an observation period of 2–6 hours after mild episodes and 24 hours after more severe episodes (Tang, 2003).

Patient and Family Education

Prevention of re-exposure to the allergen is essential.

Determining the cause of anaphylaxis, if uncertain, may require numerous diagnostic studies. Previous tolerance of a substance does not rule it out as the trigger. Direct skin testing and radioallergosorbent testing are available for some antigens.

Nursing Management
Assessment

Assess the child for respiratory distress, hypotension, tachycardia, and edema.

Assess breath sounds for wheezing.

Assess all vital signs.

Monitor urine output hourly.

Assess peripheral pulses.

Monitor oxygen saturation.

Assess skin temperature, color, and moisture.

Implementation

Emergency management of anaphylaxis is the administration of epinephrine, oxygen, and fluids.

Maintain the child on bedrest immediately after anaphylaxis until the observation period has subsided.

Provide the child and family the opportunity to express anxiety and concerns.

For home care, partner with the family to assure that the child and family members can properly administer epinephrine.

Emphasize to the family that the child should always wear a medical identification tag and should always have an EpiPen immediately available for emergencies.

Assure that the childcare providers or school officials can recognize the signs and symptoms of anaphylaxis and can appropriately administer epinephrine.

Instruct the child and family to activate the emergency medical system (9-1-1) after epinephrine is administered. The medication is available via prescription as an EpiPen or EpiPen Jr. Auto-Injector. The dosage required by the child is determined by the primary healthcare provider or immunologist.

Latex Allergy

Latex allergy is caused by an immunoglobulin E–mediated response that develops after repeated exposure to latex. A reaction to latex products can be manifested as an irritant reaction of the skin with redness, inflammation, and blisters (type IV delayed hypersensitivity) or type I hypersensitivity, which is immediate and often has systemic manifestations (e.g., itchy eyes, asthma, or anaphylaxis).

Children most at risk for latex allergy include those with myelodysplasia and congenital urinary tract anomalies. Persons who have had repeated surgeries are also at higher risk owing to high exposure to latex during surgery. Healthcare personnel are also at risk for latex allergy because of exposure in the workplace (Box 18–4).

Nursing Management
Assessment
Assess children and adolescents at high risk for signs and symptoms of latex allergy.

For allergy testing for latex, the radioallergosorbent test (RAST) is most often used.

Intervention
When a positive skin test has occurred or when the child has had a reaction to latex, all latex products must be removed from the allergic individual's environment.

Alternative products, such as nonlatex gloves and catheters, must be used when providing healthcare.

Box 18–4   Measures to Protect Against Latex Allergy

Healthcare personnel are at high risk of developing latex allergy because of intense exposure to products containing latex. An estimated 8–12% of healthcare workers are latex sensitive. You can protect yourself by using the following measures:

- Decrease exposure by using alternative products when available (use synthetic rubber, polyethylene, nitrile, neoprene, and vinyl gloves).
- Use powder-free gloves if using latex gloves (the powder has high amounts of latex that can be inhaled).
- Avoid use of oil-based hand creams and lotions before putting on latex gloves, as these preparations break down the latex.
- When symptoms of sensitivity to latex occur on exposure (rash, hives, nasal congestion, conjunctivitis, cough, or wheeze), contact the employee health department of your facility.
- If severely allergic, avoid all contact and wear a medical identification bracelet.
- Contact the National Institute for Occupational Safety and Health at 800-346-4647 or the American Nurses Association at 800-637-0323 for more information.

Emphasize to the family that the child with latex allergy should also wear a medical-alert identification bracelet at all times.

Educate families about the need to have an epinephrine kit readily available at home and school.

Be alert for any signs of hypersensitivity when the child is receiving healthcare, and be prepared with drugs and equipment to treat anaphylaxis.

Emphasize to parents and children that many everyday products contain latex, including latex balloons, condoms, and many toys.

19. ALTERATIONS IN HEMATOLOGIC FUNCTION

An understanding and application of the normal blood values in children are needed when caring for children with alterations in hematologic function (Table 19–1).

IRON DEFICIENCY ANEMIA

Iron deficiency anemia is the most common type of anemia and nutritional deficiency among children (Carley, 2003). This can result from a variety of causes, including the following:

- Anemia secondary to blood loss
- Malabsorption
- Poor nutritional intake
- Increased metabolic demands; for example, growth spurts

Clinical Manifestations (Acute)

Pallor

Fatigue

Irritability

Clinical Manifestations (Chronic)

Nail deformities

Growth retardation

Muscle weakness

Developmental delay

Tachycardia

Headache

Systolic murmur

Decreased learning ability

Decreased alertness

Decreased attention span

Pica

Diagnostic Tests

Clinical presentation

Section III: Body Systems

Table 19–1 Normal Blood Values in Children

Test	Normal Value*
Red blood cell	$3.89–4.96 \times 10^{12}$/L
Hemoglobin	10.2–13.4 g/dL
Hematocrit	31.7–39.3%
Mean corpuscular volume	72.7–86.5 micrometers^3
Mean corpuscular hemoglobin	24.1–29.4 pg
Mean corpuscular hemoglobin concentration	32.4–35.3%
Reticulocyte count	0.8–2.2%
White blood cell	$5.4–11.0 \times 10^9$/L
Differential	
Neutrophils	34.3–72.9%
Eosinophils	2.4–4.8%
Basophils	1%
Lymphocytes	13.5–52.8%
Atypical lymphocytes	2.6–5.6%
Monocytes	3.5–13.4%

*All values are for the 2- to 12-year-old child.
Note: Data from Soldin, S. J., Brugnara, C., & Wong, E. C. (2003). Pediatric reference ranges (4th ed.). Washington, DC: AACC Press.

Laboratory studies: hematocrit, hemoglobin, mean corpuscular hemoglobin, microscopic analysis, and serum iron-binding capacity and reticulocyte count.

Red blood cells are microcytic and hypochromic (Cook, 2000).

See Table 19–1 and Chapter 5 for normal blood values.

Clinical Therapy

Supplemental iron preparations

Diet high in foods with high amounts of iron

Decreased intake of cow's milk

Nursing Management
Assessment

Begin screening between 6 months and 1 year.

Review laboratory findings.

Make height and weight comparisons for the child across time.

Perform developmental screening tests for developmental delay.

Obtain diet history.

Implementation

Family-centered care focusing on prevention, dietary management, medication therapy, and follow-up

Intervention

Dietary Management

Long-term treatment focusing on the following is preferred for iron deficiency anemia:

- Planning a diet with foods rich in iron
- Iron-fortified formulas and cereals for infants
- Eliminating cow's milk feeding during infancy to prevent bleeding and loss of iron from gut
- Finger foods rich in iron for toddlers depending on age, such as meats, raisins, dates, and fruits with stones
- Encouraging foods high in vitamin C (enhances iron absorption) and protein (often contains iron)

Medication Therapy

Iron preparations are administered to correct the anemia. Ferrous sulfate should be administered with the following:

- On an empty stomach if possible
- With vitamin C
- With a straw to avoid staining teeth
- Without dairy foods, antacids, or whole grains
- With small amounts of appropriate food choices if necessary

Side effects of iron sulfate exist and must be communicated by parents to healthcare providers:

- Black, tarry stools
- Constipation
- Gastrointestinal discomfort
- Foul aftertaste

Monitor for signs and symptoms of iron overload, including the following:

- Abdominal pain
- Vomiting
- Bloody diarrhea

Severe overdose may be fatal: Keep iron preparations securely locked away from children.

Patient and Family Education

Medication administration and secure storage

Dietary management

Partnering with families to provide specific dietary information at various ages (Lesperance, Wu, & Bernstein, 2002):

- Birth:
  - Encourage breastfeeding exclusively for 4–6 months after birth and continued breastfeeding until 12 months.
  - For infants who are not breastfed, recommend only iron-fortified formula.
  - For breastfed infants who were premature or low birth weight, administer 2–4 mg/kg/day of iron drops to a maximum of 15/mg/day (according to primary healthcare provider) and return for screening for anemia before 6 months.
- Age 4–9 months:
  - Recommend starting iron-fortified infant cereal by 4–6 months.
  - Recommend two or more servings per day of iron-fortified infant cereal to meet iron requirements.
  - Recommend one feeding per day of foods rich in vitamin C (fruits and vegetables) to improve iron absorption.
- Age 9–12 months:
  - Begin introducing plain pureed meats.
  - Discourage introduction of cow's milk before 12 months of age.
  - Refer for screening if the infant is at risk for iron deficiency.
- Age 1–5 years:
  - Encourage intake of iron-rich foods (fortified cereals, lean meat, poultry, grains, dried peas and beans, dark green vegetables).
  - Limit milk consumption to 16–24 oz per day.
  - Refer for screening if the child is at risk for iron deficiency.
- Age 6 years and older:
  - Encourage intake of iron-rich foods (lean meat, fish, poultry, fortified cereals, grains, dried peas and beans, dark green vegetables, raisins).
  - Female adolescents who begin menstruation are at increased risk for iron deficiency and should be screened if indicated.

NORMOCYTIC ANEMIA

Normocytic anemia is anemia in which cells are of normal shape and size but decreased in number. This condition is treated by correcting the cause, which can be any of the following:

- Hemorrhage
- Disease-induced inflammation
- Disseminated intravascular coagulation
- Glucose-6-phosphate dehydrogenase deficiency
- Hemolytic uremic syndrome
- Anemia of chronic disease, including inflammatory conditions, infections, and neoplasms
    - Examples of infections that can cause anemia are *Haemophilus influenzae* type b, human immunodeficiency virus/acquired immunodeficiency syndrome, orbital cellulitis meningitis, and septic arthritis.
    - Examples of inflammatory causes of anemia are arthritis, cancers, and chronic heart or liver disease.

SICKLE CELL DISEASE

Sickle cell disease is a genetic autosomal recessive disorder primarily affecting African Americans. The disease is characterized by an abnormal replacement of hemoglobin with hemoglobin S with the propensity to sickle during deoxygenation. Sickling may be triggered by fever and emotional or physical stress. Sickled cells can resume a normal shape when rehydrated or reoxygenated but then have a fragile membrane and shortened life span (Tanyi, 2003). Sickle cell crises are acute exacerbations of the disease that cause increased blood viscosity from sickled cells due to hypoxia or low oxygen tension. Generally, the child has become severely dehydrated or febrile to precipitate the crisis.

Clinical Manifestations

Pain

Sickle cell crisis, including vaso-occlusive crisis, splenic sequestration, or aplastic crisis

See Box 19–1 for the precipitating factors contributing to sickle cell crisis.

Diagnostic Tests

Initial diagnosis from cord blood using hemoglobin electrophoresis

Sickledex for quick screening for those older than age 6 months

| Box 19–1 | Precipitating Factors Contributing to Sickle Cell Crisis |

Fever
Dehydration
Altitude
Extremes in temperature
Vomiting
Emotional distress
Fatigue

Alcohol consumption
Pregnancy
Elevated hemoglobin levels
Elevated reticulocyte counts
Excessive exercise or physical activity
Acidosis

Complete blood count

Reticulocyte count

Clinical Therapy

Management for the child focuses on pain control, hydration, oxygenation, prevention/treatment of infection, and reduction of energy expenditure.

Parenteral analgesia such as morphine.

Oral and intravenous fluid replacement.

Oxygen administration.

Daily prophylactic antibiotics.

Transfusions of normal red blood cells.

Nursing Management

The focus of nursing management is identification of children at risk, early recognition and prevention of crisis, promotion of growth and development, prevention of complications, and family support.

Assessment

Detailed client history.

Developmental milestones.

Pain.

Psychosocial assessment, including self-concept and self-esteem, body image, and social interactions.

Family resources.

Remain alert for signs of complications associated with sickle cell anemia.

Implementation

Nursing management for the child in crisis focuses on promoting tissue perfusion, promoting hydration, controlling pain, preventing infection, ensuring proper nutrition, preventing complications, and providing support to the child and family.

Interventions

Promote increased tissue perfusion with transfusions and activity monitoring.

Promote hydration orally and intravenously.

Manage pain with appropriate analgesics and other measures.

Prevent infection with antibiotic prophylaxis and prompt recognition of infection.

Ensure a high protein and high calorie diet.

Prevent complications of crisis, observing for worsening anemia/shock.

Provide emotional support for client and family.

Provide assistance with discharge planning and home care needs.

Patient and Family Education

Provide information on the disease and treatments.

Assess knowledge on potential crisis situations and when to seek medical attention.

Partner with family to explore resources.

Discuss signs of dehydration.

Provide information on red blood cell infusion therapy and use of deferoxamine (Desferal) for iron overload.

Assist the family with information for care of the child at school.

Refer family for genetic counseling as needed.

Assist with resources for financial and emotional support for this chronic disease.

Expected Outcomes for the Child and Family with Sickle Cell Disease

Management of pain

Maintenance of adequate hydration

Absence of side effects of the disease to multiple organs

Prompt identification of complications

Maintenance of normal growth and development

Support for the family to deal with the chronic nature of the disease and care

THALASSEMIAS

Thalassemias most often occur in people of Mediterranean descent and are a group of inherited blood disorders of hemoglobin synthesis. These blood disorders cause mild to severe anemia and are classified in types of β-thalassemias and α-thalassemias. The most common type is β-thalassemia major, also known as *Cooley's anemia*.

β-Thalassemia stems from a defective hemoglobin chain resulting in impaired production of the beta chain of hemoglobin A. In α-thalassemia, the defect occurs on the alpha chain of the adult hemoglobin. The severity of both disorders depends on the number of defective genes. The three types of β-thalassemia are the following:

- Thalassemia minor, or thalassemia trait, producing mild anemia
- Thalassemia intermedia, producing moderate anemia
- Thalassemia major, producing anemia requiring transfusions

The three types of α-thalassemia are the following:

- Alpha trait, a defect in a single alpha chain–forming gene
- α-Thalassemia minor, a defect with two genes
- α-Thalassemia major, a fatal defect in all four alpha chain–forming genes

Clinical Manifestations of β-Thalassemia

Structurally impaired shortened life span of red blood cells.

Pallor.

Failure to thrive.

Hepatosplenomegaly.

Severe anemia (hemoglobin of less than 6 g/dL).

Chronic hypoxia.

Lethargy.

Exercise intolerance.

Anorexia.

Headache.

Bone pain.

See CM 19–1 for clinical manifestations of β-thalassemia.

CM 19–1 Clinical Manifestations of β-Thalassemia

Body Organs	Clinical Manifestations	Clinical Therapy
Red blood cells (anemia)	Hypochromic and microcytic changes Folic acid deficiency Frequent epistaxis	Hypertransfusion program. Administer folic acid and increase dietary consumption of folic acid and vitamin C.
Skeletal changes	Osteoporosis Delayed growth Susceptibility to pathologic fractures Facial deformities: enlarged head, prominent forehead due to frontal and parietal bossing, prominent cheek bones, broadened and depressed bridge of nose, enlarged maxilla with protruding front teeth, eyes with mongolian slant and epicanthal fold	Assess growth and plot on chart—monitor for delays in growth. Teach safety precautions to avoid fractures.
Heart	Chronic congestive heart failure Myocardial fibrosis Murmurs	Monitor for signs of congestive heart failure. Electrocardiogram and echocardiogram may be conducted to assess heart function.
Liver/gallbladder	Hepatomegaly Hepatic insufficiency	Magnetic resonance imaging or computed tomography scans may be conducted to evaluate liver and gallbladder.

(continued)

CM 19–1 Clinical Manifestations of β-Thalassemia (Continued)

Body Organs	Clinical Manifestations	Clinical Therapy
Liver/gallbladder (*continued*)		Liver biopsy may be performed.
Spleen	Splenomegaly	Magnetic resonance imaging or computed tomography scans may be conducted to evaluate spleen.
Endocrine system	Delayed sexual maturation Fibrotic pancreas, resulting in diabetes mellitus	Assess sexual maturation using the Tanner staging.
Skin	Darkening of skin	Assess for skin changes.

Clinical Manifestations of α-Thalassemia

Similar to but milder than those of β-thalassemia

Diagnostic Tests

Hemoglobin electrophoresis

Complete blood count

Prenatal testing using chorionic villus sampling or amniocentesis

Chest x-ray

Liver computed tomography, magnetic resonance imaging, biopsy

Clinical Therapy

Supportive, involving transfusions of normal cells every 3–4 weeks

Treatment of iron overload with Desferal

Potential splenectomy

Hematopoietic stem cell transplantation (HSCT) in newly diagnosed cases

Diet for age high in folic acid and ascorbic acid and low in iron

Nursing Management

Nursing management is focused on the care surrounding transfusion therapy and support of the child and family with a chronic, life-threatening illness. Genetic counseling is recommended.

Assessment

Assess for classic manifestations listed previously.

Heart and breath sounds.

Respiratory effort.

Signs of infection.

Signs of iron overload: abdominal pain, vomiting and bloody diarrhea.

Implementation

Most care for the child may be done at home. Home care nurses can provide the needed transfusions and injections of Desferal. Parents are provided with necessary information for treatment, complications, and follow-up treatment for the child. Age-appropriate care in school and at home is a lifelong commitment for the nurse and the family.

Evaluation

Expected outcomes for the child with thalassemia include the following:

- The child is free of infection.
- The child and family demonstrate understanding of the treatment regimen and signs of potential complications.
- The child participates in age-appropriate, safe activities without undo fatigue.
- The child demonstrates a positive body image.
- The child demonstrates effective tissue perfusion.

APLASTIC ANEMIA

Aplastic anemia is a congenital or acquired condition that results from failure of the bone marrow to produce adequate numbers of circulating blood cells. Acquired types may result from infection, congenital conditions, toxins, or malignancies (Derivan & Ferrante, 2000).

Clinical Manifestations

Thrombocytopenia

Anemia

Neutropenia

Bleeding

Purpura

Weakness

Bloody stools

Epistaxis

Retinal bleeding

Tachycardia

Death related to hemorrhage, sepsis, and malignancy

Diagnostic Tests
Complete blood count

Serum iron

Bone marrow aspiration

Clinical Therapy
Determine risk factors.

Supportive treatment of transfusions, including packed cells, platelets, and granulocytes.

Immunosuppressive therapy.

Antibiotics if confirmed infection.

HSCT.

Nursing Management
Prevent bleeding.

Administer and monitor blood transfusions.

Prevent infection.

Encourage mobility as tolerated.

Educate parents and child about disorder.

Provide emotional support.

Conserve patient energy.

Observe for complications associated with transfusions.

Assist family with resources related to life-threatening disease.

CLOTTING DISORDERS
Clotting disorders include both hereditary and acquired disorders resulting in various bleeding tendencies. Hereditary disorders include hemophilia and von Willebrand disease. Acquired disorders include disseminated intravascular coagulation and idiopathic thrombocytopenic purpura.

Hemophilia
Hemophilia is defined as a group of hereditary bleeding disorders resulting from specific clotting factor deficiencies. Types of hemo-

philia include hemophilia A (factor VIII deficiency), hemophilia B (factor IX deficiency), also known as *Christmas disease*, and hemophilia C (factor XI deficiency) (Curry, 2004).

Clinical Manifestations

Spontaneous bleeding

Hemarthrosis (bleeding into a joint space)

Deep tissue hemorrhage

Limited motion

Pain

Tenderness and joint swelling

Bone changes

Contractures

Disabling joint deformities

Easy bruising

Nosebleeds

Hematuria

Bleeding after tooth extractions, minor trauma, or minor surgical procedures

Diagnostic Tests

Chorionic villa sampling.

Amniocentesis.

Client history.

Physical examination.

Laboratory tests for factor VIII or IX.

Prolonged activated partial prothrombin time.

Prothrombin time.

Thrombin time.

Fibrinogen and platelet count.

See Table 19–2 for diagnostic tests for clotting disorders.

Clinical Therapy

Factor replacement therapy with cryoprecipitate

Table 19–2　Diagnostic Tests for Clotting Disorders

Test	Normal Value	
Bleeding time	2–9 min	
Fibrinogen	200–500 mg/dL (5.9–14.7 micromole/L)	
Partial thromboplastin time	42–54 sec	
Platelet count ($\times 10^9$/L)	Males	Females
Newborns	164–351	234–346
1–2 months	275–567	295–615
2–6 months	275–566	288–598
6 months–2 years	219–452	229–465
2–6 years	204–405	204–402
6–12 years	194–364	183–369
12–18 years	165–332	185–335
>18 years	143–320	171–326
Prothrombin time	11–15 sec	
Thrombin time	12–16 sec	

Prompt and adequate treatment to prevent serious bleeding episodes

For mild hemophilia, desmopressin acetate to increase factor VIII activity

Transfusions of the missing clotting factor

Nursing Management

Important nursing care focuses on identifying the child with hemophilia and implementing measures to prevent serious bleeding events through collaboration with the child and family.

Assessment

Alert for signs and symptoms that indicate bleeding

Achievement of expected growth and development stages

Assessment of child's and family's coping strategies

Thorough medical history

Physical assessment with focus on joints

Pain

Presence of hematuria

Evidence of ecchymosis or petechia

Family resources

Implementation

The goals of nursing care include the prevention and control of bleeding episodes, limiting joint involvement, managing pain, and providing support to the child and family. Short- and long-term interventions are necessary.

Patient and Family Education

Safe and age-appropriate toys

Adapted home environment

Bleeding episode education

Seeking medical attention

Medical identification tag

Preparation and administration of factor concentrate

Individual school health plan

Physical rehabilitation as needed for joint deformities

Evaluation

Expected outcomes for the child include the following:

- Prevention of injury
- Maintenance of joint mobility
- Management of pain
- Promotion of normal growth and development
- Adequate knowledge of family to provide necessary care
- Support for family members in dealing with this chronic disease

Disseminated Intravascular Coagulation

Disseminated intravascular coagulation is a life-threatening clotting disorder occurring as a complication of serious illnesses such as hypoxia, shock, trauma, burns, liver disease, necrotizing enterocolitis, cancer, and viruses.

Clinical Manifestations

Bleeding ranging from minor oozing to frank hemorrhage

Factor depletion

Thrombocytopenia

Diagnostic Tests

Prothrombin time

Partial thromboplastin time

Fibrin-fibrinogen split products

Clinical Therapy

Identification and treatment of underlying disorder

Administering fluids

Replacement of depleted coagulation factors with fresh frozen plasma, fibrinogen, and platelets

Heparin (controversial)

Oxygen

Monitor oxygen saturation and arterial blood gases

Nursing Management
Critical nursing care focuses on the assessment of bleeding and administration of prescribed therapies.

Assessment
Petechiae

Ecchymoses

Oozing

Presence of blood in stool

Vital signs

Level of consciousness

Intake and output

Hematuria

Blood urea nitrogen and serum creatinine

Implementation

Institute bleeding control precautions.

Monitor for signs of bleeding.

Administer replacement blood products.

Monitor vital signs frequently.

Monitor for signs of shock.

Monitor oxygen saturation and arterial blood gases.

Report any signs of complications.

Idiopathic Thrombocytopenic Purpura
Idiopathic thrombocytopenic purpura is the most common bleeding disorder in children between 2 and 10 years of age. Also called *autoimmune thrombocytopenic purpura*, this disorder is characterized by an increased destruction of platelets in the spleen. The disorder

usually follows a virus such as measles or chickenpox (Bolton-Maggs, 2000); it is caused by the binding of autoantibodies to platelet antigens.

Clinical Manifestations

Bleeding due to platelet loss from gums, nosebleeds, urine, and stools

Multiple ecchymoses

Petechiae

Purpura

Diagnostic Tests

Decreased platelet count (less than 20,000–30,000 µL/dL).

Antiplatelet antibodies in the peripheral blood.

Antinuclear antibodies may be present.

Direct and indirect Coombs' test to detect antibodies.

Bone marrow aspiration to rule out leukemia.

Clinical Therapy

Clinical therapy is dependent on platelet count.

Corticosteroids for platelet counts of less than 50,000 µL/dL.

Patients with platelet counts of less than 20,000 µL/dL and minor purpura are administered intravenous immunoglobulin.

Platelet administration only if hemorrhaging occurs.

Splenectomy may be indicated to prevent destruction in spleen.

Spontaneous remission is seen in 90% of children with idiopathic thrombocytopenic purpura.

Nursing Management

Nursing care focuses on controlling and preventing the number of bleeding episodes.

Assess for evidence of bleeding, including petechiae and purpura.

Assess for hepatosplenomegaly.

Monitor for nosebleeds, oozing at intravenous sites, gastrointestinal bleeding, and indications of intracranial bleeding such as vomiting and seizures.

Preventative measures teaching parents to avoid aspirin, to avoid activities that may increase injury, and to recognize signs and symptoms of bleeding.

Meningococcemia

Meningococcemia is thought to be a result of endotoxins of *Neisseria meningitidis*. This rapidly progressing disease has a mortality rate of 17% to 60% and almost 100% in children who experience shock and coma (Smillova & Walker, 2000). The bacteria rapidly multiply, and the endotoxins from the bacteria are thought to impair protein C, which causes thrombosis formation.

Clinical Manifestations

Onset is sudden.

Respiratory infection is followed by high fever, petechial rash, massive skin and mucosal hemorrhage, hypotension, disseminated intravascular coagulation, and shock.

Vomiting, abdominal pain, headache, lethargy, and myalgia (Smillova & Walker, 2000).

Symptoms can progress to a critical level within 12–48 hours of onset.

Coagulopathy, microvascular thrombosis, and secondary hemorrhages.

Pulmonary edema with increased respiratory effort.

Ischemia of digits and limbs due to decreased cardiac output, microthrombi, vasoconstriction, and disseminated intravascular coagulation, which may result in gangrene and amputation.

Diagnostic Tests

Blood cultures revealing *N. meningitidis*

Idiopathic thrombocytopenia

Lumbar puncture to determine presence of organisms in cerebrospinal fluid

Clinical Therapy

Respiratory isolation to prevent spread of infection

Antibiotics—penicillin or third-generation cephalosporin

Removal of sources of infection

Multisystem shock management

Prompt recognition and treatment with antibiotics

Fluid volume replacement to support blood pressure and correct hypovolemic shock

Treatment of septic shock with constant critical monitoring

Treatment of disseminated intravascular coagulation

Nursing Management
Assessment
Thorough assessment of all body systems.

Level of consciousness changes.

Urinary output to evaluate renal function.

Alterations in tissue perfusions.

Oxygen saturation levels and blood gas values.

Assess for indications of seizure activity.

Implementation
Manage fluids.

Maintain respiratory support.

Administer intravenous fluids for replacement, administration of antibiotics, treatment of hypovolemia and maintenance of blood pressure.

Maintain meticulous skin care for integrity.

Provide nutritional support.

Prevent further infections.

Maintain ventilator support and arterial lines if present.

Implement seizure precautions.

Support child and family with information, resource allocation, and follow-up care.

Hematopoietic Stem Cell Transplantation (HSCT)
HSCT, once referred to as *bone marrow transplant*, has been used for many diseases such as severe combined immunodeficiency disease, aplastic anemia, and leukemia. Sources of stem cells not only include bone marrow, but also peripheral blood and cord blood. Because these cells tolerate freezing for several years, they may be obtained and cryopreserved for later use (Trigg, 2004).

There are three types of HSCT:

1. In autologous transplantation, the child's own marrow is taken, stored, and reinfused as needed.
2. In isogenic transplantation, the marrow is taken from an identical twin.
3. In allogeneic transplantation, the donor, usually a sibling, has a compatible human leukocyte antigen.

Clinical Therapy

Pretransplant phase:

- Evaluation of child, human leukocyte antigen typing, evaluation of organ function, and laboratory studies
- High doses of chemotherapy and possibly total body radiation to destroy circulating blood cells and the diseased bone marrow
- Strict isolation in a special negative pressure environment for 10 days

Transplant phase:

- Intravenous infusion with donor stem cells.
- If successful, cells will migrate to bone marrow and transplant marrow will start producing hematopoietic blood cells in approximately 2–4 weeks.

Post-transplant phase:

- Pancytopenia lasts for several weeks after transplant.
- Major risks are infection, anemia, and bleeding.
- Transfusions may be required.
- Total parenteral nutrition may be required for some children.
- Those not receiving syngeneic transplants require immunosuppressive agents to prevent graft-versus-host disease.

Nursing Management

Assessment

Monitor for this multisystem disorder by assessing skin, mucous membranes, gastrointestinal function, respiratory function, cardiac function, and hydration status.

Conduct frequent assessment, including signs of graft-versus-host disease.

Implementation

Child and parent support, with assessment of resources and use of support groups

At-home/discharge preparation

Follow-up appointments

Re-entry into school

Reasons for seeking medical treatment

20. ALTERATIONS IN CELLULAR GROWTH

CHILDHOOD CANCER
Clinical Manifestations

Each type of childhood cancer signals its presence differently. Because many of the presenting signs and symptoms of cancer are typical of common childhood illnesses, a delay in diagnosis can occur. In some cases, no symptoms are noted until the cancer is advanced. Children more commonly present with **metastases** (spread of the cancer to a site other than its origin) at time of diagnosis than do adults due to this difficulty in recognition of the disease. Some of the common presenting symptoms of cancer are the following:

Pain may be the result of a neoplasm either directly or indirectly affecting nerve receptors through obstruction, inflammation, tissue damage, stretching of visceral tissue, or invasion of susceptible tissue.

Cachexia is a syndrome characterized by anorexia, weight loss, anemia, asthenia (weakness), and early satiety (feeling of being full).

Anemia may be experienced during times of chronic bleeding or iron deficiency. In chronic illness, the body uses iron poorly. Anemia is also present in cancers of the bone marrow when the number of red blood cells (RBCs) is reduced, in part because of the presence of large numbers of other bone marrow products. Treatment of cancer often promotes further anemia.

Infection is usually a result of an altered or immature immune system. In addition, infection occurs when bone marrow cancers inhibit maturation of normal immune system cells. Infection may also occur in children who are treated with corticosteroids. Because their immune response is altered, the normal signs of infection may not appear.

Bruising can occur if the bone marrow cannot produce enough platelets; bleeding after even minor trauma can then lead to ecchymosis.

Neurologic symptoms may result from impingement on the brain or nervous system. Signs of increased intracranial pressure, decreased or altered consciousness, eye abnormalities, or other neurologic or behavioral changes may be evident.

Palpable mass may be present for certain cancers. This is most commonly abdominal but may be mediastinal or in the neck or other sites.

A variety of other symptoms can occur depending on the location of the cancer. Subcutaneous nodules may appear if leukocytosis is present, superior vena cava syndrome or respiratory difficulty can occur with mediastinal tumors (e.g., neuroblastoma), and enlarged lymph nodes are common with lymphomas (Bleyer, 2004).

During treatment for cancer, a number of complications and oncologic emergencies can occur:

Metabolic emergencies result from the lysis (dissolving or decomposing) of tumor cells, a process called *tumor lysis syndrome*. This cell destruction releases high levels of uric acid, potassium, and phosphates into the blood. Low levels of sodium and calcium occur and metabolic acidosis results. This syndrome is seen most commonly in children with Burkitt's lymphoma and acute lymphocytic leukemia (Baggott, Kelly, Fochtman, et al., 2002). A second type of metabolic emergency is septic shock. During periods of immune suppression, the child is vulnerable to overwhelming infection, resulting in circulatory failure, hypothermia or hyperthermia, tachypnea, mental changes, inadequate tissue perfusion, and hypotension. A third type of metabolic emergency occurs when large amounts of bone are destroyed by treatment, resulting in hypercalcemia (elevated calcium in the serum). Some children develop syndrome of inappropriate antidiuretic hormone and have excessive release of antidiuretic hormone. The resulting decreased urinary output leads to water intoxication.

Hematologic emergencies result from bone marrow suppression or infiltration of brain and respiratory tissue with high numbers of leukemic blast cells (hyperleukocytosis). Bone marrow suppression results in anemia and thrombocytopenia (decreased platelets) with resultant coagulation disturbance and hemorrhage. Disseminated intravascular coagulation occurs in some children and is a life-threatening complication. Gastrointestinal and central nervous system bleeding (strokes) is common. Disruption of normal white blood cell (WBC) production and resulting hyperleukocytosis can lead to obstruction of small blood vessels throughout the body.

Space-occupying lesions can present with a variety of clinical manifestations. Extensive tumor growth may result in spinal cord compression, increased intracranial pressure, brain herniation, seizures, massive hepatomegaly, cardiac and respiratory complications, and superior vena cava syndrome (obstruction of the superior vena cava by tumor).

Diagnostic Tests

Complete blood count to include the following:

- RBC, WBC, platelets [complete blood count (CBC) with differential].
- Hemoglobin and hematocrit.
- RBC indices such as mean corpuscular volume, mean corpuscular hemoglobin concentration, and mean corpuscular hemoglobin.
- WBC indices include the percent of all five types of WBCs (basophils, eosinophils, monocytes, lymphocytes, neutrophils).
- Absolute neutrophil count uses both the segmented (mature neutrophils) and bands (immature neutrophils) as a measure of the body's infection fighting capability; calculated by adding percentage of segmented neutrophils to percentage of bands and then multiplying this percentage by the WBC count.
- Serum chemistry, which includes electrolytes, including sodium, potassium, chloride, calcium, magnesium, phosphorus, carbon dioxide.
- Other studies may include renal function studies such as blood urea nitrogen and creatinine; liver studies such as total bilirubin, alanine aminotransferase, aspirate aminotransferase, lactic dehydrogenase, and blood urea nitrogen.
- Certain substances, or markers, are elevated with some specific tumors—for example, alpha-fetoprotein level may be elevated in liver tumors; vanillylmandelic acid and homovanillic acid levels may be elevated in adrenal tumors; and elevated catecholamines are found in neuroblastoma.

Bone marrow aspiration

Bone marrow biopsy

Lumbar puncture

Radiographic examination

Magnetic resonance imaging (MRI)

Computed tomography (CT)

Ultrasound

Histologic or laboratory analysis of tumor cells after biopsy of tumor

Additional studies for certain cancers such as pulmonary function tests; echocardiograms; nuclear medicine scans with radioactive isotopes, such as gallium or iodine; bone scan with technetium 99m; or positron emission tomography and single-photon emission CT, which combine nuclear medicine with CT (Leonard, 2002)

Urinalysis

Clinical Therapy

A *protocol* is a plan of action for treatment that is based on the results of staging: type of cancer, its location, the particular cell type, and its degree of spread.

Surgery is used to remove or debulk (reduce the size of) a solid tumor; it is also used to determine the stage and type of cancer.

Chemotherapy is the administration of specific drugs that kill both normal and cancerous cells (Table 20–1).

Table 20–1 Medications Used for Cancer Chemotherapy

Medication	Action/Indication	Nursing Implications
Cell cycle–specific agents		
Antimetabolites: 5-azacytidine, 5-fluorouracil, 6-mercaptopurine, 6-thioguanine, cytosine arabinoside (cytarabine), hydroxyurea, methotrexate	Work at synthesis phase of cell division; interfere with function of nucleic acid; inhibit DNA or RNA synthesis.	Most common side effects are nausea and vomiting, myelosuppression, stomatitis. Specific agents such as methotrexate and cytarabine can cause neurologic toxicity with high doses. Consult drug books and package inserts for detailed list of side effects. Obtain baseline CBC, liver function, renal function. Monitor I&O and body weight. Ensure hydration and output levels ordered by oncologist. Monitor VS and cardiovascular and respiratory function. Watch for bleeding and signs of infection.

(continued)

Table 20–1 Medications Used for Cancer Chemotherapy (Continued)

Medication	Action/Indication	Nursing Implications
		Monitor carefully during administration for signs of anaphylaxis.
Vinca alkaloids: etoposide, teniposide, irinotecan, paclitaxel, vinblastine, vincristine	Act during mitosis; bind with cell proteins to inhibit nucleic acid and protein synthesis.	Common side effects include nausea and vomiting, abdominal cramping and diarrhea, constipation, paralytic ileus, hair loss, hypotension or hypertension, peripheral neuropathy, and neurologic toxicity (latter especially with vinblastine and vincristine). Obtain baseline blood work. Consult specific drug information for period of maximum myelosuppressive effect. Be alert for bruising, infection, and other signs of myelosuppression. Monitor carefully during administration for signs of anaphylaxis.
Miscellaneous—G_1 phase activity: L-asparaginase	Causes depletion of asparagine which is needed by cancer cells; makes cell in G phase vulnerable to other agents; interferes with prosynthesis. Used in combination with other agents in leukemia and other cancers.	Administered intravenously. Major side effects are severe nausea and vomiting, hypersensitivity, renal failure, myelosuppression, acid–base imbalance. CBC, serum amylase, glucose, coagulation factors, bone marrow function, liver function tests performed before therapy and twice weekly. Monitor I&O, neurologic status, gastrointestinal symptoms, abdominal pain.

(continued)

Table 20–1 Medications Used for Cancer Chemotherapy (Continued)

Medication	Action/Indication	Nursing Implications
Miscellaneous—G_2 phase activity: etoposide	Works at G_2 phase; binds cellular proteins to cause metaphase arrest; also acts on S phase of DNA synthesis. Used with other agents, particularly in recurrent disease.	Administered orally and intravenously. Common side effects are nausea and vomiting, myelosuppression, hair loss, diarrhea. Can cause anaphylaxis; hypotension and intravenous site pain with rapid infusion. Perform baseline CBC, liver and renal function tests. Check intravenous site frequently because extravasation can cause necrosis. Monitor VS during infusion, and stop drug if hypotension occurs.
Cell cycle–nonspecific agents		
Alkylating agents: cyclophosphamide, carboplatin, cisplatin, busulfan, chlorambucil, ifosfamide, thiotepa, mechlorethamine, melphalan, procarbazine, dacarbazine	Substitute an alkyl group for a hydrogen atom, leading to blockage of DNA replication. Used for treatment of many cancers, either alone or in conjunction with other agents.	Most are administered orally and/or intravenously. Array of side effects depending on specific drug. Some common side effects are nausea and vomiting, diarrhea, myelosuppression, hair loss, neuropathies, pulmonary toxicity, renal damage; secondary tumors later in life associated with some agents. Obtain CBC and full blood work before and during treatment. Monitor for side effects of the specific agents administered. Ensure generous hydration and monitor I&O. Teach family the importance of long-term monitoring for secondary tumors.

(continued)

Table 20–1 Medications Used for Cancer Chemotherapy (Continued)

Medication	Action/Indication	Nursing Implications
Antibiotics: doxorubicin, mitomycin C, dactinomycin, bleomycin, daunorubicin, idarubicin, mitoxantrone	Interfere with nucleic acid, inhibiting DNA or RNA synthesis. Used in combination with other agents to treat leukemia and other childhood cancers.	Most are administered intravenously. Common side effects include nausea and vomiting, myelosuppression, oral ulcers, skin and pulmonary toxicity. Several have cumulative dose toxicity, such as cardiac abnormalities (doxorubicin) and skin/pulmonary complications (bleomycin); total dose the child has received must be monitored. Obtain baseline CBC and other blood studies and monitor throughout therapy. Monitor VS, lung function, cardiac function, neurologic status throughout and after therapy. Be alert for signs of myelosuppression and mucosal ulcers.
Nitrosoureas: carmustine, lomustine	Cross breakage in DNA strands so that DNA and RNA replication cannot occur. Used in lymphomas and other childhood cancers. Can cross blood–brain barrier.	Administered orally (lomustine) or intravenously (carmustine). Major side effect is myelosuppression. Others include pulmonary fibrosis, eye infarction, skin changes, hair loss, nausea and vomiting. Obtain baseline and periodic CBC and other studies. Monitor pulmonary function, skin, and signs of infection or bleeding.
Hormones: prednisone, prednisolone, dexamethasone	Analogue of hydrocortisone; anti-inflammatory; delayed and depressed immune response. Used in conjunction with other agents for many types of childhood cancer.	Often administered orally. Numerous side effects, including edema, moon face, mood lability, increased appetite, disturbed sleep, immunosuppression, disturbed glucose control, osteoporosis.

(continued)

Table 20–1   Medications Used for Cancer
Chemotherapy (Continued)

Medication	Action/Indication	Nursing Implications
		Teach child and family the effects of the drug. Minimize exposure to persons with infection. Monitor for infections in all systems. Monitor weight regularly. Take VS. Teach to take as directed. Drug must be tapered slowly at end of therapy.
Topoisomerase I inhibitor: irinotecan, mitoxantrone, topotecan	Inhibit the enzyme topoisomerase I in the cell nucleus, relaxing DNA and preventing its duplication. Used in conjunction with other agents to treat acute lymphoblastic leukemia and other childhood cancers.	Administered intravenously. Topotecan can be given intrathecally. Common side effects include nausea and vomiting, diarrhea, fever, dehydration, myelosuppression. Can alter liver function and cause skin changes. Obtain baseline and periodic CBC and other studies, including liver function. Monitor for signs of myelosuppression, gastrointestinal distress, change in liver function.

CBC, complete blood count; I&O, input and output; VS, vital signs.

Other drugs used in the treatment of children with cancer include colony-stimulating factors, antiemetics, and nutritional supplements (Table 20–2).

Radiation therapy involves the use of unstable isotopes that release varying levels of energy to cause breaks in the DNA molecule and thereby destroy cells.

Biotherapy is the use of biologic retooling and molecular intervention to produce targeted cancer therapy (Arceci & Cripe, 2002); examples include biologic retooling such as development of antibodies that are tumor-specific to certain cancers, use of drugs that stimulate the body's own immune response, cancer vaccines, gene therapy, and molecular targeting.

Hematopoietic stem cell transplantation (HSCT).

Section III: Body Systems

Alterations in Cellular Growth **345**

Table 20–2   Colony-Stimulating Factors

Medication	Action/Indication	Nursing Implications
Epoetin alfa (human recombinant erythropoietin)	This glycoprotein stimulates the bone marrow in red blood cell formation; useful when numbers of red blood cells are low due to chemotherapy effects.	Give subcutaneously or intravenously. Do not shake, and do not use if discolored or particles are present. Single-dose vials only, so discard any solution that is not used. Obtain blood tests before therapy and periodically after; improvement in hematocrit should be seen in 7–14 days. Monitor blood pressure before and during therapy, as hypertension can result. Monitor for change in neurologic response and headache; both seizures and strokes are possible side effects.
Filgrastim (Neupogen) and pegfilgrastim (Neulasta)	This human granulocyte colony-stimulating factor increases production of neutrophils by the bone marrow.	Administered subcutaneously and intravenously; prepare as directed for intravenous infusion to prevent its absorption by intravenous tubing. Single-dose vials only, so discard any solution that is not used. Incompatible with many medications; check package insert; do not give within 24 hours before or after chemotherapy drugs or their effect may be decreased. Obtain baseline and twice-weekly complete blood count. Monitor for side effects such as bone pain and heart arrhythmias; report fevers, and be alert for other signs of infection when neutrophil count is low.

(continued)

Table 20–2   Colony-Stimulating Factors (Continued)

Medication	Action/Indication	Nursing Implications
Oprelvekin (Neumega)	A hematopoietic growth factor, interleukin-11, that increases platelet count; useful in low platelet count due to chemotherapy effects on bone marrow.	Administered subcutaneously. Single-dose vials only, so discard any solution that is not used. Obtain baseline complete blood count and platelet count; monitor platelets throughout treatment. Monitor for side effects such as edema, fever, central nervous system changes, tachycardia, respiratory problems, and skin rash. Take daily weights and monitor for fluid retention.

Complementary therapies such as nutritional supplements, oral herbal supplements, touch therapy, and mind/body interventions.

In cases that cannot be successfully treated, the focus of healthcare is palliative care, providing comfort and emotional support for the terminally ill child and family.

Nursing Management
Assessment
History to identify cancer contains several components:

- Complete a genogram to identify any family history of cancer.
- Ask about history of exposure to known carcinogens, such as whether a parent works in an industry with substances such as chemicals or asbestos that might remain on clothing worn home, whether the child has been treated with radiation or chemotherapy for a previous cancer, and if the child has an identified condition such as Down syndrome or has any recognized congenital anomalies.

Physiologic assessment must be thorough when cancer or potential cancer is diagnosed:

- When the child has some symptoms of cancer, evaluation for anemia, frequent infections, bleeding disorders, loss of weight, fatigue, pain, and changes in mental health and neurologic status should be performed.

- Height and weight should be carefully measured and compared with prior findings for the child; nutrition intake history may be pertinent.
- Assess hydration status and the tumor site if it is visible.
- Evaluate pain, fatigue, infections, bruising, shortness of breath, and elimination problems.
- Observe immunization status, developmental milestones, gait, and coordination, as well as any changes in mental status.
- All body systems have thorough assessment; systems needing particular attention include neurologic, respiratory, cardiac, and gastrointestinal.
- Extensive laboratory and radiologic/imaging studies are performed.

Cancer creates many emotional challenges, so thorough psychosocial assessment is needed:

- Gather information about the crisis from the perspective of the family (Hendricks-Ferguson, 2000).
- Assess the family members (and child if old enough) for their understanding and acceptance of the diagnosis.
- Evaluate if the family has told the child about the diagnosis and whether the family needs assistance in deciding how to do this (Ishibashi, 2001).
- Ask what they have told siblings and if they need suggestions, help, and support to decide how much and when to share information with the child's siblings.
- Assess the level of anxiety during healthcare visits and scheduled treatments.
- Evaluate the family's resilience and methods of coping, such as the ability to integrate relaxing and meaningful activities into family life, the use of support systems in the extended family and community, and the ability to alter expectations to take into account the child's health status.
- Evaluate the family for stressors such as illness or death of another family member, occupational changes, financial problems, relocation, and change in vacation plans.
- Evaluate the family's knowledge of the U.S. Family Leave Act, which provides for parental use of sick time to treat an ill family member; inquire if the family's insurance carrier provides for a case manager in complex health needs such as cancer.
- Assess whether faith-based affiliations and healers are meaningful for the family.

- Ask parents about complementary therapy and medications they are obtaining from other sources and using at home.
- Evaluate the child's and family's knowledge and information sources, providing them with opportunities to ask questions.
- Assess the learning style of the child and family to adapt approaches to meet their needs.
- When the treated child is returning to school, evaluate the ability of the school to accept a medically vulnerable child into the classroom.
- Drawings, colored pictures cut out by the child to form a collage, discussion, and observation are used to assess for body image changes that occur as a result of cancer and its treatment.

Developmental assessment of children should be performed regularly during treatment for cancer, at times when the child feels well, so that results are accurate.

For the child who survives cancer, ongoing assessments are essential. Evaluate the child regularly with thorough physical, psychosocial, developmental, and cognitive assessments; carefully monitor all body systems (e.g., cardiovascular; respiratory; musculoskeletal; eye, ear, nose, and throat; genitourinary); record height and weight and general growth patterns; ask about the child's interactions with peers and performance at school; be alert for signs and symptoms that could indicate a secondary tumor.

Intervention

Ensure optimal nutritional intake because approximately 30% of children with cancer are malnourished; during treatment offer frequent, small meals.

Special nutritional products may be given orally, nasogastric or nasoduodenal tube feedings may be given, or total parenteral nutrition may be necessary.

Administer antiemetic drugs to lessen nausea from chemotherapy and radiation.

Chemotherapy drugs are prepared with special techniques under laminar flow devices to minimize potential toxic effects on healthcare providers using gloves and other hazardous drug protocols; follow the guidelines of the Occupational Safety and Health Administration in "Controlling Occupational Exposure to Hazardous Drugs" (U.S. Department of Labor, 2003).

Avoid extravasation of intravenous drugs (leakage into the soft tissue around the infusion site), as permanent tissue damage can result.

Administer fluids to ensure adequate hydration during treatments.

Administer other supportive medications as ordered, such as antiemetics to control nausea, vitamin supplements, and antibiotics.

Monitor for side effects such as myelosuppression and neutropenia; treatments may include antibiotics, granulocyte colony-stimulating factors, and colony-stimulating factors (see Table 20–2).

Monitor for thrombocytopenia; protect the child from bruises, and be alert for signs of bleeding such as petechiae, nosebleeds, and dark-colored or bloody stools, and presence of blood in vomit and urine; minimize needle sticks and other intrusive procedures during periods of thrombocytopenia; platelet infusions may be needed.

Monitor for anemia; encourage high iron intake, and administer infusions as needed.

Provide good oral hygiene with a soft toothbrush, foam wand, or water irrigation device and report oral breakdown promptly.

Partner with the oncologist, dentist, and nutritionist to plan treatment strategies to protect the oral health and erupting teeth of children.

Know all side effects of specific drugs administered and monitor for them; realize that some side effects are late and may be seen after therapy is completed.

Emphasize importance of all follow-up visits scheduled in the future for monitoring of late effects.

During radiation therapy, examine the skin daily during hospitalization or weekly when making home visits; leave the marks on the skin that outline the radiation target area; avoid use of lotions, powders, and soaps on the target skin area.

Management of infections is critical; children may be hospitalized and central lines inserted for antibiotic administration; blood cultures and cultures of infected body parts help to establish the causative organisms; administer medication treatment on time and as ordered; ensure that standard precautions and transmission-based precautions are followed; monitor temperature, vital signs, and assessment of all body systems at least every 4 hours.

Use pain management techniques to keep the child comfortable during diagnostic procedures and treatments; conscious sedation and local anesthetics are commonly used.

Facilitate contact with extended family members who might be of help, religious or spiritual connections, social service agencies, and other resources such as Internet and parent-support groups.

Assist parents who are concerned about job obligations and financial concerns.

Patient and Family Education

Basic information about the disease and the purpose of the tests that will be performed is needed as soon as the diagnosis is made.

Instructions often need to be repeated, as parents may not process information the first time it is presented due to their increased stress levels.

Assist the parents to plan how and when to tell the child the diagnosis.

Help the family to identify support systems, and intervene as needed to enhance these systems.

A variety of information and teaching approaches are needed, with specifics dependent on the child's particular treatment (Box 20–1).

The child undergoing treatment for cancer needs support appropriate to his or her developmental stage and cognitive level.

Box 20–1 The Family and Cancer Treatment

Most parents are not aware of the effects of cancer treatment and how they can help children through this experience. Depending on the stage and type of treatment, there are several suggestions to make to parents:

- Children in radiation and chemotherapy are fatigued. Provide extra rest periods with shorter activity periods between them.
- Have an overnight bag ready in case the child develops a complication and needs to be taken to stay in the hospital for a few days. Several hospital stays of a few days are normal during treatment.
- When concerned about a symptom in the child, ask the care provider. Parents are often key in identifying problems early.
- Parents are usually concerned about central line care but feel more comfortable after a few days of caring for the line.
- Children may not feel hungry, and so nutritional intake is needed when they are ready to eat.
- Remember that the children are still at the normal developmental age. Treat them as a reflection of their ages, not as if they are older or younger.
- Try to maintain contact with the child's peer group and family members.
- Seek information from other parents and resources on cancer care.
- Remind parents to get time away and relax so that parental energy remains high and they are better able to deal with the child's therapy.

Talk with the child's teachers before the return to school after treatment to explain the child's condition and assist with plans to prepare the other children; role-play with the child how to tell friends about any changes in appearance.

Explore the option of summer camp for children with cancer.

The Make-a-Wish Foundation strives to make dreams come true for ill children by sponsoring them for a desired activity or outing; refer the child to this foundation if appropriate.

Ask how care has changed for the child's siblings and what they have been told about the disease; assist the family to talk with them and inform their teachers about the family stress.

Teach the parents how to ensure adequate nutritional intake, to be alert for signs of infection, to protect the child from exposure to communicable diseases during times of neutropenia, to administer medications at home, and how to handle vomiting and pain.

Teach the parents and family about symptoms that need to be treated immediately (Box 20–2).

Box 20–2   Reportable Events for Children Receiving Chemotherapy

---

Parents require verbal and written instructions about signs and symptoms to report to the child's oncologist while the child is receiving chemotherapy.

Have parents report the following events to your child's oncologist if they occur while the child is receiving chemotherapy:

- Temperature above 38°C (101°F)
- Any bleeding, such as nosebleeds, blood in stool or urine, petechiae, bruising
- Pain or discomfort with urination or defecation
- Sores in the mouth
- Vomiting or diarrhea
- Persistent pain anywhere, including headache
- Signs of infection, such as cough, fever, runny nose, tugging at ears
- Signs of infection in central lines, such as redness, drainage, or tenderness
- Exposure to communicable diseases, especially varicella (chickenpox)

Inform dentists and other healthcare providers that the child is receiving chemotherapy before procedures. Prophylactic antibiotics should be given before and after dental care.

Adapted from Bindler, R. M., & Howry, L. B. (2005). Pediatric drug guide. Upper Saddle River, NJ: Prentice Hall Health.

Assist the parents and child to deal with any obstacles to normal development and functioning.

Teach home management of a vascular access device or central line, such as a Broviac catheter; details about cleaning the site, instilling heparin in the line or reservoir, and other needed care should be demonstrated and reviewed before discharge to home.

Emphasize the need for the child and family to have fun and be as normal as possible; play or recreation is needed for all family members.

Help parents to view the child as a "normal" child who is ill for a period of time but still needs to have limits set on behavior; develop health lifestyles; and have environmental stimulation to learn to talk, read, or perform motor and cognitive tasks.

BRAIN TUMORS
Clinical Manifestations

Central nervous system or brain tumors are the most commonly occurring solid tumors in children and the second most common malignancy after leukemia.

Brain tumors in children usually occur below the roof of the cerebellum and involve the cerebellum, midbrain, and brainstem.

The most common brain tumors in children are medulloblastoma, cerebral and cerebellar astrocytoma, ependymoma (from ependymal cells lining the brain ventricles and spinal cord canal), and gliomas of the cerebrum or brainstem; less common are supratentorial embryonal tumors and craniopharyngioma.

Children with brain tumors can manifest behavioral and neurologic changes; these may occur rapidly or slowly and subtly.

Some common symptoms include headache, nausea, vomiting, dizziness, change in vision or hearing, fatigue, and mental status changes.

Presenting signs can be categorized as follows:
- Nonspecific signs related to increasing intracranial pressure
- Secondary signs related to displacement of intracranial structures
- Focal signs suggesting direct involvement of the brain and cranial nerves

Brainstem tumors can present with weight deficits and may be mistakenly diagnosed as an eating disorder of infancy and childhood (failure to thrive).

Medulloblastomas are brain tumors in the external layer of the cerebellum, accounting for 20% of childhood brain tumors, and commonly occur in children 5–6 years of age. They are fast-growing and present with symptoms such as increased intracranial pressure, manifested by increased head circumference in infants, vomiting, headache, ataxia, and vision changes.

Astrocytomas arise from glial cells and can be either above or below the area between the cerebrum and cerebellum and comprise 40% of childhood brain tumors. The presenting symptoms vary and include endocrine, vision, behavioral changes, and increased intracranial pressure and seizures (Ryan-Murray & Petriccione, 2002).

Ependymomas commonly occur in the fourth ventricle of the posterior fossa and comprise 10% of childhood brain tumors. Impaired growth, hydrocephalus, seizures, and cranial nerve impairments are the most common manifestations.

Brainstem gliomas account for 15% of childhood brain tumors and are located in the pons and typically spread into the surrounding tissue. Cranial nerve impairments, mental status changes, and motor symptoms occur (Conway, Asuncion, & DaRosso, 1999).

Diagnostic Tests

Health history and physical examination.

CT.

MRI.

Positron emission tomography.

Single-photon emission CT.

Myelography.

Angiography.

Neurophysiologic tests (electroencephalography and brainstem evoked potentials) assess sensory pathway integrity and disease- or drug-related sensory dysfunction.

Examination for serum tumor markers such as alpha-fetoprotein and human chorionic gonadotropin are sometimes helpful.

Lumbar puncture may be used to identify abnormal cells in the cerebrospinal fluid.

Bone marrow aspiration and bone scans identify any extracranial primary neoplastic growth, as cancers in other sites can metastasize to or from the brain.

Clinical Therapy

Surgery is a common treatment and may be performed to obtain a biopsy specimen, to debulk (reduce the tumor size by partial removal) or excise the tumor, or to treat any hydrocephalus that may be present.

Radiation is commonly used.

Chemotherapy can shrink and help manage some tumors; intrathecal administration of chemotherapy is useful in some cases.

HSCT is an increasingly used treatment option.

Treatment of associated symptoms such as seizures and endocrine disturbance may be needed.

Nursing Management

Assessment

Thorough neurologic examination, including measurement of head circumference and assessment of the anterior fontanel, is necessary in children younger than age 18 months.

Perform developmental screening.

Ask about the child's social interactions, school performance, and any behavior changes that have occurred.

Intervention

Close monitoring of neurologic status is needed postoperatively and during all treatments.

Administer drugs such as chemotherapy, antibiotics, steroids, and anticonvulsants as ordered.

Explain procedures and treatments, the purpose of lines, and the use of sedation to keep the child restful, and answer any questions of the family.

Ask parents about resources such as other family members, available sick leave from work, and places to stay if they live far from the hospital.

Ensure that parents can recognize signs of infection and changes in the child's neurologic status at home.

Chemotherapy or radiation often occurs on an outpatient basis; inform parents of the desired outcome and potential side effects of these treatments.

Assist the family in obtaining any special equipment they may need to care for the child at home, such as a wheelchair, bed rails, or dressings.

Once treatment is completed, encourage regular healthcare visits to monitor for sequelae of treatment or recurrence of cancer.

NEUROBLASTOMA
Clinical Manifestations

Neuroblastoma is commonly a smooth, hard, nontender mass that can occur anywhere along the sympathetic nervous system chain; a frequent location is the abdomen, although other sites are the adrenal, thoracic, and cervical areas.

Neuroblastoma is nearly unheard of after 10 years of age and is usually diagnosed in children younger than age 5 years, with the median age at diagnosis being 2 years of age (McManus & Gilchrist, 2000).

Characteristic signs are weight loss, abdominal distention, enlarged liver, irritability, fatigue, and fever.

Altered bowel and bladder function occur when the mass is retroperitoneal.

Dyspnea or infection may occur when the tumor is mediastinal.

Neck and facial edema may result from vena cava syndrome if the tumor is mediastinal and large.

Intracranial lesions may be present with periorbital ecchymosis.

Malaise, fever, and a limp can occur if there has been metastasis to the bone.

Bone marrow disease can manifest as *pancytopenia* (abnormal depression of all cellular blood components) with neutropenia (causing infections) and anemia (causing fatigue).

Metastatic spread can result in an array of symptoms affecting multiple organs.

Diagnostic Tests

Routine blood cell counts are needed, including CBC with differential.

Tumor markers include vanillylmandelic acid, homovanillic acid, dopamine, ferritin, neuron-specific enolase, lactic dehydrogenase, and a ganglioside, GD2.

Tests for initial tumor include the following:

- Tumor tissue diagnosis by light microscopy
- Biopsy of tumor cells plus laboratory evaluation showing increased urine or serum catecholamines (two separate measures, each more than three standard deviations above the norm for age)

Tests for metastases include the following:

- Bone marrow aspirate and biopsy
- Radiolabeled scanning with metaiodobenzylguanidine
- Bone scan
- Skeletal x-ray
- CT or MRI of abdomen, liver, brain, eye orbits
- MRI of spine
- Chest x-ray with added CT or MRI if x-ray shows lesions

Clinical Therapy

Surgical excision of the mass is performed and may be the only treatment in low-risk stages.

With higher risk stages, surgery is followed by chemotherapy with a combination of drugs such as the following:

- Cyclophosphamide
- Ifosfamide
- Doxorubicin
- Cisplatin
- Carboplatin
- Teniposide
- Etoposide

Radiation is often used, especially in disseminated disease.

HSCT may be performed for advanced disease, sometimes followed by the biologic modifier *cis*-retinoic acid and fenretinide (to promote apoptosis).

Nursing Management

The presenting site of the tumor, such as the neck or abdomen, is assessed by observation and inspection; palpation is contraindicated.

Document related functioning, such as bowel and bladder function.

Take vital signs to watch for elevated temperature and vital sign changes caused by a thoracic mass.

Observe gait and coordination.

Take weight and height (or length for infant) and compare with earlier percentiles for the child.

Psychosocial assessment and emotional assessment of the family are needed.

The nursing management of the child with neuroblastoma can encompass the three phases of medical treatment: chemotherapy, surgery, and radiation; see nursing management sections earlier in this chapter.

WILMS' TUMOR (NEPHROBLASTOMA)

Nephroblastoma, an intrarenal tumor that is called *Wilms' tumor*, is a common abdominal tumor of childhood and accounts for 6% to 7% of all childhood tumors (Anderson, 2004).

Wilms' tumor is usually an asymptomatic, firm, lobulated mass located to one side of the midline in the abdomen.

Hypertension caused by increased renin activity related to renal damage is reported in 25% of cases; hematuria or abdominal pain is sometimes present.

The diagnosis of Wilms' tumor is based on an ultrasound study of the abdomen and an intravenous pyelogram; CT scanning or MRI of the lungs, liver, spleen, and brain may be performed to identify any metastasis; a complete blood count is obtained, as well as blood urea nitrogen and creatinine levels; liver function tests are performed; histologic examination is performed for tissue typing once the tumor is removed.

Surgery is performed to remove the affected kidney, to examine the opposite kidney, to remove lymph nodes for examination, and to look for other sites of metastasis.

Chemotherapy or radiation therapy, alone or in combination, is sometimes used before surgery to reduce the size of the tumor.

Children with stages III and IV disease often receive vincristine, dactinomycin, and doxorubicin; cyclophosphamide is sometimes added; radiation may also follow surgery, especially in disseminated disease.

Nursing Management

Perform a thorough baseline assessment of the child; **do not palpate** the abdomen because of the potential for spreading the cancerous cells.

Monitor the child's blood pressure carefully, as hypertension is a common finding that may require treatment.

Nursing care during the postrenal surgery phase focuses on pain management and close monitoring of fluid levels; assess daily weight, intake and output (I&O), and urine specific gravity; monitor the function of the remaining kidney; take blood pressure measurements frequently to watch for signs of shock and to assess the functioning of the remaining kidney.

During the chemotherapy phase, monitor the child for side effects of drugs, the potential for infection from the central line site, and the function of the remaining kidney.

Advise parents about home care needs, administration of medications, and monitoring for drug side effects and ongoing needs for health monitoring.

OSTEOSARCOMA, OR OSTEOGENIC SARCOMA

Osteosarcoma is a rare, malignant bone tumor that occurs predominantly in adolescent boys; the tumor is usually located at the metaphysis of the distal femur, proximal tibia, or proximal humerus (Betcher, Simon, & McHard, 2002).

Common initial symptoms of osteosarcoma are pain, swelling or mass, and limp or decreased motion; pain can be referred to the hip or back, which can delay diagnosis; pulmonary metastasis may occur; other metastatic sites include kidney, adrenals, brain, and pericardium.

Diagnosis of osteosarcoma is made through radiographic studies of the affected area and bone scan; CT or MRI scans of involved bone and other potential sites are performed; a complete blood count, liver studies, and renal studies are done for clues to metastases; a blood test is included for serum alkaline phosphatase (level may be elevated), and tumor biopsy is performed to confirm the diagnosis; arteriography may be performed if limb-sparing surgery is contemplated; cardiac assessments are performed to establish baseline function before treatment with doxorubicin.

Treatment involves both surgery and chemotherapy.

Surgery is either a limb-salvage procedure or limb amputation.

Chemotherapy is started before surgery to shrink the tumor, especially in cases where limb-salvage surgery is performed. It is also given postoperatively to treat and prevent metastasis. Drugs commonly used for osteosarcoma include doxorubicin, cisplatin, ifosfamide with mesna, and methotrexate with leucovorin rescue.

Nursing Management

Assess the child's pain or discomfort, mobility, and gait; take vital signs, especially noting temperature and respirations; psychologic assessment of the child and family are needed, especially if amputation is planned; body image disturbances occur when a limb is lost, particularly with school-age children and adolescents; assess the child's understanding of the treatment and of care after surgery; find out what support systems are available for assistance.

Observe the wound postoperatively for infection and hemorrhage; assess circulation above and below the operative site; if edema is found, elevate the limb.

Perform general postsurgical care such as skin care and pain management.

Assess body image and psychosocial adaptation.

Administer chemotherapy if ordered and instruct child and family about the medications.

Ensure that physical rehabilitation is planned and refer appropriately.

Assist the child in transition back into the school system as needed.

EWING'S SARCOMA

Ewing's sarcoma is a malignant, small, round cell tumor usually involving the diaphyseal (shaft) portion of the long bones; the most common sites are the femur, pelvis, tibia, fibula, ribs, humerus, scapula, and clavicle, but any bone may be involved.

Symptoms are similar to those of osteosarcoma and may include pain, swelling, fever, an elevated WBC count, elevated erythrocyte sedimentation rate, and elevated C-reactive protein; a fracture of the affected bone may occur.

Tumor biopsy is necessary for diagnosis, as well as tests described previously for osteosarcoma.

Initial treatment for Ewing's sarcoma is chemotherapy to reduce the tumor, followed by surgical removal of the entire bone or intensive high-dose irradiation of the entire bone; limb-salvage procedures are now commonly performed rather than amputation.

Chemotherapy is always used after initial treatment, as undetectable metastases are commonly present; drugs may include vincristine, doxorubicin, cyclophosphamide, dactinomycin, etoposide, and ifosfamide.

See Osteosarcoma, or Osteogenic Sarcoma for nursing management.

LEUKEMIA
Clinical Manifestations

Leukemia, a cancer of the blood-forming organs, is the most commonly diagnosed pediatric malignancy in children younger than age 14 years; it is characterized by a proliferation of abnormal WBCs in the body.

The main types are acute lymphoblastic leukemia, acute nonlymphoblastic leukemia, and the rare chronic leukemias of childhood.

Leukemia occurs when the stem cells in the bone marrow produce immature WBCs that cannot function normally; these cells proliferate rapidly by cloning instead of normal mitosis, causing the bone marrow to fill with abnormal WBCs; the abnormal cells then spill out into the circulatory system, where they steadily replace the normally functioning WBCs; as this occurs, the protective lymphocytic functions such as cellular and humeral immunity are reduced, leaving the body vulnerable to infections; the malignant WBCs rapidly fill the bone marrow, replacing stem cells that produce erythrocytes (RBCs) and other blood products such as platelets, thereby decreasing the amount of these products in circulation.

Children with acute lymphoblastic leukemia and acute nonlymphoblastic leukemia usually have fever, pallor, overt signs of bleeding, lethargy, malaise, anorexia, and large joint or bone pain.

Petechiae, frank bleeding, and joint pain are cardinal signs of bone marrow failure.

Enlargement of the liver and spleen (hepatosplenomegaly) and changes in the lymph nodes (lymphadenopathy) are common.

If the leukemia has infiltrated the central nervous system (entered it by means of the circulatory or lymphoid system), the child may exhibit signs such as headache, vomiting, papilledema, and sixth cranial nerve palsy (inability to move the eye laterally).

The testicles, spinal cord, and bone marrow are common sites for infiltration.

Diagnostic Tests

Diagnosis is based initially on blood counts and bone marrow aspiration; blood counts reveal anemia, thrombocytopenia, and neutropenia; bone marrow aspiration reveals immature and abnormal lymphoblasts and hypercellular marrow and is the differential test (see common laboratory values in leukemia in Box 20–3).

Box 20–3	Laboratory Values in Leukemia	
	Normal	Common values in leukemia
Leukocytes	<10,000/μL	>10,000/μL
Platelets	150,000–400,000/μL	20,000–100,000/μL
Hemoglobin	12–16 g/dL	7–11 g/dL

Percent of blast cells in marrow is measured, and 25% lymphoblasts is definitive of disease (Westlake & Bertolone, 2002).

Levels of serum uric acid and electrolytes such as calcium, potassium, and phosphorus are measured.

Leukemic cells are examined and classified by FAB type; DNA analysis may provide clues about genetic changes.

Clinical Therapy

Treatment of acute lymphoblastic leukemia involves radiation and chemotherapy; radiation is used for central nervous system disease, in T-cell leukemia, and for testicular involvement.

Intensive chemotherapy with several agents is the main treatment.

HSCT transplantation is a treatment option for the child who has a relapse with acute lymphoblastic leukemia and then achieves a second remission; the transplant is given when the child is in remission.

Transplant is also used for children with acute nonlymphoblastic leukemia; they do not need to be in remission for the transplant to be performed.

Nursing Management
Assessment

Thorough physical assessment is important to ensure prompt identification of problems without injuring the child who has deficient coagulation and immune function; observe carefully for bruising and other new sites of bleeding as well as fever or other signs of infection.

Once chemotherapy has begun, closely monitor renal functioning through specific gravity, I&O, and daily weight measurement; monitor dietary intake, nausea, vomiting, and constipation; observe for mucosal sores in the mouth.

A central line is usually in place for intravenous infusion of medications, so careful assessment of the line for proper functioning and for signs of infection is needed.

Ask the parents about any behavioral changes; central nervous system infiltration can affect the child's level of consciousness, causing irritability, vomiting, and lethargy.

The intensive treatment involving frequent venipunctures, bone marrow aspirations, and lumbar punctures requires pain assessment and an evaluation of the level of knowledge and coping skills of child and family.

Intervention

Bone marrow suppression necessitates transmission-based precautions.

Perform careful handwashing; take temperature frequently; give mouth care with antibacterial mouth washes; inspect skin, mouth, rectal area, and central line site for any signs of infection.

Special attention to renal function is needed for certain drugs; hydration with intravenous fluids to attain a specific gravity of less than 1.010 prevents or reduces the severity of hematuria and potential renal damage.

Evaluate the infusion site before and frequently during infusion; although extravasation is not as common with central lines used in cancer treatment as in peripheral lines, it can occur; many chemotherapy agents are extremely toxic to tissues.

Careful monitoring of I&O is required to record intravenous fluids given during chemotherapy infusions, to assess kidney functioning, and to monitor excretion of byproducts from destroyed tumor cells; monitor specific gravity every 8 hours as well as before and during administration of the drug and when the intravenous fluids are reduced to maintenance volume levels.

Daily weight measurements are important to assist in planning adequate hydration during chemotherapy, as well as to measure nutritional status.

Drug side effects may necessitate infusion of platelets or packed RBCs.

Provide for management of pain during procedures, treatment, and general care.

Alter the environment to provide for frequent sleep periods, as the child commonly has disturbed sleep patterns.

Facilitate nutritional intake by offering frequent, small feedings of favorite foods and administering antiemetics during treatment that causes nausea.

Inspect oral mucosa and perform gentle oral hygiene.

Record stools and institute methods to prevent and treat constipation as needed.

Facilitate child and family coping; refer to support groups and encourage therapeutic play and recreation.

Alterations in Cellular Growth **363**

Recognize that cancer treatment often continues for years and the child requires ongoing assessment, treatment, and health promotion/health maintenance activities.

Patient and Family Education

Instruct parents in the prevention of infection and use nursing care measures to prevent infection.

Instruct in all details of treatment, such as expected effects and side effects of medication or chemotherapy, care of central lines, and fluid needs.

Suggest measures to child and family to enhance physical care:

- Have rest periods each day.
- Avoid areas of exposure to people with illnesses.
- Drink generous amounts of water.
- Eat a healthy diet, using frequent, small, and nutritious meals to obtain enough nutrients.
- Take medicines prescribed to decrease nausea.
- Maintain good oral hygiene with soft toothbrush and water pik.
- Avoid sun exposure and check skin each day for any signs of bruises, pressure areas, cuts, or scratches.
- Promote bowel elimination through regular dietary and toileting practices.
- Report any signs of infection, changes in condition, or other concerns.

Provide emotional care and resources:

- Be prepared for loss of hair with plans for hats, wigs, or other alternatives.
- Continue contact with friends via phone, via Internet, and in person when possible.
- Try relaxation techniques to aid in sleep and management of treatments.
- Talk with clergy, teachers, parents, counselors, friends, or other supportive people about the experience of having leukemia.
- Keep a journal to record feelings and experiences.

Assist in plans for return to school and use of tutors or other methods to provide for educational needs.

HODGKIN DISEASE

Hodgkin disease is manifested by nontender, firm lymphadenopathy, usually in the supraclavicular and cervical nodes but occasionally in the mediastinal area; a mediastinal growth can cause respiratory difficulty because of pressure on the trachea or bronchi.

Fever, night sweats, and weight loss occur in one-third of children with Hodgkin disease and are associated with a more aggressive form of the disease.

The leukocyte count and erythrocyte sedimentation rate may be elevated.

Diagnosis is based on lymph node biopsy; Reed-Sternberg cells (large cells with two nucleoli) are present.

A staging classification is used to determine disease severity; the basis for staging is data obtained from the history, physical examination, chest x-ray study (for metastasis), chest CT scan, CT or MRI scans of the retroperitoneal nodes, lymphangiogram if there is retroperitoneal involvement, laboratory studies (complete blood count, erythrocyte sedimentation rate, serum copper level, liver function tests), positron emission tomography, bone scans, and a radionuclide scan with gallium.

Bone marrow biopsy, bone scan, or a staging laparotomy may be performed in certain situations.

Chemotherapy using a four-drug combination has been found to be the most effective drug treatment. Drugs commonly used include Adriamycin (doxorubicin), bleomycin, cyclophosphamide, dacarbazine, etoposide, mechlorethamine, methotrexate, prednisone, procarbazine, and vinblastine.

Radiation is commonly added, with low doses for children who are still growing and larger doses for those who are physically mature or those whose disease is more advanced at diagnosis.

HSCT is a treatment option in children with advanced disease or relapse.

Nursing management for all soft tissue tumors is found in Retinoblastoma.

NON-HODGKIN LYMPHOMA

There are three types of pediatric non-Hodgkin lymphoma: (1) lymphoblastic lymphoma (30% to 40%), (2) small noncleaved cell (Burkitt's) lymphoma (40% to 50%), and (3) large cell lymphoma (15%) (Hussong, 2002).

Children with non-Hodgkin lymphoma present with fever, weight loss, and night sweats less often than those with Hodgkin disease.

The lymph glands are usually enlarged or nodular, with the most frequent sites being the cervical, axillary, inguinal, and femoral nodes; the disease may be diffuse, without nodular glands.

The anterior mediastinum is the primary site for T-cell lymphomas; tumors that occur in this area may compress the airway (causing breathing difficulty) or superior vena cava (leading to swelling of the face, neck, or arms) and can cause pain.

Jaw involvement is common in Burkitt's lymphoma.

An abdominal mass may cause pain, nausea, and vomiting.

CBC is performed; additional blood tests include renal and liver function, electrolytes, uric acid, and lactic dehydrogenase.

Bone marrow aspiration and lumbar puncture are performed.

Chest x-ray, bone scan, gallium scan, CT, and MRI can help to isolate affected body organs.

Diagnosis is confirmed by tissue biopsy.

A staging system is used to describe the tumor mass and extension to other body area; treatment is tailored to the type of cancer and its stage.

Stages I and II may be treated with drugs such as vincristine, cyclophosphamide, prednisone, and methotrexate for several months; intrathecal medication is added if head and neck cancers are present.

Stages III and IV are treated with additional drugs (up to nine total) for longer periods of time (1–2 years).

HSCT is a treatment option in children with advanced disease or relapse.

Nursing management for all soft tissue tumors is found in Retinoblastoma.

RHABDOMYOSARCOMA

Rhabdomyosarcoma is a soft tissue cancer that occurs most often in the muscles around the eyes (extraorbital); in the neck; and less commonly in the abdomen, genitourinary tract, and extremities; genitourinary, bladder, and prostate cancers are more common in children younger than age 5, whereas paratesticular and extremity cancer is more common among adolescents.

Tumors occurring close to the eye produce swelling, ptosis, visual disturbances, and eye movement abnormalities.

When the tumor occurs in the genitourinary tract, the result can be urinary obstruction, hematuria, dysuria, vaginal discharge, and a protruding vaginal mass.

Rhabdomyosarcoma occurring in the abdomen may be asymptomatic; there is rapid metastasis to the lungs, bones, bone marrow, and distant lymph nodes, with resultant multiple clinical manifestations.

Diagnosis of the mass is confirmed by CT, MRI, positron emission tomography, bone marrow aspiration, and biopsy.

CBC, renal and liver studies, and urinalysis are performed.

Lumbar puncture may be used in head and neck tumors.

A useful biologic marker, Desmin, allows differentiation of rhabdomyosarcoma from other round cell tumors.

Chest and lung CT scans are performed.

Treatment involves surgical removal of the tumor when possible.

Surgery is followed by wide-field radiation and chemotherapy with a combination of drugs such as actinomycin, cyclophosphamide, and vincristine.

Nursing management for all soft tissue tumors is found in Retinoblastoma.

RETINOBLASTOMA

Retinoblastoma is an intraocular malignancy of the retina.

The first sign of retinoblastoma is a white pupil, termed *leukokoria* or *cat's eye reflex*.

The red reflex is absent, asymmetric, or of a differing color in the affected eye.

Other symptoms may include a fixed strabismus (a constant deviation of one eye from the other), orbital inflammation, glaucoma, and heterochromia (irises of different colors).

Children at risk for retinoblastoma due to family history can be tested for the RB1 gene.

Diagnostic tests for the cancer include full ocular examination and CT or MRI scans of the eye orbit.

All children with a history of retinoblastoma in the family should be examined by an ophthalmologist after birth, at 6 weeks, every 2–3 months until 2 years and then every 4 months until 3 years, and then annually (Dulczak & Frothingham, 2002; Pakakasama & Tomlinson, 2002) to aid in early diagnosis.

Tumors are classified according to a staging system, from a very small, localized tumor (group I) to tumors involving more than half the retina and with seeding into the vitreous (group V).

Treatment for retinoblastoma may include removal of the eye (enucleation) when there is permanent retinal damage or failure to respond to other treatment.

Other surgical treatments involve cryotherapy or photocoagulation (argon laser therapy).

Radiation is nearly always used, either as the sole treatment or before surgery to shrink the tumor.

Chemotherapy is sometimes used but is often ineffective, as the drugs often fail to penetrate sufficiently into the eye; chemotherapy drugs include carboplatin, etoposide, vincristine, and cyclosporine.

Nursing Management
Assessment
Careful family histories can sometimes identify children at risk who need frequent physical examinations—for example, if a family history of retinoblastoma is present, the child should receive frequent eye examinations.

Physiologic assessment of the child with a soft tissue tumor, such as Hodgkin disease, non-Hodgkin lymphoma, rhabdomyosarcoma, and retinoblastoma, focuses on the child's general condition; accurate height and weight measurements are essential to provide a baseline against which to measure the child's growth during treatment, as well as for calculation of chemotherapeutic drug dosages.

Observe the area of the tumor, such as the face, neck, and abdomen, and describe any changes.

Monitor respiratory status if the tumor is on the face or neck; report any changes in respiratory pattern to the physician.

Avoid palpation of any tumor site or enlarged area; metastasis can be influenced by injudicious palpation and manipulation of a tumor site.

Notify the physician of a change in any lymph node or any other area of the body.

Gastrointestinal and genitourinary function can be altered by the presence of a tumor and by treatment such as chemotherapy and radiation; careful monitoring of the child's I&O measurement is essential.

Abdominal and pelvic tumors may affect defecation, so charting of all bowel movements is important; explain to the family and child why keeping accurate records is necessary.

Observe wounds closely for lack of healing as a result of chemotherapy or radiation.

Examine the mouth and extremities for wounds or ulcers.

Nutritional changes caused by treatment affect the body's ability to support healthy cells and heal wounds.

Assessment of the family's psychosocial status and coping mechanisms is an essential component of nursing care.

Assessment of body image is needed when the child has a soft tissue tumor affecting appearance of the head and neck.

Ask about symptoms of depression such as loneliness, lack of interest, anxiety, and suicidal thoughts in school-age children and adolescents.

Intervention
Children with lymphoma affecting the mediastinum may need respiratory support; position the child so that the head is elevated; administer chemotherapy drugs as ordered, maintaining adequate fluids to facilitate excretion of the resultant breakdown products; monitor the central line used for chemotherapy administration, and teach parents care of the central line when the child is at home.

For the child with a rhabdomyosarcoma involving the bladder, monitor urinary output carefully; report hematuria and painful urination; monitor the changes that occur during therapy; administer pain medications as needed, and use distraction and other techniques to decrease the child's discomfort; emphasize to parents the need for follow-up CT and MRI scans after completion of treatment.

When the child with retinoblastoma undergoes removal of the eye, the parents and child need detailed instructions on postsurgical care; demonstrate to the parents care of the socket and use of a conformer to maintain the eye socket shape; when healing is complete and the child receives a prosthetic eye, instruct parents about its insertion and care; the child can gradually be taught to take over this care when old enough; encourage periodic healthcare visits to monitor for signs of a tumor in the other eye.

Adapt developmental interventions as needed to accommodate for sensory alterations.

Attention is directed at the body changes of the cancer and its treatment; children and adolescents may need suggestions to deal with hair loss, disfigurement, and living with serious illness; referral to other children and teens with similar concerns may be helpful.

Parents of all children need help to encourage normal development in the child with cancer.

Nursing management during chemotherapy and radiation is discussed earlier in this chapter in the general sections on these treatment measures.

Patient and Family Education

Teach the family about the chemotherapy drugs and their side effects.

Teach about the care of surgically placed venous access devices.

Provide written and illustrated information about the chemotherapy protocol(s).

Provide the family with radiation and surgery education specific to the tumor treatment.

Refer the family to nutrition resources such as dietitians for ways to promote the child's adequate intake of food and fluid.

Reinforce with families the importance of long-term follow-up after treatment for a soft tissue tumor; increased risk for secondary cancers for two to three decades is possible, and early identification can help with prompt diagnosis (Metayer, Lynch, Clarke, et al., 2000).

Partner with other healthcare providers to provide instructions to families as the child transitions from oncology treatment back to the pediatrician so they understand the importance of telling all care providers about the cancer and treatment.

As children grow into teen and young adult years, help them to take over this important task in their care; recommended annual examinations include the following:
- CBC
- Physical examination with special attention to skin, abdomen, and thyroid

- Monitoring for signs of hypothyroidism and hyperthyroidism
- Neurologic and developmental examinations and monitoring of school performance
- First mammogram at 25 years for those with chest radiation
- Pap and pelvic examinations for teen and young adult women
- Mental status assessment
  (Smith, 2003)

21. Alterations in Gastrointestinal Function

STRUCTURAL DEFECTS

Cleft Lip and Palate

Description and Etiology

Cleft lip with or without cleft palate results from a failure of the maxillary processes to fuse with the elevations on the frontal prominence during the sixth week of gestation; normally, union of the upper lip is complete by the seventh week (Mitchell & Wood, 2000); fusion of the secondary palate occurs between 5 and 12 weeks of gestation.

The cause is believed to be multifactorial, involving a combination of environmental and genetic influences:

- Family history of the condition, presence of other malformations, such as tracheoesophageal fistula, maternal use of tobacco, parental age, the use of anticonvulsants or steroids during pregnancy, and infections during pregnancy; other medications that interfere with growth factors and enzymes crucial to cell differentiation and division include vitamin A, lithium, retinoids, and phenytoin (Mitchell & Wood, 2000)

Higher intake of folate appears to be protective against the defect.

Clinical Manifestations

Cleft lip may be a simple dimple in the vermilion border of the lip or a complete separation extending to the floor of the nose; the defect may be unilateral or bilateral and may occur alone or in combination with a cleft palate defect.

Cleft palate defects are less obvious when they occur without a cleft lip and may not be detected at birth unless a thorough examination of the oral cavity is performed; clefts of the hard palate form a continuous opening between the mouth and nasal cavity and may be unilateral or bilateral, involving just the soft palate or the soft and hard palate.

Diagnostic Tests

Cleft lip and palate are generally diagnosed prenatally, at birth, or during the newborn assessment by characteristic physical findings.

Because the defects are sometimes associated with other defects, diagnostic studies to detect ear deformities, skeletal deformities, heart defects, and genitourinary defects are conducted.

Clinical Therapy

Because speech, hearing, and dentition may be affected, coordinated care by specialists in plastic and oral surgery, audiology, speech, otolaryngology, and orthodontics is necessary.

The cleft lip is usually repaired after 10 weeks of age.

The lip is sutured together, and a stabilizing device is put in place to prevent tension on the suture line.

After surgery, the infant's elbows may be restrained to prevent flexion and resultant trauma to the facial suture lines; crying is minimized by use of pain medication and physical comforting.

Timing of the cleft palate repair depends on surgeon preference, the condition of the infant, and the size and severity of the cleft defect; most commonly, the closure is completed between 6 and 18 months of age.

Postoperative feeding protocols vary from the use of special nipples or syringes to breastfeeding.

Infants with cleft lip and cleft palate are prone to recurrent otitis media, which can lead to hearing problems, so ear infections should be promptly evaluated by a health professional with expertise in ear care and treatment.

The child who has had cleft palate repair will require orthodontic care; early visits permit assessment of tooth eruption and the need for future orthodontic work.

Nursing Management

Assessment

Assessment of the family's reactions is an integral part of care in the postpartum period.

Assess the infant's ability to feed adequately.

Perform thorough and ongoing assessments of all body systems, remaining alert for any other abnormalities.

Perform frequent growth measurements.

Assess developmental progression.

Intervention

Facilitate feeding of the infant, assisting the mother to breastfeed or providing special nursing bottles if needed.

Promote parent–infant bonding by explaining the nature of the structural defect and the procedure for correction.

Interact and speak to the infant in the parents' presence, and point out the infant's positive attributes, such as alertness, soft skin, or active movements.

Parents can also be referred to the American Cleft Palate-Craniofacial Association for information about the disorder.

Postoperative care for the infant involves vital signs; respiratory assessment; maintenance of suture line by prescribed cleansing, care to minimize crying, and positioning on back to prevent elbow flexion; pain control.

Ongoing care after surgery involves growth and developmental monitoring, careful assessment of ear infections, and referral for early dental and orthodontic care when needed.

Tracheoesophageal Atresia and Fistula
Description and Etiology

Esophageal atresia is a malformation that results from failure of the esophagus to develop as a continuous tube during the fourth and fifth weeks of gestation.

In esophageal atresia, the foregut fails to lengthen, separate, and fuse into two parallel tubes (the esophagus and trachea) during fetal development; instead, the esophagus may end in a blind pouch or develop as a pouch connected to the trachea by a fistula (tracheoesophageal fistula).

Esophageal atresia is often associated with a maternal history of polyhydramnios; associated anomalies may occur, including congenital heart defects, gastrointestinal or urinary tract anomalies, and musculoskeletal abnormalities.

Clinical Manifestations

Symptoms in the newborn include excessive salivation, drooling, and sneezing, often accompanied by the three classic signs—cyanosis, choking, and coughing.

During feeding, fluid returns through the nose and mouth; aspiration places the infant at risk for pneumonia; the abdomen may become distended secondary to air trapping.

Diagnostic Tests

Diagnosis is confirmed by attempting to pass a 5 or 8 French naso-gastric tube into the stomach; it will meet resistance and can be advanced only minimally.

Specific defects and associated anomalies are determined by radiologic examination.

Echocardiogram and abdominal ultrasound are performed.

Careful examination of the lungs is needed.

A delay in diagnosis can be fatal because ingested fluid or secretions may enter the lungs and lead to pneumonia.

Clinical Therapy

A nasogastric tube is inserted to suction the upper pouch.

Intravenous antibiotics and fluids are begun, and surgery is performed as soon as the infant is stable; the first stage usually involves ligation of the fistula and insertion of a gastrostomy tube, whereas, in the second stage, the two ends of the esophagus are reconnected, if possible.

Nursing Management

Assessment

The nurse should be alert for the signs and symptoms in the immediate newborn period.

Assess for difficulty feeding and excessive drooling.

Assess for the classic signs of choking, coughing, and cyanosis.

Assess for respiratory distress, and assess the lung sounds carefully.

Esophageal atresia is a surgical emergency; the infant requires close observation and intervention to maintain a patent airway in the preoperative period.

Intervention

Surgical intervention for a newborn is a stressful situation for the parents and family; the parents require emotional support throughout the infant's hospitalization.

Eliciting questions and allowing parents to participate in the infant's care, especially feeding (when permitted), can facilitate bonding and help to prepare parents for care of the infant after discharge.

Preoperatively, suction is readily available to remove any secretions that accumulate in the nasopharyngeal airway; place the infant with the head of the bed slightly elevated to minimize aspiration of secretions into the trachea; continuous or low-intermittent suction via a nasogastric tube is used to remove secretions from the blind pouch; oral fluids are withheld, and the infant is maintained with fluids administered intravenously or through an umbilical artery catheter.

Postoperatively, gastrostomy drainage is maintained, and intravenous fluids and antibiotics are administered; total parenteral nutrition (TPN) may be required until gastrostomy or oral feedings are tolerated; monitoring and assessment of feeding tolerance are ongoing; feedings are introduced slowly and in small amounts; assess for respiratory difficulty during reintroduction of feedings.

Monitor weight and growth and developmental achievements throughout the entire treatment period.

Collaborate with the parents regarding home care needs, and teach them about gastrostomy tube care and feeding, signs of infection, and how to prevent postoperative complications.

Pyloric Stenosis

Pyloric stenosis (also called *hypertrophic pyloric stenosis*) is a hypertrophy of the circular muscle of the pyloric canal causing obstruction.

The exact cause of pyloric stenosis is unknown, although immature function or absence of pyloric ganglion cells has been suggested (Letton, 2001).

Hypertrophy of the circular pylorus muscle results in stenosis of the passage between the stomach and the duodenum, partially obstructing the lumen of the stomach; the lumen becomes inflamed and edematous, which narrows the gastric outlet opening until the obstruction becomes complete; forceful vomiting becomes evident.

As the obstruction progresses, the infant becomes dehydrated and electrolytes are depleted, resulting in metabolic imbalances.

Manifestations usually become evident 2–8 weeks after birth, with peak incidence at 3–5 weeks; initially, the infant appears well or regurgitates slightly after feedings; as the obstruction progresses, the vomiting becomes projectile.

The infant generally appears hungry, especially after emesis; appears irritable and lethargic; fails to gain weight; and has fewer and smaller stools.

On physical examination, visible peristaltic waves across the abdomen and an olive-sized mass in the right upper quadrant may be evident; some infants have bloody gastric vomitus related to the mucosal erosion caused by gastritis or esophagitis.

An abdominal ultrasound is the most common study performed to confirm the diagnosis of pyloric stenosis.

Serum electrolyte and acid-base measurements are used to determine the degree of dehydration, electrolyte imbalance, and anemia; they reveal hypochloremia, metabolic alkalosis, and hyperbilirubinemia.

Surgical correction (pyloromyotomy) is the treatment of choice; open pyloromyotomy is performed through a periumbilical incision or through a small, transverse, upper abdominal incision, or laparoscopic pyloromyotomy is now used.

Nurses assess for signs and symptoms that may indicate the disorder; observe the infant's abdomen for the presence of peristaltic waves and auscultate bowel sounds that may be hyperactive; palpation reveals an olive-shaped mass in the right upper quadrant of the abdomen, especially when the stomach is empty such as after a vomiting episode.

Preoperatively, assess the infant's history of vomiting, vital signs, weight, and nutritional status; assess skin turgor, fontanels, urinary output, weigh diapers, capillary refill, and mucous membranes to determine whether hydration is adequate; measure vomitus and describe vomiting episodes; be alert for signs of an electrolyte imbalance, particularly low levels of serum chloride, sodium, potassium, and an elevated pH.

Maintain nothing-by-mouth (NPO) status, and administer intravenous fluids preoperatively.

Monitor intake and output (including vomitus), blood urea nitrogen, creatinine, and urine specific gravity; maintain patency of nasogastric tube, and measure aspirated content.

Postoperatively, maintain hydration status, monitor the surgical site for intactness and signs of infection, provide pain relief, initiate feedings as ordered, and support the family in learning about the disorder and home care needed on discharge.

Intussusception

Intussusception occurs when one portion of the intestine prolapses and then invaginates or telescopes into another; the most common site of intussusception is the ileocecal valve.

The etiology of intussusception is multifactorial; viral infection, use of medications that influence gut motility, and the body's inflammatory mediators, such as cytokine, nitric oxide, and prostaglandins, are all associated with increased rates of intussusception (Spiro, Arnold, & Barbone, 2003).

Decreased intestinal motility results, followed by impaired blood circulation to the intestinal tract involved; a proximal portion of the intestine invaginates into another portion of the intestine, typically in the direction of peristalsis; the walls of the intestine rub together, and the mesentery becomes compressed, resulting in inflammation, edema, obstruction, and decreased blood flow; telescoping of the intestine obstructs the passage of stool.

If uncorrected, intussusception can lead to life-threatening complications associated with necrosis, perforation, hemorrhage, peritonitis, and increasing pain.

Vomiting and passage of brown or reddish stool occur; a long, cylindrical palpable mass may be present in the upper right quadrant or mid-upper abdomen, and rectal bleeding may occur (Klein, Kapoor, & Shugerman, 2004).

Diagnosis is made on the basis of the history and confirmed by radiographs and ultrasound of the abdomen; stool for guaiac is performed.

Oxygen, saline, and aqueous contrast material may also be used to reduce the intussusception; if reduction of the intussusception does not occur with these methods, surgical intervention to reduce the invaginated bowel and remove any necrotic tissue is necessary.

Preoperative nursing assessment includes vital signs, monitoring for abdominal distention, and auscultating for bowel sounds every 4 hours; monitor intravenous intake, urine output, and measure any vomitus; assess for number and characteristics of stools.

Monitor fluid and electrolyte status, and maintain patent nasogastric tube.

Postoperative care focuses on monitoring for early signs of infection, managing the child's pain, and maintaining nasogastric tube patency; feeding protocols usually include clear liquid feeding or breastfeeding after bowel sounds are present with an advance to half-strength milk and other foods as the infant or child tolerates them.

Gastroschisis

Gastroschisis is a congenital defect of the ventral abdominal wall, characterized by herniation of abdominal viscera outside the abdominal cavity through a defect in the abdominal wall to the side (most often to the right) of the umbilicus.

The cause of gastroschisis is multifactorial and involves vascular disruption of the fetal mesenteric vessels; it is more common in infants of young mothers, particularly with a history of low socioeconomic status, smoking, and poor nutritional status; some over-the-counter medications, including ephedrine and phenylpropanolamine, have also been implicated (Salihu, Boos, & Schmidt, 2002; Weir, 2003).

Diagnosis is confirmed by prenatal ultrasound or at birth; it is associated with elevation of maternal serum alpha-fetoprotein (MSAFP); routine prenatal ultrasonography and determination of MSAFP levels permit early diagnosis and mobilization of the multidisciplinary team of obstetricians, geneticists, neonatologists, and pediatric surgeons needed to manage the congenital anomalies.

The immediate action at birth is to protect the exposed abdominal contents from injury by application of warm, sterile, saline-soaked dressings over defect; temperature regulation is needed for the neonate because heat is lost through exposed viscera, and fluids are required to replace fluid losses through viscera; blood cultures are performed before administering antibiotics; an orogastric or nasogastric tube may be inserted to prevent distention; a thorough examination is performed to rule out cardiac and other abnormalities.

Clinical therapy has usually consisted of urgent surgical reduction; current trends are to suture a prosthetic silo around the defect; this permits gradual return of the intestines to the abdominal cavity over 5–10 days as the cavity slowly enlarges (Weir, 2003).

Nursing care of the neonate centers on protecting the sac or protruding organs, preventing hypothermia, preventing and identifying infection, providing preoperative and postoperative care, and supporting the family.

Monitor temperature and other vital signs, ensure a patent gastrostomy tube, manage nutrition and pain control, and foster the family's contact and bonding with the infant.

Omphalocele

Omphalocele is a congenital malformation in which intra-abdominal contents herniate through the umbilical cord.

The defect results from failure of the abdominal contents, such as intestines and liver, to return to the abdomen when the abdominal wall begins to close by the 11th week of gestation; unlike gastroschisis, the tissues are covered by a translucent sac (peritoneum) into which the umbilical cord inserts.

The defect can involve any abdominal organ; however, the large or small intestine, stomach, liver, gallbladder, pancreas, spleen, urinary bladder, or internal genitalia are most common.

Omphalocele is often associated with other congenital anomalies, such as cardiac defects; genitourinary anomalies; trisomy 13, 18, or 21; craniofacial abnormalities; and diaphragmatic abnormalities (Weir, 2003).

Diagnosis is confirmed by prenatal ultrasound or at birth; it is associated with elevation of MSAFP; routine prenatal ultrasonography and determination of MSAFP levels permit early diagnosis and mobilization of the multidisciplinary team of obstetricians, geneticists, neonatologists, and pediatric surgeons needed to manage the congenital anomalies.

See Gastroschisis, earlier, for clinical therapy and nursing management summary.

Anorectal Malformations

Anal stenosis, a thickened and constricted anal wall, is treated by anal dilatation; ribbon-like stools are characteristic until the anus is dilated.

In anal atresia, perineal inspection at birth reveals the absent anal opening; failure to pass meconium is diagnostic for the condition.

Anal atresia is characterized as *high* or *low*, depending on where the rectum ends, either above the levator muscle or partially descending through this muscle and ending near the perineal floor; the rectum often ends in a fistula; in high anal atresia, the fistula often ends in the prostatic urethra in males and in the vagina in females; neonates with a low type of anal atresia usually have a well-formed sacrum, a prominent midline groove, and a prominent anal dimple.

Anal atresia requires surgical correction to preserve bowel, urinary, and sexual function; a colostomy is initially performed in neonates with high anal atresia; low lesions, including those with perineal fistulas, are corrected electively when the infant's condition is stable.

Ultrasound and lower gastrointestinal radiographic studies are used to confirm the diagnosis and demonstrate the extent of the anomaly; physical examination of all body systems is performed to identify any associated abnormalities.

Some anal stenoses can be treated with dilation alone; anal atresia requires reconstructive surgery.

Nursing care focuses on newborn assessment of anal patency, preoperative and postoperative care, and supporting the family.

During the initial newborn assessment, the perineal area is inspected for a poorly developed anal dimple or sacral anomalies; observe and record passage of meconium.

Once the diagnosis is made, monitor the child's intake, output, and cardiorespiratory functioning.

Provide postoperative care as required, advancing the diet as indicated, and instructing parents on necessary home care.

If a temporary colostomy is performed, teach parents how to care for the ostomy site.

OSTOMY

An *intestinal ostomy* is an opening, or stoma, into the small or large intestine that diverts fecal matter to provide an outlet when a distal surgical anastomosis, obstruction, or nonfunctioning structures prevent normal elimination.

Depending on the integrity and function of anatomic structures, the ostomy may be temporary or permanent.

Infants and small children with imperforate anus, necrotizing enterocolitis, Hirschsprung disease, volvulus, or intussusception may require a temporary or permanent colostomy or ileostomy; ostomies may also be indicated for children with inflammatory bowel disease, intestinal tumors, or abdominal trauma.

When assessing the family and child approaching ostomy surgery, it is important for the nurse to determine their ability to understand and accept the physical changes that occur. Preoperative education focuses on educating the child and family and preparing them for postoperative management.

Discuss how the appliance looks, and explain the purpose of the pouch in developmentally appropriate terms.

Section III: Body Systems

Provide examples of pouches and other stoma equipment.

Encourage the parents and child to touch and manipulate all equipment; a younger child can be shown how to place a pouch on a doll; older children can practice placing a pouch on their skin.

Postoperative care of a child with an ostomy is similar to that for any child who undergoes abdominal surgery, including pain management, monitoring for signs of infection, skin inspection, and careful assessment of vital signs and respiratory function.

Management of the stoma may be coordinated by an ostomy nurse or nurse case manager.

Once healing has occurred, assess the stoma, quality and amount of fecal matter, skin condition, and adherence of the pouch; evaluate the understanding and ability of the family to care for the ostomy.

HERNIAS
Diaphragmatic Hernia
In a *diaphragmatic hernia*, abdominal contents protrude into the thoracic cavity through an opening in the diaphragm; sites of herniation include the substernal space, posterolateral region, and the esophageal hiatus.

A diaphragmatic hernia is a life-threatening condition.

Severe respiratory distress occurs shortly after birth; as the infant cries, abdominal organs extend into the thorax, decreasing the size of the thoracic cavity; the infant becomes dyspneic, with nasal flaring, tachypnea, retractions, and cyanosis.

Characteristic findings include a barrel-shaped chest, sunken abdomen, and diminished or absent breath sounds on affected side; pneumothorax may occur.

Bowel sounds may be auscultated over the chest; heart tones may be auscultated on the right side of the chest.

Congenital diaphragmatic hernia may be diagnosed in utero by ultrasound; if not identified prenatally, the condition is first identified postnatally by physical signs and symptoms; confirmation is made by chest radiologic examination; magnetic resonance imaging is helpful in confirming the diagnosis and in determining the position of organs in the chest and abdomen (Hedrick, Crombleholme, Flake, et al., 2004).

When a diaphragmatic hernia is diagnosed in utero, close prenatal observation and delivery at a facility with the capability of extracorporeal membrane oxygenation is recommended (Hedrick et al., 2004).

At the time of delivery, immediate respiratory support is essential.

The infant is positioned with the head and thorax higher than the abdomen to facilitate downward movement of abdominal organs.

Endotracheal intubation and ventilator support are necessary to manage respiratory compromise.

A nasogastric tube is inserted to decompress the stomach.

Intravenous fluids are administered through an umbilical artery catheter.

Once the infant's condition is stabilized, surgery is performed to correct the defect.

Nursing care in the neonatal intensive care unit centers on maintaining ventilatory support of the infant, preoperative preparation, postoperative care, and supporting the family during this life-threatening event.

Continuous monitoring of vital signs is performed.

Maintain intravenous fluid administration.

Promote decreased stimulation to keep the infant calm and thus maintain low abdominal pressure.

Keep parents informed about the infant's condition, and provide emotional support before and after surgery; allow them to see and touch the infant if possible.

Postoperative care includes positioning the infant on the affected side to facilitate expansion of the lung on the unaffected side, observing closely for signs of infection, maintaining respiratory support, and carefully monitoring fluid and electrolyte balance.

Cluster nursing care of infant to minimize exertion.

Partner with parents to encourage their participation in the infant's care to promote parent–infant attachment.

Before discharge, instruct parents in care of incision, prevention of infection, and feeding techniques.

Umbilical Hernia

An umbilical hernia results from imperfect closure or weakness of the umbilical muscle ring; the condition is often associated with diastasis recti (lateral separation of the abdominal muscles).

The hernia appears as a soft swelling covered by skin; the size varies among individuals.

The herniated area protrudes with coughing, crying, or straining during a bowel movement; contents of the hernia include omentum or portions of the small intestine.

Most defects resolve spontaneously by 3–4 years of age as the muscular ring closes.

Surgery by laparoscope or open repair is indicated in cases of strangulation (closure of the umbilical ring around a portion of the bowel, preventing it from moving back into the abdomen), increased protrusion of the hernia after the age of 2 years, or little or no improvement in a large defect after the age of 4 years.

Nursing management involves providing information and support.

Instruct parents not to apply tape, straps, or coins to reduce the hernia because they can cause strangulation of the hernia.

If surgery is required, it is usually performed in a short-stay unit; provide general postoperative care.

Teach parents how to care for the surgical site, to monitor for bleeding, and to recognize signs of infection; reinforce the importance of returning for follow-up evaluation.

DISORDERS OF MOTILITY
Gastroesophageal Reflux and Gastroesophageal Reflux Disease
Description and Etiology

Gastroesophageal reflux (GER) is the return of gastric contents into the esophagus and is the result of relaxation of the lower esophageal sphincter.

Gastroesophageal reflux disease is a more serious manifestation of GER; it is a pathologic process in infants manifested by poor weight gain, esophagitis, neurobehavioral changes, and persistent respiratory symptoms or complications (Arguin & Swartz, 2004).

Three mechanisms allow reflux of the gastric contents across the esophagogastric junction and into the esophagus:

1. Transient lower esophageal sphincter relaxations
2. Hypotensive or incompetent lower esophageal sphincter
3. Anatomic disruption of the esophagogastric junction

Clinical Manifestations

Manifestations vary from an occasional burp to persistent emesis and failure to thrive.

Postprandial regurgitation is the most common sign of GER in infants. The regurgitation ranges from spitting to forceful vomiting (Sondheimer, 2003).

Children with GER are frequently hungry and irritable; they lose weight and experience failure to thrive; there may be a history of vomiting and frequent upper respiratory infections; apparent life-threatening events and cyanotic episodes may be reported.

Manifestations of respiratory problems associated with GER include cyanosis, wheezing, stridor, chronic cough, and recurrent croup.

Diagnostic Tests

Diagnosis is confirmed by a thorough history of the child's feeding patterns and by diagnostic evaluation using contrast upper gastrointestinal series (barium fluoroscopy), upper gastrointestinal endoscopy with esophageal biopsy, pH probe monitoring (insertion of a small catheter into the esophagus through the nose that is left in place for 18–24 hours to measure pH and, thus, determine number of reflux episodes), or gastroesophageal scintigraphy (radionuclide scanning to evaluate gastric emptying) (Jung, 2001; Murray & Christie, 2000).

Laboratory studies may reveal anemia secondary to blood loss.

Testing for cow's milk protein allergy, including cutaneous tests, eosinophil smears of the nasal mucosa, immunoglobulin G antilactoglobulin levels, and intestinal biopsy, is generally performed because there is a high association between GER and cow's milk allergy (Arguin & Swartz, 2004).

Clinical Therapy

Generally, feeding modification, thickened feeds, frequent burping during feeding, and positioning with the upper body in the vertical position during and after feeding are effective management for milder cases.

Treatment for severe cases of gastroesophageal reflux disease, such as those with persistent vomiting with failure to thrive, chronic esophagitis, esophageal strictures, or chronic pulmonary disease (Sondheimer, 2003), may include surgery to create a valve mechanism by wrapping the greater curvature of the stomach (fundus) around the distal esophagus (Nissen fundoplication).

Medications, such as histamine 2 (H_2) receptor antagonists, proton pump inhibitors, and antacids, may be helpful for some infants and children.

Nursing Management

Assessment

Collect history on the amount of feedings and the feeding techniques used by the family.

Ask about amount, frequency, and type of vomiting.

Perform careful assessment of all body systems with particular attention to gastrointestinal and respiratory systems.

Monitor length and weight, and place ongoing measurements on growth grids.

Intervention

Infants receiving oral feedings are administered smaller feedings; elevate the head of the bed to prevent aspiration; if the child has difficulty maintaining this position, a Tracy harness or reflux board may be used.

If the child has a gastrostomy tube, maintain skin integrity around the stoma site; secure the tube so that the infant cannot dislodge or pull on it.

Administer medications as ordered, remaining alert for expected side effects.

Prepare the child for diagnostic tests.

Provide postoperative care for the child undergoing surgery.

Family Education

Instruct parents how to feed and position the infant, and provide comfort and emotional support.

Partner with parents, and encourage them to hold and cuddle the infant during all feedings.

Show parents how to keep the upper body elevated, and discourage use of infant seats.

Caution the family that the enlarged nipple now has the capacity to deliver too much formula too fast for the infant and may produce a choking hazard.

Providing the infant with a pacifier helps to meet nonnutritive sucking needs.

Teach parents how to suction the nose and mouth if vomiting occurs.

Teach administration and side effects of any medications.

Constipation

Constipation is characterized by pebble-like, hard stools for a majority of bowel movements for at least 2 weeks; firm stools at least two times per week for 2 weeks; and no evidence of structural, endocrine, or metabolic disease.

Constipation may be caused by an underlying disease, diet, or psychological factor; it may result from defects in filling or, more commonly, emptying of the rectum.

Pathologic causes of defective filling include ineffective colonic propulsive activity, caused by hypothyroidism or use of medication, and obstruction; other causes include a structural anomaly (stricture or stenosis) or an aganglionic segment (Hirschsprung disease).

If the rectum fails to fill, stasis leads to excessive drying of the stools; emptying of the rectum depends on the defecation reflex; lesions of the spinal cord, weakness of the abdominal muscles, local lesions blocking sphincter relaxation, and a desire to avoid painful stools all may impede attempts to defecate.

Constipation in the newborn can indicate an obstructed large bowel, such as with Hirschsprung disease or anorectal anomaly with anal stenosis (Clayden & Keshtgar, 2003).

Constipation during infancy is commonly seen as a result of mismanagement of diet; however, the disorder is generally easily managed with dietary changes.

Dietary and fluid management are the treatments of choice for constipation that has no underlying pathologic cause.

Constipation in young infants can usually be corrected by increasing the amount of fluids or adding 2 oz of pear or apple juice to daily intake; increasing physical activity and fluid intake may be effective for some children.

Removing constipating foods (bananas, rice, and cheese) from the child's diet often decreases the constipation; increasing the child's intake of high-fiber foods (whole grain breads, raw fruits, and raw vegetables) and fluids also promotes bowel elimination.

A single glycerin suppository or enema may be required to remove hard stool.

The nurse assesses the child's diet history; obtain a description of bowel patterns and habits from parents.

Palpate the abdomen, and assess the child's abdomen for firmness or tenderness and the presence of palpable mass (retained stool); auscultate for bowel sounds.

If a digital rectal examination is performed, assess for presence of stool in rectum; assess for hemorrhoids, anal fissures, or other abnormalities of the abdomen or perineum.

Partner with the family and teach parents dietary measures to promote regularity of bowel movements; children can be given a high-fiber diet that includes fruits and vegetables and adequate fluids.

Hirschsprung Disease

Hirschsprung disease, also known as *congenital aganglionic megacolon*, is a congenital anomaly in which inadequate motility causes mechanical obstruction of the intestine.

The RET proto-oncogene is a major gene for the disease (Howard, 2001), and a failure of the migration of neural crest cells (from which cells forming ganglia arise) during the embryonic stage has been implicated (Thompson, 2001).

The absence of autonomic parasympathetic ganglion cells in the colon prevents peristalsis at that portion of the intestine, resulting in the accumulation of intestinal contents and abdominal distention; the presence of trapped stool in the colon continues to build up, causing expansion of the colon to larger than normal, hence the name *megacolon*.

In newborns, symptoms include failure to pass meconium, refusal to suck, abdominal distention, and bile-stained emesis.

In the older child, symptoms may include failure to gain weight and delayed growth; the child may have a history of abdominal distention, severe constipation alternating with diarrhea (frequent, watery stools), and vomiting.

The stool may be normal size or have a ribbon-like appearance.

Diagnosis is made on the basis of the clinical criteria and history; bowel patterns; anorectal manometry; radiographic contrast studies, such as barium enema; and rectal biopsy for presence or absence of ganglion cells (Swenson, 2002).

Abdominal radiograph and barium contrasts reveal a distended small bowel and proximal colon with an empty rectum.

Rectal biopsy reveals the presence of aganglionic cells.

Anorectal manometry demonstrates absence of relaxation of the internal sphincter in response to rectal distention.

Treatment in infancy involves surgical removal of the aganglionic bowel with end-to-end anastomosis to the anal canal (Thompson, 2001).

For the child with a milder defect, management may involve dietary modification, stool softeners, and isotonic irrigations to prevent impaction until the child is toilet trained.

Nursing assessment in the newborn period includes careful observation for the passage of meconium; assess the newborn for refusal to suck, abdominal distention, and bile-stained emesis.

When the disease is diagnosed later in infancy or in childhood, obtain a thorough history of weight gain, nutritional intake, and bowel elimination habits; assess the child's growth and developmental achievements.

Assess the child for abdominal distention, severe constipation alternating with diarrhea (frequent, watery stools), and vomiting; note the appearance of the stool.

Teach parents the need for chronic care over time; regular bowel movements are important to promote adequate elimination and prevent obstruction.

Teach parents how to prevent skin breakdown in the rectal area by changing diapers frequently, cleansing the area carefully, and applying protective ointment at each diaper change.

If surgical correction is necessary, nursing care includes monitoring for infection, managing pain, maintaining hydration, measuring abdominal circumference to detect any distention, and providing support to the child and family.

Parents require instruction in ostomy care in those cases when the child has a colostomy.

Gastroenteritis

Gastroenteritis (acute diarrhea) is an inflammation of the stomach and intestines that may be accompanied by vomiting and diarrhea.

Viral and bacterial infections are the most common cause of gastroenteritis.

Dehydration is the most common serious outcome of gastroenteritis in children; see Chapter 14 for a thorough discussion of dehydration treatment and nursing care.

INTESTINAL PARASITIC DISORDERS

Intestinal parasitic disorders occur most frequently in tropic regions; outbreaks take place in areas where water is not treated, food is incorrectly prepared, or people live in crowded conditions with poor sanitation.

In the United States and Canada, outbreaks of diseases caused by protozoa or helminths (worms) are increasing.

Young children, especially those in childcare, are most at risk of infection; they often lack good hygiene practices and are more likely to put objects and their hands into their mouths.

The most common intestinal parasitic disorders are summarized in Table 21–1, and common medication treatments are outlined in Table 21–2.

INFLAMMATORY DISORDERS
Peptic Ulcer

A *peptic ulcer* is an erosion of the mucosal tissue in the lower end of the esophagus, in the stomach (usually along the lesser curvature), or in the duodenum.

Many cases of ulcer are caused by *Helicobacter pylori*, a gram-negative rod that is transmitted by the fecal–oral or oral–oral route.

Primary ulcers occur in previously healthy children, whereas secondary ulcers occur in those with prior disease, such as cancer or burns, or those receiving medications, such as salicylates, nonsteroidal anti-inflammatory drugs, or corticosteroids.

The most common symptom is abdominal pain (burning) associated with an empty stomach, which may awaken the child at night; vomit-

Table 21–1   Clinical Manifestations of Common Intestinal Parasitic Disorders

Parasitic Infection	Transmission, Life Cycle, Pathogenesis	Clinical Manifestations	Clinical Therapy	Comments
Giardiasis Organism: protozoan *Giardia lamblia* *Giardia lamblia*	Transmission is through person-to-person contact, unfiltered water, improperly prepared infected food, and contact with animals. Cysts are ingested and passed into the duodenum and proximal jejunum, where they begin actively feeding. They are excreted in the stool.	May be asymptomatic *Infants:* diarrhea, vomiting, anorexia, failure to thrive *Older children:* abdominal cramps; intermittent loose, foul-smelling watery, pale, and greasy stools	Available medications include furazolidone and quinacrine. Furazolidone has fewer side effects than quinacrine but is more expensive. Metronidazole is also effective but is not licensed in the United States for treatment of giardiasis.	Most common intestinal parasitic organism in the United States. Infection may resolve spontaneously in 4–6 weeks without treatment. Parents or caregivers should wear gloves when handling diapers or stool of parasite-infected infant or child.

(continued)

Alterations in Gastrointestinal Function **391**

Table 21–1   Clinical Manifestations of Common Intestinal Parasitic Disorders (Continued)

Parasitic Infection	Transmission, Life Cycle, Pathogenesis	Clinical Manifestations	Clinical Therapy	Comments
Enterobiasis (pinworm) Organism: nematode *Enterobius vermicularis* 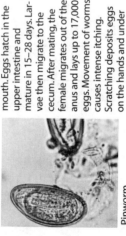 Pinworm	Transmission is from discharged eggs inhaled or carried from hand to mouth. Eggs hatch in the upper intestine and mature in 15–28 days. Larvae then migrate to the cecum. After mating, the female migrates out of the anus and lays up to 17,000 eggs. Movement of worms causes intense itching. Scratching deposits eggs on the hands and under the nails.	Intense perianal itching, irritability, restlessness, and short attention span; in females, can migrate to the vagina and urethra to cause infection. Itching intensifies at night when the female comes to the anal opening to lay eggs.	Available medications include mebendazole, pyrantel pamoate, and piperazine citrate. The child and all household members should be treated at the same time. Treatment may be repeated in 2–3 weeks.	Most common helminthic infection in the United States. Transmission is increased in crowded conditions such as housing developments, schools, and childcare centers.

Ascariasis (roundworm) Organism: nematode *Ascaris lumbricoides*	Transmission is from discharged eggs carried from hand to mouth. Adult lays eggs in small intestine. Eggs are excreted in stool, where they incubate for 2–3 weeks. Swallowed eggs hatch in the small intestine. Larvae may penetrate intestinal villi, entering the portal vein and liver, then moving to the lung. Larvae that ascend to upper respiratory tract are swallowed and proceed to the small intestine, where they repeat the cycle.	Mild infection may be asymptomatic. Severe infection may result in intestinal obstruction, peritonitis, obstructive jaundice, and lung involvement.	Available anthelminthic medications include mebendazole, pyrantel pamoate, or piperazine citrate. Stools should be examined 2 weeks after treatment and monthly for 3 months. Family members and contacts of the child should be treated if indicated. If the child has intestinal obstruction, treatment may include administering piperazine through a nasogastric tube and duodenal scion. Obstructing worms sometimes have to be surgically removed.	Most common in warm climates. Primarily affects children 1–4 years of age.

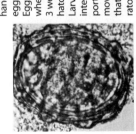

Roundworm

(continued)

Table 21–1 Clinical Manifestations of Common Intestinal Parasitic Disorders (Continued)

Parasitic Infection	Transmission, Life Cycle, Pathogenesis	Clinical Manifestations	Clinical Therapy	Comments
Hookworm disease Organism: nematode *Necator americanus* Hookworm	Transmission is through direct contact with infected soil containing larvae. Worms live in the small intestine and feed on villi, causing bleeding. Eggs are deposited in the bowel and excreted in feces. Eggs hatch in damp shaded soil. Larvae attach to and penetrate the skin then enter the bloodstream, migrating to the lungs. Larvae then migrate to the upper respiratory passages and are swallowed.	In healthy individuals, mild infection seldom causes problems. More severe infection may result in anemia and malnutrition. Presence of larvae on the skin may cause burning and itching, followed by redness and papular eruption.	Available medications include mebendazole and pyrantel pamoate. Stools should be examined 2 weeks after treatment and monthly for 3 months. Family members and contacts of the child should be treated if indicated.	Children should wear shoes when outdoors, although other unprotected areas of the skin may still come in contact with larvae.

Strongyloidiasis
(threadworm)

Organism: nematode
Strongyloides stercoralis

Transmission is from the ingestion of discharged larvae in the soil. Life cycle is similar to that of the hookworm, except the threadworm does not attach to the intestinal mucosa, and feeding larvae (rather than eggs) may be deposited in the soil.

Mild infection may be asymptomatic. Severe infection may result in abdominal pain and distention, nausea, vomiting, and diarrhea. Stools may be large and pale, with mucus. Severe infection may lead to a nutritional deficiency.

Available medications include thiabendazole or mebendazole. Treatment may need to be repeated if symptoms recur after treatment. Family members and contacts of the child should be examined and treated if indicated.

Most common in older children and adolescents.

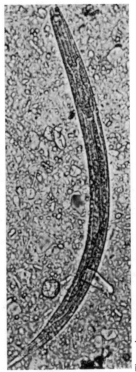

Threadworm

(continued)

Table 21-1   Clinical Manifestations of Common Intestinal Parasitic Disorders (Continued)

Parasitic Infection	Transmission, Life Cycle, Pathogenesis	Clinical Manifestations	Clinical Therapy	Comments
Visceral larva migrans (toxocariasis) Organism: nematode *Toxocara canis* or *T. cati*, commonly found in dogs and cats	Transmission through the ingestion of eggs in the soil. Ingested eggs hatch in the intestine. Mobile larvae then migrate to the liver and eventually to all major organs (including the brain). Once migration is complete, they encapsulate in dense fibrous tissue.	Most cases are asymptomatic. Affected children may have a low-grade fever and recurrent upper airway diseases. Severe symptoms include hepatomegaly, pulmonary infiltration, and neurologic disturbances. In all cases there is a hypereosinophilia of the blood.	There is no specific treatment. Corticosteroids have been used in severe cases. Thiabendazole has been recommended, but efficacy is not established (infection usually resolves spontaneously).	Most common in toddlers. Deworm household pets monthly if indicated. Keep children away from areas contaminated with animal droppings.

Note: *Giardia lamblia* courtesy of Centers for Disease Control and Prevention. Atlanta, GA; pinworm (p. 718), roundworm (p. 714), hookworm (p. 719), and threadworm (p. 721) from A. M. Rudolph, J. I. E. Hoffman, & C. D. Rudolph. (1996). Rudolph's pediatrics (20th ed.). Stamford, CT: Appleton & Lange, with permission.

Table 21–2   Medications Used to Treat Intestinal Parasitic Infections

Medication	Indications	Nursing Implications

Furazolidone	Used in treatment of
	  Giardiasis
	  Enterobacter aerogenes
	  Escherichia coli
	  Proteus
	  Salmonella
	  Shigella
	  Staphylococcus
	  Vibrio cholerae
		Protect medication from heat and light exposure.
		Monitor for side effects:
		  Abdominal pain
		  Nausea, vomiting
		  Diarrhea
		  Fever
		  Hypotension
		  Headache
		  Dizziness
		  Hypoglycemia

Mebendazole	Used in treatment of
	  Pinworm
	  Roundworm
	  Hookworm
	  Threadworm
	  Whipworm
		Tablets may be chewed and swallowed or crushed and mixed with food.
		Monitor for side effects:
		  Abdominal pain
		  Diarrhea
		  Fever

Pyrantel pamoate	Used in treatment of
	  Pinworm
	  Roundworm
	  Hookworm
		Oral suspension should be shaken well before administration.
		Administer with milk or fruit juices.
		Monitor for side effects:
		  Headache
		  Anorexia
		  Nausea
		  Vomiting
		  Diarrhea

Thiabendazole	Used in treatment of
	  Threadworm
	  Pinworm
	  Roundworm
	  Hookworm
		Administer after meals.
		Chewable tablets must be chewed thoroughly
		Shake suspension well.
		Monitor for side effects:
		  Dizziness
		  Anorexia
		  Nausea
		  Vomiting
		  Diarrhea
		  Pruritus
		  Hematuria

Note: Data from R. M. Bindler, & L. B. Howry. (2005). Pediatric drugs & nursing implications. (3rd ed.). Upper Saddler River, NJ: Prentice Hall Health.

ing and pain after meals, anemia, occult blood in stools, and abdominal distention may also be present.

Diagnosis is based on the history and radiologic studies.

H. pylori can be diagnosed by culture of the organism taken via gastroscopy or measurement of *H. pylori* antigens in stool specimens; a urea breath test is effective (Kirschner, 2001) because the organism hydrolyzes urea.

When *H. pylori* is the causative agent, antimicrobial agents, such as bismuth salts, tetracycline, and metronidazole combination, are given.

Other drug combinations, such as antacids in liquid form (Maalox, Mylanta) and histamine antagonists (ranitidine, cimetidine, and famotidine), are also used.

The nurse assesses the child for abdominal pain, vomiting, and abdominal distention.

Monitor red blood cell (RBC) count, hemoglobin, and hematocrit.

Assess for family history of *H. pylori* infection.

Partner with the family and explain that antibiotics must be administered as scheduled.

Caution parents to avoid aspirin products, which irritate the gastric mucosa; if an antipyretic or pain medication is needed, acetaminophen is administered.

Because psychological stress can contribute to peptic ulcer disease, the parents and child should be assisted to identify sources of stress in the child's life.

Assess coping mechanisms and provide referral for psychological counseling, if appropriate.

Teach relaxation techniques, and recommend community classes on yoga or other stress reduction.

Appendicitis

Appendicitis is an inflammation of the vermiform appendix, the small sac near the end of the cecum.

Appendicitis almost always results from an obstruction in the appendiceal lumen causing edema. Obstructions include fecalith (hard fecal mass), parasitic infestations, stenosis, hyperplasia of lymphoid tissue, or a tumor.

Continued secretion of mucus after acute obstruction of the lumen increases pressure, causing ischemia, cellular death, necrosis, and ulceration; as edema increases, the vascular supply to the appendix is compromised, increasing the permeability of the appendix; bacteria then invade the appendix, causing further inflammation.

At onset, symptoms include periumbilical cramps, abdominal tenderness, and fever; pain may be described throughout the abdomen, with periumbilical pain common.

As the inflammation progresses, pain in the right lower abdomen becomes constant. Pain is often most intense at McBurney's point, halfway between the anterior superior iliac crest and the umbilicus.

Symptoms progress to include guarding, rigidity, nausea, vomiting, onset of pain before vomiting, anorexia, and rebound tenderness after palpation over the right lower quadrant.

Rovsing's sign (indirect tenderness) and psoas sign (pain induced by flexion of the hip) may also be observed (Paulson, Kalady, & Pappas, 2003).

Diarrhea or constipation may be present; as appendicitis progresses, the child remains motionless, usually in a side-lying position with knees flexed.

An elevated white blood cell count (above 15,000/mm^3) may occur but occurs less often in young children than in teens.

Treatment of acute appendicitis involves immediate surgical removal (appendectomy), either through laparoscopic or open method (Vegunta, Ali, Wallace, et al., 2004).

Preoperatively, the child is kept NPO; intravenous fluids and electrolytes are administered; antibiotics are administered if the appendix is ruptured or the child is at high risk for infection; a nasogastric tube may be inserted before or after surgery.

Postoperatively, intravenous fluids and antibiotics (if prescribed) are continued; if the appendix has ruptured before surgery, a Penrose drain is inserted and the wound may not be completely sutured.

Preoperatively, the nurse performs a detailed assessment of the child's pain to differentiate appendicitis from other illnesses.

Allow the child to assume any position that promotes comfort; administer analgesics routinely as ordered, and note results of medications; ask the family what might be comforting for the child, such as music, gently stroking the back, or having family present.

Assess fluid-volume status every 2 hours; assess skin turgor, eyes, and mucous membranes for signs of dehydration; monitor intake and output, and assess vital signs.

Once bowel sounds return, offer water in small amounts followed by other clear fluids and advancing to a regular diet as tolerated.

For many children, appendicitis may be the reason for their first hospitalization and only experience with healthcare personnel beyond their usual provider; the nurse must elicit a history, perform a physical examination, coordinate diagnostic tests, and prepare the child for surgery in a short period of time; emotional support is essential for the child and parents.

Encourage the child to deep breathe postoperatively by blowing bubbles or use of incentive spirometry.

Assess vital signs, and observe the abdominal incision every 4 hours for redness, edema, or drainage; if a drain is present, assess drainage for color, consistency, and amount.

Administer antibiotics as prescribed.

Necrotizing Enterocolitis
Description and Etiology
The etiology of necrotizing enterocolitis is most often seen in premature infants and is multifactorial; causes include intestinal ischemia, bacterial or viral infection (a result of the premature infant's decreased immune response and greater risk for infection), and immaturity of the gastrointestinal mucosa (a result of the premature infant's decreased amount of gastric acid and proteolytic enzymes and underdeveloped protective intestinal mucin layer) (Kliegman & Willoughby, 2005).

Vascular compromise, leading to hypoxia and ischemia, causes a reduced blood flow to the bowel, leading to necrosis of the bowel mucosa; the damaged bowel stops secreting protective enzymes, allowing gas-forming bacteria to invade the necrotic tissue; this bacterial invasion further damages the intestinal mucosa by releasing bacterial toxins and gas, causing abdominal-distention disease sites, most commonly the terminal ileum and colon.

Necrosis of the bowel can lead to intestinal perforation and sepsis, making this a life-threatening condition.

Clinical Manifestations

Manifestations generally occur between 3 and 14 days of life but can occur as early as the first day of life and as late as 3 months of age.

The infant may initially show signs of feeding intolerance (increased gastric residuals, vomiting, irritability, and abdominal distention).

The abdomen is mildly distended initially, progressing to severe distention.

Bloody diarrhea.

Decreased urine output.

Bile-stained emesis.

A characteristic clinical triad of abdominal distention, bilious vomiting, and bloody stools.

Signs of sepsis, such as hypothermia, hypotension, bradycardia, lethargy, and apnea.

Long-term complications of necrotizing enterocolitis may include short bowel syndrome, strictures, and cholestasis; abdominal perforation can lead to sepsis, shock, and death.

Diagnostic Tests

Diagnosis is made on the basis of characteristic clinical manifestations and the presence of free peritoneal gas, dilated bowel loops, bowel distention, and bowel wall thickening on abdominal x-rays.

Stools and emesis are monitored for occult blood.

Laboratory data reveal anemia, leukopenia, leukocytosis, thrombocytopenia, electrolyte imbalance, and metabolic or respiratory acidosis.

Blood cultures are performed to identify invasive organisms.

Clinical Therapy

Requires prompt intervention.

Therapy begins with discontinuation of all enteral feedings.

A nasogastric or orogastric tube is inserted and maintained on low suction to prevent gastric distention, and intravenous fluids are started.

TPN may be initiated through a central line.

Antibiotics are administered prophylactically or to treat sepsis.

Perforation or necrosis of the bowel necessitates surgical resection of the bowel; an ileostomy or colostomy may be performed in some cases.

All cases of necrotizing enterocolitis are treated with strict enteric precautions to prevent the spread of infection to other premature infants on the unit.

Early aggressive enteral formula feedings of premature infants are avoided because of the increased incidence of the disease in these cases; human milk has been shown to be protective against the disease, so breastfeeding or feeding the mother's expressed milk is the feeding method of choice for all premature infants.

New treatments are being attempted with probiotics—live and beneficial microorganisms that promote normal gut flora; *Lactobacillus acidophilus* and *Bifidobacterium infantis* are examples of organisms that can be administered by special formula.

Nursing Management

Assessment

Observe for feeding intolerance by aspirating gastric residual (if the infant is receiving enteral feedings).

Measure abdominal circumference, and assess bowel sounds in the premature or high-risk infant every 4–8 hours; even minimal changes in circumference can indicate necrotizing enterocolitis and should be reported to the primary care provider.

Careful monitoring of vital signs, intake, and output is essential to detect any complications.

Intervention

Maintaining fluid and electrolyte balance is essential; provide intravenous fluids, probiotics, or feedings as ordered.

Provide comfort by holding and cuddling an infant who is NPO, and offer a pacifier to meet nonnutritive sucking needs.

Careful assessments for infection and maintenance of skin integrity are essential.

Parents require emotional support, reassurance, and help in bonding with their infant. They are coping with the birth of an infant who is critically ill; make appropriate referrals for support as indicated.

Once the infant is discharged, frequent follow-up care is needed; encourage regular healthcare visits for monitoring growth, development, and nutritional intake, and to receive preventive care such as immunizations.

Partner with the parents to establish home care routine.

If TPN is administered at home, the parents will need education regarding proper administration of TPN and how to care for the central line.

Instruct parents in administration of medications.

If the infant required an ostomy, teach parents proper care of the stoma.

Meckel's Diverticulum

Meckel's diverticulum is the most common congenital anomaly of the gastrointestinal tract and is the most common cause of lower-gastrointestinal bleeding in children (Sadovsky, 2001).

The defect results when the omphalomesenteric duct, which connects the midgut to the yolk sac during embryonic development, fails to atrophy; instead, an outpouching of the ileum remains, usually located near the ileocecal valve; the pouch contains gastric or pancreatic tissue, which secretes acid, causing irritation and ulceration.

Clinical manifestations usually appear by 2 years of age; they include abdominal pain, nausea and vomiting, rectal bleeding, abdominal distention, peritonitis, and diarrhea (Neidlinger, Madan, & Wright, 2001).

The child may develop symptoms of intussusception, incarcerated hernia, volvulus, or intestinal obstruction.

Diagnosis of Meckel's diverticulum is based on the history; radionuclide imaging and scanning can usually detect the gastric tissue, confirming the diagnosis; laparoscopy may be performed to confirm diagnosis.

Treatment is surgical excision of the diverticulum and removal of any involved bowel via resection using either open or laparoscopic techniques (Sadovsky, 2001).

Preoperatively, the nurse maintains an intravenous infusion to correct fluid and electrolyte imbalances.

Monitor intake and output.

Observe for rectal bleeding, and test stools for occult blood.

Maintain the child on bedrest.

Assess vital signs every 2 hours, and monitor for signs of shock.

Perform postsurgical abdominal care, including pain relief; administration of intravenous solutions; and monitoring abdominal sounds, respiratory system, and skin.

At the time of discharge, parents need instructions on caring for the surgical site, preventing infection, reintroduction of fluids and food, providing an adequate diet, and administering prescribed medications.

Recurrent Abdominal Pain

Recurrent abdominal pain is a frequent problem among young children and adolescents, particularly girls of school age.

The pain is generally located in the periumbilical area and occurs on a regular basis.

A thorough history and physical examination are necessary to rule out organic causes.

Laboratory studies, such as a complete blood count, may be ordered to rule out other illness; gastrointestinal studies may be performed in an outpatient setting.

When no organic cause can be identified, treatment of recurrent abdominal pain focuses on providing outlets for the release of stress within the family and in other settings in the child's life, enhancing the child's coping methods, and promoting dietary changes that encourage regular bowel movements.

Cognitive behavioral therapies, such as relaxation techniques, have proven effective because they reduce autonomic arousal and muscle tension (Hyman & Danda, 2004).

Inflammatory Bowel Disease

Inflammatory bowel disease encompasses two distinct chronic disorders, Crohn's disease and ulcerative colitis, which have similar symptoms and treatment.

Both diseases involve faulty regulation of the immune response of the intestinal mucosa in individuals who are genetically predisposed and have a genetic trigger (Gokhale, 2001).

See Table 21–3 for contrasts in manifestation of the two disorders.

Diagnosis centers on evaluating the cause and identifying the extent of involved bowel and differentiating an infectious process (organisms, e.g., *Shigella* and *Salmonella*) from inflammatory bowel disease.

Table 21–3   Comparison of Ulcerative Colitis and Crohn's Disease

	Ulcerative Colitis	Crohn's Disease
Type of lesions	Continuous, superficial involvement	Segmental, transmural (through the wall) involvement
Clinical manifestations		
Anal or perianal lesions	Rare	Common
Anorexia	Mild to moderate	Can be severe
Diarrhea	Often severe	Moderate
Growth retardation	Mild	Significant
Pain	Present	Common
Rectal bleeding	Present	Absent
Weight loss	Moderate	Severe
Risk of cancer	Slightly increased	Greatly increased

Laboratory studies help to identify related nutritional, electrolyte, and blood abnormalities.

Anemia is common; an elevated erythrocyte sedimentation rate, elevated C-reactive protein, hypoalbuminemia, and thrombocytosis are other possible findings.

Stools are positive for occult blood.

Antineutrophil cytoplasmic antibodies may be detected in serum studies.

Perinuclear highlighting of those autoantibodies (perinuclear antineutrophil cytoplasmic antibodies) is associated with ulcerative colitis and Crohn's disease.

Radiologic studies, such as upper gastrointestinal series, may reveal deep ulcerations in the terminal ileum, a cobblestone appearance, or a narrowing in the small bowel, and fistulas may also be detected.

A colonoscopy allows for direct visualization of the gastrointestinal tract surface; a biopsy conducted during colonoscopy confirms the diagnosis of inflammatory bowel disease and is useful in determining the extent and severity of inflammation (Baron, 2002).

Medications, such as aminosalicylates, corticosteroids, and immunosuppressants, are commonly used in treatment.

Nursing management occurs mainly in the community and home and focuses on helping the child and family adjust to the emotional impact of a chronic disease, administering medications and diet therapy, monitoring nutritional status, monitoring growth status, and providing appropriate referrals.

Assess for abdominal distention, tenderness, and pain; monitor bowel sounds and stool pattern; measure abdominal girth.

Body image is often a concern for children and adolescents with inflammatory bowel disease because of disease effects and medication side effects; offer referrals for counseling, and help the child identify his or her own strengths.

Providing adequate stress reduction may be helpful in control of inflammatory bowel disease; collaborate with the parents to teach young children relaxation techniques, such as deep breathing, progressive tensing and relaxing of muscles, and visualization of favorite places; encourage busy school-age children and teens to have quiet and restful times each day, in addition to physical activity periods.

DISORDERS OF MALABSORPTION
Short Bowel Syndrome

Short bowel syndrome is a decreased ability to absorb and digest a regular diet because of a shortened intestine.

The signs and symptoms of weight loss and malabsorption of fluids and micro- and macronutrients occur after surgical intestinal resection of a portion of the intestines (Scolapio, 2002).

During the first 3 months after bowel resection, watery diarrhea is common; in the transition period, the remaining bowel usually increases its absorptive surface area and partially compensates for the absent intestine.

The infant or young child requires nutritional support initially to provide sufficient nutrients for adequate growth and development; a combination of TPN via central line and oral fluids may be required.

Once the bowel begins to recover, enteral feedings may be started; these include a high-fat, low-carbohydrate diet with added stimulants for mucosal growth hormones (gastrin, insulin, enteroglucagon, and growth hormone); careful management of nucleotide, glutamine, polyamine, and fatty-acid components in enteral feedings can also encourage growth of normal intestinal mucosa.

The section of the intestine that is resected also determines the vitamin and nutrient deficiencies of the child with short bowel syndrome.

When the ileum is resected, bile salts, fluids, and electrolyte absorption decrease, so diarrhea can result; loss of ileum also leads to steatorrhea and fat-soluble vitamins.

When the colon is resected, fluid and electrolyte management is impaired.

Resection of the jejunum is compensated for effectively by the remaining bowel (Jakubik, Colfer, & Grossman, 2000).

Adaptation of the diet to facilitate absorption may include use of amino acids and peptides rather than protein and use of medium-chain triglycerides rather than other sources of fat [American Academy of Pediatrics (AAP), 2004a].

Nursing care focuses on meeting the child's nutritional and fluid needs and teaching parents how to care for the child at home during the lengthy recovery period.

Celiac Disease
Description and Etiology
Celiac disease, or gluten-sensitive enteropathy, is a chronic malabsorption syndrome; a genetic factor is believed to play a role in etiology.

Celiac disease is an immunologic disorder (Zelnik, Pacht, Obeid, et al., 2004) characterized by intolerance for gluten, a protein found in wheat, barley, rye, and oats.

Inability to digest glutenin and gliadin (protein fractions) results in the accumulation of the amino acid glutamine, which is toxic to mucosal cells in the intestine; damage to the villi ultimately impairs the absorptive process in the small intestine.

Clinical Manifestations
In the early stages, celiac disease affects fat absorption, resulting in excretion of large quantities of fat in the stools (steatorrhea); stools are greasy, foul smelling, frothy, and excessive.

As changes in the villi continue, the absorption of protein; carbohydrates; calcium; iron; folate; and vitamins A, D, E, K, and B_{12} become impaired.

The classic features of celiac disease in infancy include chronic diarrhea, malabsorption syndrome, failure to thrive, and abdominal pains (Zelnik et al., 2004).

The child also exhibits vomiting, irritability, anemia, hypotonia, and ulcers of the mouth.

If diagnosis is delayed, the child begins to show evidence of protein deficiency (wasted musculature, abdominal distention), delayed dentition, and changes in bone density.

Complications associated with the disorder include hypocalcemia, osteoporosis, osteomalacia, and rickets.

Diagnostic Tests

Diagnosis is confirmed through measurement of fecal fat content, duodenal biopsy, and improvement with removal of gluten products from the diet.

Serum screening tests are more often being used successfully for diagnosis; immunoglobulin A antiendomysial antibodies and immunoglobulin A antitissue transglutaminase antibodies are commonly used (Murdock & Johnston, 2005).

Clinical Therapy

Management of the disease is total exclusion of gluten from the diet for life; barley, wheat, and rye are completely eliminated, and symptoms generally improve within a few days to weeks.

The intestinal villi return to normal in approximately 6 months.

Growth should improve steadily, and height and weight should reach normal range within 1 year.

Vitamin supplementation may be needed for a period of time if the child has become malnourished.

Nursing Management

Assessment

Assess the child for vomiting, irritability, anemia, hypotonia, and ulcers of the mouth.

Assess growth pattern and developmental achievements.

Ask the family about the child's bowel elimination patterns.

Observe stools for amount and characteristics.

Intervention

Partner with the parents to establish a nutritional plan for the child.

Offer the parents a thorough explanation of the disease process, and emphasize that dietary changes must be continued even though the child has improved.

Provide the parents and child with a list of foods that can be consumed, including fruits, meats, rice, and vegetables, including corn.

Arrange periodic visits to a dietitian.

Perform regular physical assessments, nutritional monitoring, growth measurement, and developmental screening.

Assist the family to work with the school so that the diet can be successfully integrated into that setting.

HEPATIC DISORDERS
Hyperbilirubinemia
Description and Etiology

Bilirubin is a yellow pigment produced from the breakdown of RBCs.

Newborns have more RBCs per kilogram of weight than adults, and, because the lifespan of the RBC is shorter in newborns than in adults, they are at risk for producing more bilirubin than their livers are capable of metabolizing, thus causing hyperbilirubinemia and resultant jaundice.

The majority of newborns experience some degree of jaundice in the first week of life, but it is usually self-limiting and resolves quickly; the term newborn's bilirubin level usually peaks between the third and fifth day of life (Shaw, 2003).

Two types of jaundice can occur in the newborn—physiologic and pathologic.

Physiologic jaundice is normal and occurs in 50–60% of term newborns (Cash, 2004); jaundice is usually visible 2–4 days after birth and lasts until day 6; peak bilirubin concentration reaches 6–7 mg/dL.

Preterm newborns are more susceptible to hyperbilirubinemia with 63% reaching bilirubin levels of 10–19 mg/dL (Shaw, 2003).

Pathologic jaundice can occur from conditions, such as neonatal sepsis, intestinal obstruction, or polycythemia (Blackburn, 2003), or from blood group incompatibility between the mother and the fetus.

See Box 21–1 for risk factors contributing to hyperbilirubinemia.

Box 21–1	Clinical Risk Factors for Development of Severe Hyperbilirubinemia

Important risk factors for severe hyperbilirubinemia in infants at more than 35 weeks' gestation include breastfeeding, gestation less than 38 weeks, hyperbilirubinemia in a sibling, and visible jaundice before discharge (AAP, 2004b).

Additional risk factors for development of severe hyperbilirubinemia include

- Bilirubin level higher than normal before hospital discharge
- Visible jaundice in the first 24 hours of life
- Blood group incompatibility or known hemolytic disease, such as glucose-6-phosphate dehydrogenase deficiency
- Significant bruising or cephalohematoma
- Problems with breastfeeding, especially if accompanied by excessive weight loss
- East Asian race

A term infant who is formula feeding is at very low risk of developing severe hyperbilirubinemia (AAP 2004b).

Clinical Manifestations

Newborn jaundice is first evident on the face and then progresses to the trunk and finally to the extremities.

Clinical manifestations of acute bilirubin encephalopathy include lethargy, hypotonia, and poor sucking ability (AAP, 2004a).

These symptoms progress to irritability and hypertonia (backward arching of the neck and trunk), possibly accompanied by fever and high-pitched cry alternating with drowsiness and hypotonia. In the advanced phase, which probably denotes irreversible brain damage, the infant demonstrates pronounced hypertonia, shrill cry, no feeding, apnea, fever, coma, seizures, and death (AAP, 2004a).

Diagnostic Tests

A blood test, performed by heelstick or venipuncture, measures total serum bilirubin (TSB) in the newborn; if phototherapy is already in progress, the TSB should be drawn with the phototherapy lights turned off because phototherapy lights can alter TSB results (Shaw, 2003).

A transcutaneous bilirubin measurement device is recommended as a noninvasive way to estimate TSB in babies whose TSB is less than 15 mg/dL; transcutaneous bilirubin generally provides measurements within 2–3 mg/dL of the TSB and can replace the blood test to measure TSB before phototherapy is initiated; phototherapy *bleaches* the skin, making transcutaneous measurement unreliable after phototherapy is initiated (AAP, 2004b).

Depending on risk factors and clinical history, additional laboratory tests may include blood typing and Rh factor and Coombs' test; Coombs' test looks for maternal antibodies coating the newborn's RBCs; a direct positive Coombs' test indicates Rh incompatibility but not necessarily ABO incompatibility (Shaw, 2003).

A complete blood count with differential and smear may be done to look for spherocytes (RBCs that are smaller and more fragile than normal RBCs) and to assess presence of infection.

Urinalysis, urine culture, and cerebrospinal fluid are obtained if history or presentation suggests sepsis.

If exchange transfusion is potential, a type and crossmatch is ordered (AAP, 2004b).

Clinical Therapy
Phototherapy most effectively reduces serum bilirubin in newborns with nonhemolytic jaundice.

Phototherapy is thought to reduce the amount of indirect or unconjugated bilirubin in the baby's bloodstream by promoting excretion via the intestines and kidneys; phototherapy exposes the infant's skin to blue light at certain wavelengths, which changes bilirubin into water-soluble and excretable forms; phototherapy also facilitates excretion of unconjugated bilirubin through the liver and speeds passage through the bowel (Shaw, 2003).

Many newborns with hyperbilirubinemia are also mildly dehydrated; frequent breastfeeding (every 2–3 hours) is recommended; in some instances, supplemental fluid intake in the form of milk-based formula may be used to improve hydration and inhibit the enterohepatic circulation of bilirubin.

When intensive phototherapy fails to decrease TSB and/or TSB rises to recommended levels for exchange, or if the newborn exhibits signs of intermediate to advanced stages of acute bilirubin encephalopathy, an exchange transfusion is indicated.

Pharmacologic therapy with the drug tin-mesoporphyrin may become more common in the future; this drug inhibits the production of heme oxygenase and can prevent or treat hyperbilirubinemia.

Nursing Management
The nurse plays a critical role in identifying the newborn at risk, providing parent education and support, and providing nursing care to the newborn undergoing treatment for hyperbilirubinemia; the nurse coordinates communication among all members of the newborn's care team, including physicians, laboratory personnel, and parents.

Assessment
The nurse assesses the newborn for jaundice each time vital signs are assessed and no less than every 8–12 hours (AAP, 2004b).

To assess the presence of jaundice in the newborn, the nurse presses the newborn's skin with digital pressure, revealing the color of the subcutaneous tissue.

Visual estimation of bilirubin levels can lead to errors, however, and is used only to assess the need for further investigation (AAP, 2004b).

If the nurse suspects the presence of jaundice, a transcutaneous bilirubin measurement or TSB level is indicated and it is reported to the newborn's primary care provider and documented in the chart.

Assess feeding ability and state of hydration.

Implementation

Maintain phototherapy for infants receiving it.

Foster breastfeeding and adequate hydration.

Provide verbal and written information about jaundice to parents and what conditions warrant immediate medical care after discharge.

Schedule and encourage parents to keep initial newborn visit to pediatric healthcare home.

Biliary Atresia

Biliary atresia is the pathologic closure or absence of hepatic or common bile ducts at any point from the porta hepatic to the duodenum (Kotb, Kotb, Sheba, et al., 2001).

The disorder leads to cholestasis, fibrosis, and cirrhosis (Kelly, 2002).

It is the most common pediatric liver disease necessitating transplantation and the most common cause of infant jaundice.

The cause of biliary atresia is unknown.

Absence or blockage of the extrahepatic bile ducts results in blocked bile flow from the liver to the duodenum; this altered bile flow soon causes inflammation and fibrotic changes in the liver.

In addition to blockage, the disease can also be caused by hepatocellular dysfunction.

Lack of bile acids interferes with digestion of fat and absorption of fat-soluble vitamins A, D, E, and K, resulting in steatorrhea and nutritional deficiencies.

Jaundice is detected approximately 2 or 3 weeks after birth; bilirubin levels increase, accompanied by abdominal distention and hepatomegaly.

As the disease progresses, splenomegaly occurs.

The infant experiences easy bruising, prolonged bleeding time, and intense itching.

Stools are puttylike in consistency and white or clay colored because of the absence of bile pigments.

Excretion of bilirubin and bile salts results in tea-colored urine.

Failure to thrive and malnutrition occur as the destructive changes of the disease progress.

Diagnosis is based on the history, physical examination, and laboratory evaluation; laboratory findings reveal elevated bilirubin levels, elevated serum aminotransferase and alkaline phosphatase values, prolonged prothrombin time, and increased ammonia levels.

Abdominal ultrasound is used to rule out other causes.

Percutaneous liver biopsy suggests biliary atresia, and an exploratory laparotomy confirms the diagnosis (Kotb et al., 2001).

Treatment involves surgery to attempt correction of the obstruction (hepatoportoenterostomy) and supportive care.

Supportive treatment is directed at managing the bleeding tendencies by administering oral vitamin K, preventing rickets through vitamin D supplementation, controlling itching and irritability with cholestyramine and antihistamines, and promoting adequate nutrition; low-dose oral antibiotics are administered to prevent cholangitis (Kelly, 2002).

Liver transplantation may be required for survival.

Nursing care includes preoperative and postoperative care, supporting the family, educating the family about home care, and preparing the family for organ transplantation.

Weigh the infant daily; administer TPN; intralipids; and fat-soluble vitamins A, D, E, and K as prescribed.

Diagnosis of this potentially fatal disorder can be devastating to parents; provide emotional support, and offer frequent explanations of tests during the initial diagnostic evaluation.

Intensive care during surgery and transplantation is needed, accompanied with chronic care to support the child's growth and prevention of organ rejection.

Hepatitis
Description and Etiology

Hepatitis is an inflammation of the liver caused by a viral infection.

Hepatitis may occur as an acute or chronic disease.

Acute hepatitis is rapid in onset and, if untreated, may develop into chronic hepatitis.

The most frequently diagnosed causative organisms are hepatitis A virus, hepatitis B virus, hepatitis C virus, hepatitis D virus, and hepatitis E virus. Other types of non-A and non-B have been identified, such as hepatitis G.

See Table 21–4 for descriptions about the various types of hepatitis.

The liver's response to injury by the viruses that cause hepatitis leads to invasion of the parenchymal cells by the virus, resulting in local degeneration and necrosis.

Subsequent infiltration of the parenchyma by lymphocytes, macrophages, plasma cells, eosinophils, and neutrophils causes inflammation that blocks biliary drainage into the intestine.

Impaired bile excretion causes a buildup of bile in the blood, urine, and skin (jaundice).

Structural changes in the parenchymal cells account for other altered liver functions.

Regeneration of parenchymal cells occurs within 3 months, and most children recover completely.

In some children, however, a progressive and total destruction of the hepatic parenchyma, known as *acute fulminating hepatitis*, develops; children with this form of the disease require a liver transplant.

Another complication, chronic active hepatitis, may lead to scarring of the liver and progressive deterioration of liver function.

In some persons, especially those who develop chronic hepatitis, liver cancers and cirrhosis can develop.

Clinical Manifestations

Nausea, vomiting, anorexia, malaise, fatigue, right upper quadrant pain, hepatosplenomegaly, and fever commonly occur.

Initial symptoms are followed by an icteric phase when jaundice occurs; darkening of urine, clay-colored stools, and the characteristic yellowing of the skin and sclera are observed.

Table 21–4   Comparison of Major Hepatitis Types

Type	Incubation	% Icteric	% Who Become Chronic Carriers	Clinical Features
Hepatitis A	4 weeks (10–50 days)			More acute onset; frequently sub-clinical in young children
Children <5 years		<5	0	
Adults		50–75	0	
Hepatitis B (HBV)	1–6 months			Extrahepatic manifestations more common
Infants		<5	>90	
Adults		20–60	5–10	
Hepatitis C	6–7 weeks			Frequently manifests without jaundice; predisposes to hepatocellular carcinoma
All ages		20–30	≥60	
Hepatitis D	2–8 weeks			Most common viral cause of fulminant hepatitis
Coinfection with HBV		Not known	<5	
Superinfection of HBV carrier			>80	
Hepatitis E	2–9 weeks			Severe in pregnant women; high mortality and fetal loss
All ages		~10	0	

Note: Adapted from B. Holst, & D. Ritter. (2001). Managing viral hepatitis. Clinician Reviews, 11, 51–62.

Diagnostic Tests

Diagnosis is often made on the basis of a thorough history and physical examination.

A history of exposure to persons with the disease is significant.

Physical examination reveals a tender, enlarged liver; abdominal pain; and flulike symptoms.

Laboratory evaluation includes serologic testing to detect the presence of antigens and antibodies to hepatitis A virus, hepatitis B virus, hepatitis C virus, or hepatitis D virus, and liver function studies.

Serum glutamic oxaloacetic transaminase, serum glutamic pyruvic transaminase, and bilirubin are elevated.

Clinical Therapy

The spread of viral infections can be interrupted by elimination of the virus from the infected population, institution of proper hygiene, and passive or active immunization (Table 21–5).

Active immunization for hepatitis A, a two-dose series, is recommended for all persons at risk of acquiring and transmitting the disease, and for all children in certain states of the United States.

Immunization for hepatitis B, a three-dose series, is recommended for all children and at-risk adults; the first dose is given within 12 hours of birth to the infant born to an infected mother or to a mother with unknown status (see Chapters 8 and 13 for further information about immunizations).

Management of the illness includes bedrest, hydration, and adequate nutrition during the flulike phase; if prothrombin times are increased, vitamin K is administered.

Nursing Management

Nursing care focuses on immunizing against hepatitis A and B, preventing the spread of infection, providing fluid and nutritional support, promoting growth and development, reducing risk of complications, and providing care for the child.

Table 21–5 Transmission, Immunization, and Prophylaxis for Hepatitis

Type	Primary Transmission	Immunization Available	Prophylaxis
Hepatitis A	Fecal–oral	Yes	Immune serum globulin
			Hepatitis A vaccine
Hepatitis B	Blood products IV drug use In utero Sexual activity	Yes	Hepatitis B immune globulin Hepatitis B vaccine
Hepatitis C	Blood products Sexual activity IV drug use Body piercing	No	None
Hepatitis D	Blood products IV drug use In utero Sexual activity	No	Hepatitis B vaccine
Hepatitis E	Fecal–oral	No	None

Cirrhosis (End-Stage Liver Disease)

Cirrhosis is a degenerative disease process that results in fibrotic changes and fatty infiltration in the liver; it can occur in children of any age as the end stage of several disorders, including biliary atresia (Kelly, 2002).

The diffuse destruction and regeneration of the hepatic parenchymal cells result in an increase in fibrous connective tissue and disorganization of the liver structure.

When the disease process results from obstruction, as in biliary atresia, jaundice is an initial sign that intensifies with progression of the disease.

In other diseases that cause cirrhosis, jaundice may be a late sign, intermittent, or absent.

Steatorrhea is frequently present and can lead to rickets, hemorrhage, and failure to gain weight.

Anemia can occur as a result of chronic blood loss from the gastrointestinal tract.

Pruritus is common, particularly in children with biliary malformations.

Clubbing of the digits and cyanosis are other common findings.

Diagnostic evaluation is based on the child's history of infection or disease with liver involvement.

Physical examination may reveal jaundice, skin changes, ascites, and hemodynamic changes.

Laboratory evaluation reveals abnormal liver function tests.

A liver biopsy may help to determine the extent of the parenchymal damage.

Medical management focuses on treating the child's symptoms and achieving optimal nutritional status and growth.

Liver transplant is often the treatment of choice.

Clinical manifestations include ascites, hepatic encephalopathy, and hemorrhage from esophageal varices.

Nursing care focuses on monitoring physiologic and psychosocial changes to identify early signs of end-stage hepatic failure.

Monitor vital signs frequently.

Daily weight measurement is performed to assess for fluid retention.

Close monitoring of electrolytes and liver function test results helps determine the need for fluid-replacement therapy.

Measure abdominal girth daily.

Careful administration of medications and monitoring for side effects are necessary because drug metabolism is altered in liver disorders.

If ascites is present, provide a low-sodium, low-protein diet and restrict fluids.

Parents of a child with cirrhosis are coping with a life-threatening disorder, and their anxiety and stress are high; the child may be waiting for a liver transplantation that represents the only hope for recovery; provide support to parents, and encourage them to verbalize their fears and concerns.

INJURIES TO THE GASTROINTESTINAL SYSTEM
Abdominal Trauma
Description and Etiology

Abdominal injuries may be caused by blunt or penetrating trauma; the type of injury determines the extent of organ damage.

Low-velocity trauma—for example, when a child strikes the handlebars of a bicycle—usually results in single-organ injury.

High-velocity blunt trauma, which may occur in motor vehicle crashes, usually involves multiple organs.

Solid organs, such as the liver and spleen, are more vulnerable to injury than hollow organs, such as the stomach, intestines, and bladder.

Motor vehicle crashes are the most common and also the most preventable unintentional injury in children (National Safety Council, 2003); on impact, small children who are held on a parent's lap or improperly restrained in a safety seat can easily become airborne, striking objects or being thrown from the car; when older children involved in severe crashes are wearing only lap belts, injury to the hollow organs may result.

Bicycles are another cause of abdominal injuries in children; bicycle accidents account for 5–14% of blunt abdominal trauma in children (Lam, Eunson, Munro, et al., 2001); such injuries commonly occur when the child strikes the handlebars during a fall or sudden stop or is struck by a car.

Child abuse is another major cause of abdominal trauma.

Injury to the abdominal organs can result in hemorrhage and organ necrosis.

Digestive enzymes and/or bacterial contents of the bowel may be released into the peritoneum.

Clinical Manifestations

Clinical manifestations of abdominal injury include pain, abdominal distention, muscle guarding, decreased or absent bowel sounds, nausea and vomiting, hypotension, hypovolemia, and shock.

Diagnostic Tests

Suspected abdominal trauma in a child necessitates a thorough history and physical examination; the description of the event should be compared with the child's signs and symptoms.

A computed tomography scan is performed to assess for internal bleeding and air in the abdomen.

Focused abdominal sonography for trauma is more specific and can demonstrate the presence or absence of pericardial fluid, abdominal fluid, and some parenchymal injuries (Schulman, 2003).

Baseline laboratory studies, including blood type and cross-match, are done.

Peritoneal lavage may be performed; during peritoneal lavage, a dialysis catheter is inserted into the abdominal cavity, and normal saline or lactated Ringer's solution is instilled; the fluid is then drained and analyzed for the presence of RBCs, amylase, and bacteria, which could indicate organ damage.

A urinary catheter may be inserted to check for the presence of blood and bladder rupture.

Clinical Therapy

Treatment of an abdominal, liver, or spleen injury takes place in the pediatric intensive care unit and focuses on preventing or managing hemorrhage and monitoring for signs of shock.

An intravenous infusion is initiated for fluid maintenance and to provide access for blood products.

The child is kept NPO, and a nasogastric tube is inserted.

Blood transfusions and pharmacologic management are used to treat blood loss.

Serial hematocrit levels are monitored to identify continued bleeding.

Exploratory laparotomy is sometimes warranted to treat hollow organ injuries or to repair liver or spleen lacerations when bleeding is not controlled.

Nursing Management
Assessment

Nursing care includes initial and ongoing assessments of the child's condition.

Initial assessment includes assessing the abdomen for bruising, pain, guarding, rebound tenderness, distention, and absence of bowel sounds (Schulman, 2003).

Monitor vital signs every hour or more frequently as warranted.

Measurement of abdominal circumference (to detect distention), intake and output monitoring, serial hematocrit levels, and auscultation of bowel sounds are also performed hourly.

Assess for increasing severity of pain, fever, and loss of bowel sounds, which may indicate a previously undiagnosed bowel or hollow-organ injury (Schulman, 2003); back pain may indicate retroperitoneal bleeding.

Monitor white blood cell count, amylase, and alkaline phosphatase; notify the primary healthcare provider of any changes.

Assess for increasing heart rate, hypotension, dyspnea, and other changes that may indicate shock.

Intervention

The child and parents are usually fearful and anxious when the child is admitted to the hospital; if the injury was preventable, parents may have feelings of guilt or anger; provide emotional support.

Administer fluids and blood products as prescribed.

Maintain nasogastric tube, if present.

Prepare the child and parents for surgery if necessary.

Provide postoperative care, including pain control; vital sign measurement; and respiratory, cardiovascular, and gastrointestinal system evaluations.

Once the child's condition is stabilized, nursing care shifts to preventive teaching; partner with the child and parents to ensure their understanding of safety measures to prevent future injuries.

INGESTION OF FOREIGN SUBSTANCES
Ingestion of Poisons
Poisonings are the second leading cause of unintentional home injury death and account for nearly one-third of all unintentional home injuries (Home Safety Council, 2004).

Common causes of poisonings include medications, caustics and cleaning agents, cosmetics, plants, hydrocarbons, insecticides, and pesticides.

The leaves, stems, or flowers of many common household and garden plants are poisonous—examples include Boston ivy, poinsettia, philodendron, lily of the valley, daffodil (bulbs), azalea, and rhododendron.

Nail care products, mothballs, weed and bug killers, and rodent killers are other potential hazards.

Although 75% of poisons are ingested, other routes of contamination include dermal, inhalation, and ocular (Litovitz, Klein-Schwartz, White, et al., 2000).

The manifestations of poisoning depend on the toxin (see Table 21–6 for clinical manifestations and therapy for common poisons).

Blood and urine toxicology screens, arterial blood gases, and electrolytes are performed when a child ingests a poison; testing of vomitus for presence of medication or other poisonings may be helpful in determining the amount ingested.

In the emergency department, the child's vital signs and level of consciousness are assessed, and specific information about the poison is obtained from the parent (Box 21–2 summarizes emergency management for poisoning).

Nursing Management
Nursing care focuses on initial emergent care and stabilization of the child with poisoning, followed by family education to reduce the risk of repeated poisoning.

Take a history from the family about the child's suspected ingestion substance, time, amount, and symptoms.

Initial assessment focuses on airway, vital signs, and neurologic status.

Assess drooling, diaphoresis, and increased or depressed respirations.

Assess for wheezing, respiratory distress, or stridor.

Table 21-6 Clinical Manifestations of Commonly Ingested Toxic Agents

Type	Sources	Clinical Manifestations	Clinical Therapy
Corrosives (strong acids and alkaline products that cause chemical burns of mucosal surfaces)	Batteries Household cleaners Clinitest tablets Denture cleaners Bleach Toilet bowl cleaners	Severe burning pain in mouth, throat, or stomach; swelling of mucous membranes; edema of lips, tongue, and pharynx (respiratory obstruction); violent vomiting; hemoptysis; drooling; inability to clear secretions; signs of shock, anxiety, and agitation	Do not induce vomiting! Dilute toxin with water to prevent further damage. Give activated charcoal.
Hydrocarbons (organic compounds that contain carbon and hydrogen; most are distillates of petroleum)	Gasoline Kerosene Furniture polish Lighter fluid Paint thinners	Gagging Choking Coughing Nausea Vomiting Alteration in sensorium (lethargy) Weakness Respiratory symptoms of pulmonary involvement, tachypnea, cyanosis, retractions, grunting	Do not induce vomiting! (Aspiration of hydrocarbons places child at high risk for pneumonia.) Use gastric lavage if severe central nervous system and respiratory impairment are present. Use of activated charcoal is controversial. Provide supportive care. Decontaminate skin by removing clothing and cleansing skin.
Acetaminophen	Many over-the-counter products	Nausea Vomiting Sweating	Give activated charcoal. Gastric lavage has limited use.

	Pallor	Administer charcoal or NAC [concentrated form of acetylcysteine (Mucomyst)], which binds with the metabolite, preventing absorption and protecting the liver.
	Hepatic involvement (pain in upper right quadrant, jaundice, confusion, stupor, coagulation abnormalities)	
Salicylate	Products containing aspirin	Nausea	Depends on amount ingested.
		Disorientation	Give activated charcoal.
		Vomiting	Gastric lavage has limited use.
		Dehydration	Administer IV sodium bicarbonate, fluids, and vitamin K.
		Diaphoresis	
		Hyperpnea	
		Hyperpyrexia	
		Bleeding tendencies	
		Oliguria	
		Tinnitus	
		Convulsions	
		Coma	
Mercury	Broken thermometers	Tremors	Similar to that for lead poisoning (see Lead Poisoning).
	Chemicals	Memory loss	
	Paints	Insomnia	
	Pesticides	Weight loss	
	Fungicides	Diarrhea	
		Anorexia	
		Gingivitis	

(continued)

Alterations in Gastrointestinal Function **423**

Table 21–6 Clinical Manifestations of Commonly Ingested Toxic Agents (Continued)

Type	Sources	Clinical Manifestations	Clinical Therapy
Iron	Multiple vitamin supplements	Vomiting Hematemesis Diarrhea Bloody stools Abdominal pain Metabolic acidosis Shock Seizures Coma	Give activated charcoal. Gastric lavage has limited use. Administer IV fluids and sodium bicarbonate. Deferoxamine chelation therapy.

Assess for decreased responsiveness and seizure activity.

Assess heart rate, skin color, capillary refill, peripheral and central pulses, and blood pressure.

Assess pupils (abnormally large or pinpoint pupils may be observed).

Assess mouth, lips, and tongue for corrosive burns or edema.

Assess breath for unusual odor.

Assess the child for vomiting and diarrhea.

Assess vomitus for presence of medication or other ingested substances.

Determine the child's height and weight.

See Box 21–2 for nursing care needed.

Box 21–2 Emergency Management for Poisoning

1. Stabilize the child. Assess ABCs (airway, breathing, and circulation). Provide ventilatory and oxygen support.
2. Perform a rapid physical examination, start an IV infusion, draw blood for toxicology screen, and apply a cardiac monitor.
3. Obtain a history of the ingestion, including substance ingested, where child was found, by whom, position, when the child was found, how long unsupervised, history of depression or suicide, allergies, and any other medical problems.
4. Reverse or eliminate the toxic substance using the appropriate method:
   a. Antidotes and agonists
      - Acetylcysteine (Mucomyst; for acetaminophen poisoning)
      - Digibind (for digoxin poisoning)
      - Naloxone (Narcan; for opioid overdose)
      - Flumazenil (Romazicon; for benzodiazepine overdose)
   b. Gastric lavage
      - A gastric tube is inserted through the mouth.
      - Normal saline solution is instilled and aspirated until the return is clear.
      - Contraindicated in children who have ingested alkaline corrosive substances, as insertion of the tube may cause esophageal perforation.
   c. Activated charcoal
      - Used in children who have ingested acids to decrease continued damage and potential perforation of stomach and intestines.

- Given to absorb and remove any remaining particles of toxic substances.
- Usual dosage administration is 1g/kg of body weight.
- A commercial preparation of activated charcoal is administered orally or through a gastric tube.
- Available as a ready-to-drink solution in an opaque container.
- May be mixed with apple juice or soda if protocol allows to encourage consumption.
- A covered cup and straw are used when giving orally to prevent the child from seeing the black liquid and to minimize spillage.
- Activated charcoal is administered only if the child is not vomiting, because aspiration of charcoal is damaging to lung tissue.
- Should not be administered for ingestion of caustic substances or hydrocarbons.

   d. Cathartics
- Hasten excretion of a toxic substance and minimize absorption. The most commonly used cathartic is magnesium sulfate.

Note: Syrup of ipecac. The use of ipecac is no longer recommended because it may not remove all poison and can be harmful in some situations. Encourage parents to remove it from their homes.

5. Other measures depend on the child's condition, the nature of the ingested substance, and the time since ingestion. May include diuresis, fluid loading, cooling or warming measures, anticonvulsive measures, antiarrhythmic therapy, hemodialysis, or exchange transfusions.
6. The child's total condition is constantly evaluated to maintain airway, breathing, and circulation. Therapeutic management is adjusted as needed to treat evolving condition.
7. Consider the emotional status of the family. Provide information about the child, involve them in care when possible, and arrange for support persons and services to be available to them.

Once immediate care has been provided, nursing care shifts to providing emotional support and preventing recurrence.

Instruct all families to keep the toll-free number for the American Association of Poison Control Centers close to phones (1-800-222-1222).

Families with children require instructions for avoiding childhood poisoning. Teach family members these interventions to help avoid childhood poisonings:

- Place household cleaners, medications, vitamins, and other potentially poisonous substances out of the reach of children or in locked cabinets.
- Use warning stickers, such as Mr. Yuk, on all containers.
- Buy products with childproof caps.
- Store products in their original containers.
- Never place household cleansers or other products in food or beverage containers.
- Remove all houseplants from the child's play areas.
- Put the poison control center phone number by every phone in the house.
- Use caution when visiting other settings that are not childproofed (e.g., grandparents' homes). Remember that visitors may have pills in their purses or pockets that are easily accessible.

Ingestion of Foreign Objects

Children ingest a variety of foreign objects, including coins, pins, parts of toys, batteries, and bones from foods.

If the foreign body is lodged in the esophagus, they may present with substernal pain, drooling, and dysphagia; some children may exhibit respiratory symptoms, including wheezing or coughing.

Complications include perforation of the intestinal tract and development of strictures at the site of a retained foreign body.

Radiographs of the neck, chest, esophagus, and abdomen are useful tools in verifying ingestion and to identify the location of the object; endoscopic examination and retrieval of the ingested foreign body may be necessary.

Nursing care centers on supporting the child, collaborative assistance in the identification and removal of the foreign body, and teaching the child and family measures to reduce reoccurrence.

Lead Poisoning

Lead poisoning is an excessive accumulation of lead in the blood.

Approximately 310,000 children from 1 to 5 years of age in the United States are at risk for exposure to harmful lead levels. 1.6% Have a level of ≥10 mg/dL; many of these children are poor and live in older houses in inner cities (Morbidity and Mortality Weekly Report, 2005).

Even children with levels below 10 mg/dL may experience cognitive defects due to lead exposure.

| Box 21–3 | Sources of Lead Exposure |

Sources of lead exposure include the following:

- Lead-based paint
- Soil and dust
- Drinking water from coolers with lead-soldered or lead-lined tanks, from lead-soldered teapots, or from lead pipes or lead-soldered pipes
- Food grown in contaminated soil, stored in lead-soldered cans or leaded crystal, or prepared in improperly fired pottery
- Parental occupations and hobbies that involve exposure to lead (e.g., plumbing, battery manufacturing, highway construction, furniture re-finishing, stained glass work, and pottery making)
- Airborne lead in areas surrounding smelters and battery manufacturing plants

Lead in paint is the most common source of lead exposure for pre-school children; children are also exposed to lead when they ingest contaminated food, water, and soil or when they inhale dust contaminated with lead (see Box 21–3 for sources of lead).

Lead interferes with normal cell function, primarily of the nervous system, blood cells, and kidneys, and adversely affects the metabolism of vitamin D and calcium (see Table 21–7 for clinical manifestations of lead poisoning).

Once in the body, lead accumulates in the blood, soft tissues (kidney, bone marrow, liver, and brain), bones, and teeth; lead that is absorbed by

Table 21–7 Clinical Manifestations of Lead Poisoning

Mild Toxicity (10–15 mcg/dL)	Moderate Toxicity (16–69 mcg/dL)	Severe Toxicity (≥70 mcg/dL)
Myalgia or paresthesia	Arthralgia	Paresis or paralysis
Mild fatigue	General fatigue	Encephalopathy may lead abruptly to seizures, changes in consciousness, coma, and death
Irritability, lethargy	Difficulty concentrating	
Occasional abdominal discomfort	Muscular exhaustibility	
	Tremor	Lead line (blue-black) on gingival tissue
	Headache	
	Diffuse abdominal pain	Colic (intermittent, severe abdominal cramps)
	Vomiting	
	Weight loss	
	Constipation	
	Anemia	

Note: Adapted from Agency for Toxic Substances and Disease Registry. (1990). Lead toxicity. Case studies in environmental medicine (p. 11). Atlanta: Agency for Toxic Substances and Disease Registry.

the bones and teeth is released slowly, so exposure to even small doses over time can result in dangerously high levels of lead in the body.

The Centers for Disease Control and Prevention now recommends screening children at high risk, with reduced screening for those at low risk. In addition, all children enrolled in Medicaid should be tested, with follow-up management and care (Advisory Committee on Childhood Lead Poisoning Prevention, 2000); a blood lead (Pb-B) level is the most useful screening and diagnostic test for lead exposure.

A complete blood count reveals anemia; iron deficiency is assessed by serum iron, total iron-binding capacity, and serum ferritin levels.

Urinalysis, blood urea nitrogen, and creatine are performed to assess for renal damage.

Abdominal radiograph reveals lead if present.

A Pb-B below 10 mg/dL is considered acceptable, although it may still not screen out all children with impaired development due to lead.

An environmental history should be obtained for children with Pb-B levels between 10 and 19 mg/dL to identify removable sources of lead; follow-up testing is required.

Children with Pb-B levels between 20 and 69 mg/dL require a full medical evaluation, including a detailed environmental and behavioral history, physical examination, and tests for iron deficiency; interventions to remove sources of lead from the child's environment are necessary.

For levels above 25 mg/dL, chelation therapy is also administered.

Children with Pb-B levels greater than 70 mg/dL are critically ill from lead poisoning and require immediate chelation therapy and interventions to provide a lead-free environment.

Chelation therapy involves the administration of an agent that binds with lead, increasing its rate of excretion from the body.

Calcium disodium ethylenediamine tetraacetate ($CaNa_2$ EDTA), dimercaprol (BAL), D-penicillamine, or succimer may be used.

Children with Pb-B levels between 25 and 69 mg/dL receive $CaNa_2$ EDTA for 5–7 days, followed by a rest period and then a second chelation treatment.

Children with Pb-B levels greater than 70 mg/dL are given dimercaprol and $CaNa_2$ EDTA, followed by a rest period and a second chelation treatment using $CaNa_2$ EDTA alone.

Long-term follow-up of children receiving chelation therapy is essential; the child should never be discharged unless a lead-free home environment has been ensured.

Nurses often work with state and local health officials to plan screening for children at high risk of lead exposure.

Educate parents about sources of lead in the environment and techniques to reduce exposure; emphasize the importance of housekeeping interventions to reduce exposure to lead dust; this includes damp mopping of hard surfaces, floors, windowsills, and baseboards; washing the child's hands and face before meals; and frequent washing of toys and pacifiers.

Teach parents the importance of including foods high in iron and calcium in the child's diet to counteract losses of these minerals associated with lead exposure.

Be sure that parents understand the importance of follow-up testing of lead levels.

If the child is developmentally delayed, refer the family to an infant stimulation or child development program.

22. ALTERATIONS IN GENITOURINARY FUNCTION

URINARY SYSTEM CONDITIONS
Bladder Exstrophy

Failure of the abdominal wall to fuse during fetal development results in extrusion of the bladder wall through the lower abdominal wall. The rectus muscles and symphysis pubis are widely separated. The bladder becomes inflamed with exposure to air and trauma during delivery. Renal damage may result from infection or obstruction. The abnormal bladder epithelium is prone to neoplasms.

Clinical Manifestations

The bladder mucosa appears as a mass of bright-red tissue exposed through an abdominal opening, and urine continually leaks from an open urethra. Females may have a split clitoris, separated labia, or absent vagina. Males may have a short, stubby penis; dorsal chordee; and a ventral prepuce. Epispadias and bilateral inguinal hernias may be present.

Diagnostic Testing

Diagnosis by prenatal ultrasound or physical assessment

Urinalysis, urine culture; see Table 22–1 for usual urinalysis findings

Radiologic imaging

Clinical Therapy

Surgical reconstruction is performed in several stages to address all defects.

- Closure of the bladder and abdominal wall is performed, usually within 24–48 hours after birth. Insertion of a suprapubic catheter and bilateral ureteral stents create a urinary diversion to promote healing. The wound and pelvis are immobilized to promote healing. Medication is provided to reduce urinary spasms.
- Urinary continence procedure or a urinary diversion procedure because a functional bladder cannot be reconstructed (Surer, Ferrer, Baker, et al., 2003).
- Pelvic closure with an osteotomy; sutures and Bryant's traction or a spica cast.

Table 22–1   Normal Freshly Voided Urinalysis Results

Macroscopic Examination	Normal Results
Color	Pale yellow, clear
Odor	Ammonia-like smell
Specific gravity	≤1.010 when well hydrated
pH	4.5–8.0
Protein	Negative; <150 mg/24 hr
Glucose	<130 mg/24 hr
Ketones	Negative
Bilirubin	Negative

Microscopic Examination	Normal Results
Red blood cells	0–5 per high-powered field (HPF)
White blood cells	<2 per HPF
Casts (hyaline)	1 per every 10–20 low-powered fields
Crystals	None

Note: Data from J. C. Liao, & B. M. Churchill (2001). Pediatric urine testing. Pediatric Clinics of North America, 48(6), 1425–1440.

- Reconstruction of bladder neck and ureteral reimplantation.
- Repair epispadias to create functional and normal-appearing genitalia.

Nursing Management
Assessment
Before surgery, monitor urine output and serum and urine chemistries to assess renal function and hydration. Weigh the newborn daily.

Assess family support systems and coping mechanisms.

After surgery, routinely record urine output from each tube every 2–4 hours; note any signs of tube obstruction (change in urine output, urine or blood draining from the urethral meatus, or increased intensity of bladder spasms). Assess pain.

Assess for wound dehiscence and bladder prolapse. Monitor lower limb peripheral circulation if a spica cast is used.

Implementation
Prevent the umbilical cord clamp from injuring the bladder mucosa.

Protect the bladder mucosa with a sterile saline-soaked dressing covered in sterile plastic wrap. Use a skin sealant to protect the skin from leaking urine.

After surgery, use aseptic technique for wound care, and monitor for signs of infection. Avoid abduction of the infant's legs to reduce stress on the surgical area.

Promote comfort by administering pain medications and antispasmodic agents. Administer antibiotics as prescribed.

Provide emotional support to parents, and promote parent–infant bonding through bathing and feeding.

Patient and Family Education

Teach parents to change dressings and to diaper the infant.

Educate parents to identify signs and symptoms of infection (cloudy urine, increased temperature, purulent drainage, foul odor from the incision, increased fussiness, or decreased feeding), and report them to the healthcare provider.

Discuss the need for follow-up visits to assess urinary function and to plan the next stages of surgery.

Teach parents to initiate toilet training at the appropriate age for bowel movements, even if urinary continence is not yet achieved.

Discuss ways to promote the child's self-esteem and self-confidence with sexual identity and function.

Enuresis

Enuresis is repeated involuntary voiding by a child who has reached 5–6 years at which time day and night bladder control is expected. Structural or neurologic pathology is uncommon. Nocturnal enuresis occurs with high frequency in children whose parents have a history of bedwetting. Other causes are illness, preoccupation with concerns or stress, and obstructive sleep apnea.

Primary enuresis—child has never had a dry night; due to maturational delay and small functional bladder.

Intermittent enuresis—child has occasional nights or periods of dryness.

Secondary enuresis—has been reliably dry for 6–12 months, bedwetting begins owing to stress, infections, or sleep disorders.

Clinical Manifestations

Diurnal enuresis—daytime frequency, urgency, constant dribbling, and involuntary loss of bladder control

Nocturnal enuresis—bedwetting

Diagnostic Testing

Urinalysis and urine culture

Functional bladder capacity and urine flow measurement

Bladder sonogram to measure postvoid residual

Clinical Therapy

A spontaneous cure rate occurs in approximately 15% of children each year, with or without intervention.

At 6–7 years, a multitreatment approach uses fluid intake management, bladder training, enuresis alarms, and positive reinforcement. Foods believed to contribute to enuresis (caffeine, milk, chocolate, and citrus) may be avoided.

Medications, such as desmopressin acetate, oxybutynin, and imipramine, may be used. See Table 22–2.

Nursing Management

Assessment

Review the child's urine and bowel elimination patterns, developmental milestones, toilet training history, and urinary symptoms.

Inspect the child's lower spine for signs of occult spina bifida (fistulas, sacral dimples, or tufts of hair). Identify potential stressors that may contribute to enuresis.

Identify how much of a problem the enuresis is to the child and family. Are the parents and child equally motivated to resolve the problem?

Implementation

Educate the child and parents about bladder control development and the causes and treatment of enuresis. Ensure that they understand that the wetting cannot be controlled.

When the parents and child are motivated and ready, strategies for parents to implement include promoting regular stools, providing most of fluid intake during the morning and afternoon, having the child double void before bed, offering praise and encouragement to the child, and maintaining a calendar to document progress.

Discuss the use of an enuresis alarm to determine whether the child and parents are willing to use it long term (10–12 weeks) until the child becomes consistently dry.

Discuss ways to reduce stressors on the child or to help the child cope with the stressors.

Hypospadias and Epispadias

Congenital anomalies in which the urethral meatus has an abnormal location on the penis resulting from failure of the urethral folds to fuse completely over the urethral groove. Hypospadias often occurs

Table 22–2 Medications Used in the Treatment of Enuresis

Medication	Action/Indication	Nursing Implication
Desmopressin acetate Oral or nasal administration	A vasopressin with an antidiuretic effect. It reduces urine production for 8–12 hours after dosing.	Reserved for times when the child is away from home for a sleepover or camp. Tablet form has a more consistent dose. Sit the child upright so that nasal medication stays on nasal mucosa and not down the throat. One-half of dose is administered to each nostril. Monitor blood pressure during initial dose-regulating period. Teach family to weigh the child daily and report weight gain.
Oxybutynin (Ditropan) Oral administration, extended-release tablet available	Relaxes smooth muscle of the bladder that increases bladder capacity and delays the initial desire to void.	Monitor for effects on nocturia, urinary frequency, urge incontinence, and completeness of bladder emptying. May cause dry mouth. May be taken with food.
Imipramine (Tofranil) Oral administration	Tricyclic antidepressant. Anticholinergic activity and nervous system stimulation, leading to earlier arousal to full bladder sensation.	Monitor for mood changes, fatigue, and sleep–arousal patterns. Be alert to associated dangers of overdoses. Administer dose 1 hour before bedtime, or one-half dose is given in afternoon and one-half at bedtime. Give with food to lessen gastrointestinal irritation. Weigh child twice a week, and monitor for edema. Avoid over-the-counter medications. Avoid exposure to strong sunlight. Effectiveness of drug may decrease with continued use.

Note: Data from R. Mercer. (2003). Dry at night: Treating nocturnal enuresis. Advance for Nurse Practitioners, 11, 26–32; and B. A. Wilson, M. T. Shannon, & C. L. Stang. (2004). Nurse's drug guide. Upper Saddle River, NJ: Prentice Hall.

with congenital inguinal hernias, undescended testes, and chordee. Most cases of epispadias occur with bladder exstrophy.

Clinical Manifestations

Hypospadias—the urethral meatus may be located anywhere along the ventral surface of the penis, from the perineum to the tip of the glans; chordee (curvature of the penis), and an incomplete or hooded foreskin may also be present.

Epispadias—the urethral meatus is located anywhere on the dorsal surface of the penis and may be at the level of the bladder neck.

Diagnostic Testing

Diagnosis by prenatal ultrasound or by physical examination

Urinalysis and urine culture

Testing for a chromosome abnormality or problem in androgen metabolism when the meatus is located on the perineum or scrotum

Clinical Therapy

Surgical correction of the structural defect is performed during the first year of life. The infant *should not be circumcised* because the foreskin tissue may be used for surgical repair.

A caudal nerve block is often used for initial postoperative pain relief. Anticholinergic medications (e.g., oxybutynin or hyoscyamine) are used to relieve bladder spasms.

A urethral stent is placed to maintain patency of the new urethral canal. A suprapubic or urethral urinary drainage catheter may be inserted to let urine flow without tension on the urethral sutures.

Nursing Management

Assessment

Assess the newborn for urine stream, exit site, and angle of urination.

Assess family support systems and coping mechanisms when the newborn is diagnosed with this defect. Assess the older child's anxiety about surgery and fear of mutilation.

After surgery, monitor for penile swelling, dysuria, bleeding at the surgical site, infection, and evidence of pain.

Implementation

Educate the parents to reduce anxiety concerning the future appearance and functioning of the penis. Use dolls and pictures to explain the procedure to an older child.

Protect the surgical site from injury, and ensure that the stent or catheter is not removed.

Encourage fluid intake and document intake and output hourly to detect postoperative urinary complications (kinks in the tubing or obstruction by sediment). Notify the physician if there is no urine output for 1 hour.

Administer medication—anticholinergics, antibiotics, and analgesics.

Patient and Family Education

Demonstrate care of the reconstructed area, including catheter or stent care, incision care, penis care, emptying of the drainage bag, and securing the catheter.

Use a double-diapering technique to protect the stent.

Do not bathe the child in the tub until the stent or catheter is removed.

Restrict the infant or toddler from activities (e.g., playing on riding toys) that put pressure on the surgical site. Avoid holding the infant or child straddled on the hip. Limit the child's activity for 2 weeks.

Encourage fluids to ensure adequate hydration. Offer fruit juice, fruit-flavored ice pops, fruit-flavored juices, flavored ice cubes, and gelatin.

Administer the *complete course* of prescribed antibiotics to avoid infection.

Observe for signs of infection—fever, swelling, redness, pain, strong-smelling urine, or change in flow of the urinary stream. The urine will be blood tinged for several days.

Call the physician if urine is seen leaking from any area other than the penis.

Obstructive Uropathy

A structural or functional obstruction in the urinary tract interferes with urine flow and results in urine backflow into the kidneys. Obstructions can occur at various sites:

- Ureteropelvic junction—obstruction may be caused by folds in the upper ureter or fibrotic stenosis
- Posterior urethral valves—a congenital membrane obstructs the posterior urethra, the most common cause of bladder outlet obstruction and severe obstructive uropathy (Cooper, Andrews, Hansen, et al., 2002)
- Narrowing at the ureterovesicular junction, a ureterocele, a ureter that inserts into an abnormal location within the urinary tract, or ureteral hypoplasia

Hydronephrosis, an accumulation of urine in the renal pelvis, results from obstruction. It compromises kidney function, resulting in hypertension, metabolic acidosis, inability to concentrate urine, urinary stasis and infection, and chronic renal failure (CRF).

Clinical Manifestations
Abdominal mass, enlarged kidney, palpable bladder

Hypertension

Urinary frequency, poor urinary stream, enuresis

Hematuria, urinary tract infection (UTI)

Pain

Failure to thrive

Diagnostic Testing
Hydronephrosis may be detected by prenatal ultrasound.

Urinalysis.

A diuretic-enhanced radionuclide scan and a voiding cystourethrogram.

Serial serum creatinine and electrolyte levels.

Arterial blood gases may reveal metabolic acidosis due to improper renal function.

Clinical Therapy
For acute obstructions, urethral or suprapubic catheterization for an obstructed posterior urethral valve until surgery (Woolf & Thiruchelvam, 2001).

Surgical correction or urinary diversion to lower the pressure in the kidney (pyeloplasty, valve repair, reconstruction, vesicostomy, or valve ablation).

In cases of urinary incontinence—clean intermittent catheterization or diversion with a temporary or permanent ostomy.

Antibiotic prophylaxis to reduce the risk for UTI.

Nursing Management
Assessment
Palpate the abdomen for a mass or distended bladder. Monitor the urine output, and observe the force of the urine stream.

Observe for peripheral edema and costovertebral angle tenderness.

Implementation

Prepare the parents and child for the surgical procedure.

After surgery, monitor vital signs, intake and output, and bladder distention.

Administer antibiotics and antispasmodics, such as oxybutynin. Administer pain medication when the epidural catheter placed for pain management is removed.

Discharge teaching includes care of the stents, catheter, or urinary diversion, as well as dressing changes. Provide information about signs of infection or obstruction and pain management.

Encourage follow-up care when signs of UTI or impaired renal functioning are noted.

Urinary Tract Infection

An infection of the upper or lower urinary tract of bacterial, viral, or fungal origin.

- A lower UTI involves the bladder and urethra.
- An upper UTI or pyelonephritis involves the ureters, renal pelvis, and renal parenchyma.

UTIs in newborns and infants may indicate an abnormality of the genitourinary tract. Renal scarring can result from hydronephrosis or the inflammatory and ischemic effects of the infection.

Usually, an organism ascends the urethra to the bladder and up toward the kidney. Causative organisms include *Escherichia coli, Staphylococcus, Klebsiella, Proteus, Pseudomonas aeruginosa, Enterobacter*, and *Enterococcus* (Santen & Altieri, 2001).

An increased risk of UTI occurs with urinary stasis, infrequent voiding, irritated perineum, constipation, masturbation, sexual abuse, and sexual activity in adolescent females.

Clinical Manifestations

Newborn—unexplained fever or no fever, failure to thrive, poor feeding, vomiting, diarrhea, strong-smelling urine, change in voiding habit, irritability

Lower UTI
- Infant—fever, diarrhea, vomiting, irritability, lethargy, foul-smelling diapers, poor feeding, failure to gain weight
- Preschooler—fever, hematuria, urgency, dysuria, frequency, cloudy urine, foul-smelling urine, dehydration, abdominal pain, enuresis

- School age—dysuria, enuresis, hematuria, strong smelling urine, diarrhea, frequency or hesitancy, mood changes, abdominal pain, suprapubic or flank pain, dehydration

Upper UTI—high fever, chills, abdominal pain, nausea, vomiting, flank pain, costovertebral angle tenderness, moderate to severe dehydration

May be asymptomatic

Diagnostic Testing

Urine culture and sensitivity collected by midstream clean-catch void, sterile catheterization, or suprapubic aspiration.

Urinalysis reveals white blood cells (WBCs) in the urine. A complete blood count reveals an elevated WBC count.

A blood culture may be obtained to assess for sepsis.

Radiologic imaging—renal and bladder sonogram and a cystogram (voiding cystourethrogram or radionuclide) to detect pyelonephritis and renal scarring (Kraus, 2001).

Clinical Therapy

Antibiotic therapy when urine samples are collected and changed as needed when culture sensitivity is available. Intravenous (IV) antibiotics and fluids if oral antibiotics are not tolerated.

Follow-up urine cultures monthly for 3 months, every 3 months for 6 months, and then annually, as future infections may be asymptomatic. Prophylactic antibiotics in cases of vesicoureteral reflux or recurrent infections.

When a structural defect exists, surgical correction may prevent recurrent UTIs.

Nursing Management

Assessment

Assess the infant for toxic appearance, fever, and poor feeding and oral intake. Assess for quality, quantity, and frequency of voiding. Observe the urinary stream. Palpate the abdomen and suprapubic and costovertebral areas for masses, tenderness, and distention. Assess for abdominal or flank pain, frequency, urgency, and dysuria. Palpate or percuss the bladder after voiding to evaluate bladder emptying. Assess vital signs.

Measure the child's height and weight, and plot on a growth curve to evaluate the growth pattern. Assess for behavioral changes, such as bedwetting and loss of bladder control.

Assess sexual activity or potential for sexual abuse in young children.

Implementation

Administer medications, promote rehydration, assess renal function, and partner with parents and older children to minimize the risk of future infection.

Encourage fluid intake to dilute the urine and flush the bladder.

Emphasize the importance of taking the full course of antibiotics.

Toilet-trained toddlers may regress and need diapers temporarily. Enuresis may occur in children who have previously been dry at night. Reassure parents that this is normal and to give support to the child.

Children with renal scarring should have their blood pressure monitored during future healthcare visits.

Parent and Family Education

Provide education to parents and children about strategies to reduce the risk for future UTIs.

Teach proper perineal hygiene. Girls should always wipe the perineum from front to back after voiding.

Encourage the child to drink plenty of fluids, but avoid caffeinated and carbonated beverages that may irritate the bladder.

Caution against tight underwear; children should wear cotton rather than nylon underwear.

Encourage the child to void more frequently and to fully empty the bladder.

Discourage bubble baths and hot tubs, which can irritate the urethra.

Encourage abstinence of sexual activity. Instruct sexually active girls to void before and after sexual intercourse to flush out bacteria introduced during intercourse.

Vesicoureteral Reflux

Backflow of urine from the bladder into the kidneys prevents complete emptying of the bladder and creates a reservoir for bacterial growth. Causes include incomplete development of the ureterovesical junction, or the ureters are abnormally inserted into the bladder. Complications include renal scarring, hypertension, and chronic kidney failure (Vogt, 2002).

Clinical Therapy

A renal ultrasound and voiding cystourethrogram reveals the defect and severity of reflux (e.g., to the ureter, renal pelvis, or dilating the ureter and renal pelvis).

Antibiotics to prevent UTIs.

Surgery to reimplant the ureters may be required.

Nursing Management

After ureteral reimplantation, monitor urine output through the Foley catheter. The urine is initially bloody and may have clots. Follow orders for irrigating the Foley catheter when urine output is diminished.

Administer IV fluids at a rate of 1.5 times maintenance to maintain a high urinary output, minimize clot formation, and overcome obstruction caused by bladder swelling (Ellsworth, Cendron, & McCullough, 2000).

Administer antibiotics, antispasmodics, and analgesics as prescribed.

Discharge teaching includes administration of antibiotics and antispasmodics, a high-fiber diet to reduce constipation, and avoidance of active play for 3 weeks. Provide guidelines to call the physician for a fever of more than 38.5°C (101.5°F), abdominal or back pain, or swelling and redness of the incision.

RENAL DISORDERS
Acute Postinfectious Glomerulonephritis

Acute postinfectious glomerulonephritis (APIGN) is an inflammation of the glomeruli of the kidneys. Usually, the child is recovering from a group A beta-hemolytic streptococcal infection of the throat or skin and then develops signs of APIGN after 8–14 days. An immune complex reaction localizes on the glomerular capillary wall, leading to inflammation and glomerular injury. Obstructed glomerular capillaries reduce the glomerular filtration rate. Increased vascular permeability allows red blood cells, red cell casts, and eventually protein molecules to be excreted. Sodium and water are retained, resulting in edema. APIGN is a significant cause of acute and chronic renal failure (ARF and CRF) in children.

Clinical Manifestations

Abrupt onset with flank or midabdominal pain, irritability, malaise, and fever; costovertebral tenderness may occur.

Microscopic or gross hematuria; dysuria; oliguria may or may not be present.

Mild periorbital and dependent edema may progress in severity to cause dyspnea, cough, ascites, crackles, and a gallop rhythm (Lang

& Towers, 2001); hypovolemia due to fluid shifting between vascular and interstitial spaces, despite obvious signs of excess fluid retention.

Acute hypertension causing encephalopathy with headache, nausea, vomiting, irritability, lethargy, and seizures.

Diagnostic Tests
Urinalysis to detect hematuria, proteinuria, leukocytes, and red and white cell casts.

Serum protein, lipid levels, blood urea nitrogen (BUN), and creatinine concentrations.

Complete blood count to detect anemia and an elevated WBC count; erythrocyte sedimentation rate, serum complement 3.

An antistreptolysin O titer and anti-DNAse B titer help document strep throat and skin infections.

A renal biopsy when clinical features are inconclusive (Lang & Towers, 2001).

Clinical Therapy
Bedrest and supportive therapy during the acute phase.

Restricted fluids, potassium, and sodium with volume overload; restricted protein intake when urine output is severely diminished.

Antihypertensive medication, such as hydralazine (Apresoline), and a diuretic, such as furosemide (Lasix) for hypertension. IV diazoxide, nitroprusside, or hydralazine for severe hypertension with cerebral dysfunction (Lang & Towers, 2001).

Antibiotics are *not* a treatment for APIGN. Antibiotics are used to treat the original infection. Family members are screened for streptococcal infections and treated as necessary.

Nursing Management
Assessment
Monitor vital signs and fluid and electrolyte status; weigh daily, and monitor intake and output. Document urine-specific gravity. Assess the urine color to detect hematuria.

Assess for periorbital and dependent edema. Measure the abdominal girth. Auscultate heart and lung sounds every shift and note respiratory effort to detect signs of fluid overload (crackles, dyspnea, and cough).

Section III: Body Systems

Monitor blood pressure. Assess for signs of encephalopathy (headache, blurred vision, vomiting, decreased level of consciousness, confusion, and convulsions).

Assess the child's and parents' level of understanding and the availability of support.

Implementation
Maintain bedrest.

Administer IV antihypertensives for severe hypertension.

Carefully plan the child's fluid intake over the entire day. Make sure parents and visitors understand the need to limit fluids.

Monitor for signs of infection, and reduce the child's exposure to infection. Limit visitors, encourage good handwashing, and screen visitors for upper respiratory infections.

Reposition the child frequently. Protect skin over bony prominences. Elevate lower extremities. Maintain proper hygiene and dry skin. Change diapers frequently.

Plan the child's diet with no added salt and low protein. Encourage the anorexic child to eat by providing favorite foods in compliance with the diet.

Support parents who blame themselves for not responding more quickly to the child's initial symptoms. Discuss the etiology of the disease and the child's treatment, and correct misconceptions.

Patient and Family Education
Educate parents about the medication regimen, potential side effects, dietary restrictions, and signs and symptoms of complications. It may require 3 weeks for hypertension and gross hematuria to resolve and longer for complete resolution of the disorder.

Educate parents to accurately assess the child's blood pressure and test urine for albumin.

Emphasize avoiding exposure of the child to individuals with upper respiratory tract infections.

Discuss plans for child's return to normal routine and activities, with periods allowed for rest.

Acute Renal Failure
The renal function abruptly diminishes and is unable to maintain electrolyte and fluid balances. ARF occurs most frequently in neo-

nates and children who are critically ill with asphyxia, shock, heart failure, and sepsis. ARF occurs in one of three ways.

Prerenal—decreased blood flow and perfusion to an otherwise normal kidney due to a systemic condition, such as hypovolemia, septic shock, or cardiac failure.

Intrarenal—primary kidney damage due to sustained hypoperfusion, infection, nephrotoxic drugs or poisons, or diseases, such as hemolytic uremic syndrome (HUS) or APIGN (Prakash, Sen, Kumar, et al., 2003).

Postrenal—obstruction of the urinary flow from both kidneys, such as posterior urethral valves or a neurogenic bladder.

Clinical Manifestations

Prerenal ARF—a healthy child suddenly develops a significant illness or injury (fever, dehydration or hypovolemia, dry mucous membranes, tachycardia, and poor peripheral perfusion)

Intrarenal and postrenal ARF—nausea, vomiting, lethargy, edema, crackles, gallop heart rhythm, gross hematuria, oliguria, and hypertension develop due to electrolyte imbalances, uremia, and fluid overload; other signs include pallor, lethargy, headache, seizures, and confusion; a flank mass may be palpated if an obstructive disorder is present

Diagnostic Tests

Urinalysis to detect hematuria, proteinuria, and red blood cell or granular casts

Blood chemistry (BUN, serum creatinine, sodium, potassium, and calcium levels); see Table 22–3

Renal ultrasound to detect hydronephrosis or other structural defects; a renal biopsy when the cause of ARF cannot be determined from other tests

Clinical Therapy

Treatment, often provided in the pediatric intensive care unit, is dependent on the cause of the ARF.

IV fluid boluses with normal saline or lactated Ringer's solution for hypovolemia; albumin may be administered when blood loss is the cause of circulatory depletion.

Diuretics are given to children with fluid overload. If response to diuretics is poor, fluid restrictions to maintain zero water balance are initiated. Intake should equal output.

Table 22–3   Diagnostic Tests for Renal Failure

Diagnostic Tests	Normal Values	Findings in Renal Failure
Urinalysis		
pH	4.5–8.0	Lowered
Osmolarity	50–1,400 mOsm/L	>500 prerenal
		<350 intrarenal
Specific gravity	1.001–1.030	High prerenal ARF
		Low intrarenal ARF
		Normal postrenal ARF
Protein	Negative	Positive
Serum chemistry*		
Potassium	3.5–5.8 mmol/L	Elevated
Sodium	135–148 mmol/L	Normal, low, or high; depends solely on the amount of water in the body
Calcium	2.2–2.7 mmol/L	Low
Phosphorus	1.23–2 mmol/L	Increased
Urea nitrogen	3.5–7.1 mmol/L	Increased
Creatinine	0.2–0.9 mmol/L	Increased
pH	7.38–7.42	Low acidic
Hemoglobin	7.27–7.49	Decreased
Hematocrit	11.0–13.3 g/dL	Decreased
Platelet count	32.7–39.3%	Decreased
	$165–332 \times 10^9$/L	Decreased
Albumin	3.5–5.2	Decreased

ARF, acute renal failure.
*Please refer to Chapter 6 for normal values for various ages.

Eliminate all sources of potassium intake. Hyperkalemia is treated with sodium polystyrene sulfonate (Kayexalate). Metabolic acidosis, hyponatremia, and hypocalcemia are also treated.

Antibiotics for infection. Avoid nephrotoxic drugs (e.g., aminoglycosides, nonsteroidal anti-inflammatory agents, cephalosporins, sulfonamides, tetracycline, and radiographic contrast dye with iodine).

Extra carbohydrate intake during the catabolic state.

Dialysis to correct severe electrolyte imbalances, manage fluid overload, and cleanse the blood of waste products.

Nursing Management
Assessment
Assess vital signs, level of consciousness, hydration status, peripheral perfusion, and signs of acute illness or injury. Assess for signs of electrolyte imbalance.

Weigh daily. Monitor urinalysis, urine culture, and blood chemistry studies. Inspect urine for color. Cloudy urine may indicate infection; tea-colored urine suggests hematuria. Assess urine-specific gravity and intake and output.

Assess the child's and parents' stressors, coping abilities, and the availability of support.

Implementation

Estimate the child's fluid status by daily weights, intake and output, and blood pressure two or three times daily. Monitor serum sodium. Aim for a stable serum sodium concentration and a decrease in body weight by 0.5–1.0% a day.

- If the child has oliguria, limit all fluid intake to replacement of insensible fluid loss (approximately one-third of the daily maintenance requirements in afebrile children).
- If serum sodium concentration rises and weight falls, insufficient fluids have been given. If the serum sodium level falls and the weight increases, excessive fluids have been given.
- Increase fluid administration by 12% for each centigrade degree of temperature elevation.

Administer antibiotics and antihypertensive agents as prescribed. Monitor drug levels. Be alert to signs of drug toxicity.

Tailor the child's diet to nutritional need and high-metabolic rate. Parenteral or enteral feeding may be used until oral feeding is possible. Sodium, potassium, and phosphorus may be restricted. See Table 22–4.

Use standard precautions and good handwashing to prevent infection.

Encourage parents to verbalize fears and assist them in working through feelings of guilt. Explain procedures and treatment measures to decrease anxiety.

Teach parents to administer medications, correctly measure the blood pressure, and identify symptoms of progressive renal failure.

Collaborate with a nutritionist to assist the family in appropriate food choices and menu planning, integrating ethnic and cultural food preferences.

Chronic Renal Failure

CRF is a progressive, irreversible reduction in renal function that leads to end-stage renal disease (ESRD), the most advanced form of CRF. Long-term complications of CRF and ESRD include hyperten-

Table 22–4   Nutritional Information for the Child with Kidney Disease

High-Sodium Content Foods	High-Potassium Content Foods	High-Phosphorus Content Foods
Soups and sauces: such as gravy, spaghetti and tomato sauce, barbecue sauce, steak sauce	*Fruit:* apricots, avocados, bananas, citrus fruits, fresh pears, nectarines, dates, figs, cantaloupe and other melons, prunes, and raisins	*Dairy products:* milk, cheese, yogurt, custard, pudding, ice cream
Processed lunch meats: bologna, ham, salami, hot dogs, etc.	*Vegetables:* celery, dried beans, lima beans, potatoes, leafy greens, spinach, tomatoes, winter squash	Dried beans, peas
		Nuts, peanut butter
Smoked meat and fish: bacon, chipped beef, corned beef, ham, lox	*Whole grains:* especially those containing bran	Chocolate
Sauerkraut, pickles, and other pickled foods	Sardines, clams	Dark cola
	Peanuts	Sausage, hot dogs
Seasonings: horseradish, soy sauce, Worcestershire sauce, meat tenderizer, and monosodium glutamate (MSG)	*Dairy products:* milk, ice cream, pudding, yogurt	
	Potassium-containing salt substitutes	

Note: Children with kidney disease have restricted diets, generally low in sodium, potassium, and phosphorus. Help families by reviewing foods to avoid or eat in very small quantities.

sion, anemia, bone disease, poor growth, and social developmental issues.

Major causes of CRF are congenital defects; obstructed urine flow and reflux; hereditary diseases, such as polycystic kidney disease (PKD); glomerular diseases; and systemic diseases, such as diabetes and lupus. As CRF progresses, metabolic acidosis occurs. Retention of excessive sodium and water leads to hypertension. Hypocalcemia and elevated phosphorus levels lead to renal osteodystrophy. Failure of the kidneys to produce erythropoietin leads to anemia.

Clinical Manifestations

Initially asymptomatic, followed by signs of pallor, headache, nausea, anorexia, fatigue, and decreased mental alertness and ability to concentrate.

Anemia leads to tachycardia, tachypnea, and dyspnea on exertion.

With disease progression, hypertension, edema, failure to thrive or short stature, osteodystrophy, delayed fine and gross motor development, and delayed sexual maturation occur. Osteodystrophy increases the child's risk for spontaneous fractures, rickets, and valgus deformity of the legs.

In ESRD, uremic symptoms develop, including nausea, vomiting, anorexia, unpleasant (uremic) breath odor, progressive anemia, uremic frost (urea crystals deposited on the skin), pruritus, malaise, headache, progressive confusion, tremors, pulmonary edema, dyspnea, and congestive heart failure.

Diagnostic Testing
The patient's glomerular filtration rate is calculated, using the serum creatinine level and the patient's height and gender stage of CRF (Hogg, Furth, Lemley, et al., 2003).

Imaging studies to identify kidney damage.

Serum electrolyte, phosphate, BUN, creatinine levels, and pH to monitor fluid and electrolyte status; see Table 22–3 for findings related to renal failure.

Clinical Therapy
The goals are to slow the progression of kidney disease, prevent complications, and promote growth and development, using a combination of dietary, fluid, and electrolyte management and hypertension control. Treatment is modified as the child's status changes.

Maximize caloric intake for growth. Restriction of dietary phosphorus, potassium, and sodium is tied to the child's electrolyte levels and fluid balance.

- Infants receive a special formula with less potassium, such as Similac 60/40, that is supplemented with extra carbohydrates, fat, and protein. Overnight enteral feedings are used to increase calories when growth is impaired.
- High-quality protein (meat, fish, poultry, and egg whites) to support growth: optimal protein intake for infants is 2.0–2.5 g/kg/day; and for older children, 1.5–2.0 g/kg/day.
- Vegetable oils, hard candy, sugar, honey, and jelly add calories to the child's diet.

Growth hormone helps some children achieve their target height.

Phosphate-binding agents, vitamin D, and calcium supplementation are used to prevent some of the bone demineralization associated with renal osteodystrophy. See Table 22–5 for other medications used in management of CRF.

Table 22–5   Medications Commonly Used by Children with Chronic Renal Failure (CRF)

Medication	Action or Indication	Nursing Considerations
Vitamin and mineral supplement (Nephrocaps)	Adds vitamins and minerals missing from a heavily restricted diet	Only prescribed vitamins should be used; over-the-counter brands may contain elements that are harmful.
Phosphate-binding agents: calcium carbonate (Tums), calcium acetate (PhosLo) or sevelamer hydrochloride (Renagel)	Reduces absorption of phosphorus from the intestines	Ensure that the phosphate-binding agent is aluminum-free.
Calcitriol (Rocaltrol)	Replaces the calcitriol that kidneys are no longer producing to keep calcium balance normal	Monitor serum calcium level. Ensure that a calcium supplement is provided.
Epoetin alfa (Epogen, Procrit)	Stimulates bone marrow to produce red blood cells, treats anemia owing to CRF	Given by IV or SC injection. Monitor blood pressure, as hypertension is an adverse effect. Monitor hematocrit and serum ferritin level according to facility guidelines.
Iron supplementation	Treats iron deficiency when epoetin alfa is prescribed	May be administered orally or by IV during hemodialysis.
Growth hormone	Used to stimulate growth in children with CRF	Record accurate height measurements at regular intervals.
Antihypertensive agents:		
Angiotensin-converting enzyme inhibitor (enalapril, lisinopril)	Used with proteinuric kidney disease because it slows the progression to ESRD	Monitor renal function and electrolyte balance.
Loop diuretics	Used when volume overload is present	

ESRD, end-stage renal disease.

Renal replacement therapy, either dialysis or renal transplant. See Renal Replacement Therapy.

Nursing Management

Assessment

Identify complications of CRF, including signs of hypertension, edema, poor growth and development, and anemia. Assess vital signs to help identify electrolyte alterations.

Perform a family assessment to help identify particular needs of the child and family. The child's socialization, body image, and psychological development are often affected. Determine any risk for nonadherence with treatments, particularly among adolescents.

Implementation
Monitor for side effects of diuretics and electrolyte imbalance (weakness, muscle cramps, dizziness, headache, and nausea and vomiting).

Use aseptic technique for all procedures and good handwashing. Monitor for signs of infection.

Provide small, frequent feedings and attractive meals, while adhering to food restrictions. See Table 22–4. Acknowledge the child's preferences in meal planning.

Plan the child's 24-hour fluid intake so the child has some fluids with meals, to take medications, and when thirsty. Use medicine cups or small cups for fluids given. Ensure that all visitors know and maintain the child's fluid restriction.

Provide emotional support and therapeutic play to the child who is often traumatized by frequent needle sticks, diagnostic procedures, and hospitalization.

Support school-age children and adolescents who are embarrassed about their appearance and perceived differences from peers.

Patient and Family Education
Provide information about the disease process, dialysis treatments, and kidney transplantation as the disease progresses. Stress the importance of long-term treatments.

Identify a consistent time within the family routine for medication administration. Educate the family about side effects of medications and complications associated with the disease.

Emphasize the need for the 23-valent pneumococcal and meningococcal vaccines. Immunization with live-virus vaccines should occur before kidney transplantation.

Promote social development and interaction with other children while attempting to reduce exposure to infection. Schedule dialysis to allow the child to participate in school.

Educate the school nurse and teachers about dialysis treatment and how to assist the child when a peritoneal dialysis exchange needs to occur during the day.

Assist in selecting clothing to cover the dialysis shunt site and to complement and enhance the child's physical appearance.

Refer to the National Kidney Foundation and local support groups.

Develop a plan for adolescents to transition from pediatric to adult services.

Hemolytic Uremic Syndrome (HUS)

HUS is an acute renal disease often linked to enterohemorrhagic *E. coli* strain O157:H7 from contaminated beef. Other organisms linked to HUS include *Shigella dysenteriae, Salmonella, Yersinia*, and *Campylobacter*. Autosomal recessive and dominant forms of HUS cause less than 5% of cases (Varade, 2000).

A toxin damages the lining of the glomerular arterioles, causing endothelial cell swelling. Fibrin deposited in the renal arterioles and capillaries causes a partial occlusion that damages red blood cells and leads to hemolytic anemia. Thrombocytopenia develops as platelets cluster in damaged vascular endothelial cells. ARF and acute tubular necrosis develops.

Clinical Manifestations

An episode of gastroenteritis with diarrhea, upper respiratory infection, or UTI precedes HUS onset by 1–2 weeks. HUS signs and symptoms include hypertension, pallor and purpura, neurologic involvement (irritability, seizures, altered level of consciousness, hallucinations, cerebral edema, posturing, or blindness), and ARF (hematuria and proteinuria, oliguria or anuria, edema and ascites).

Diagnostic Testing

Urinalysis to detect hematuria, casts, and proteinuria.

Serum BUN and creatinine are elevated. Serum albumin is decreased. Serum electrolytes reveal hyponatremia, hyperkalemia, hypocalcemia, hyperphosphatemia, and hyperglycemia (if the pancreas is affected by clot formation). Arterial blood gases reveal metabolic acidosis.

Hemoglobin, hematocrit, and platelet counts are decreased. WBCs are increased. A peripheral blood smear with fragments of red blood cells, fibrin split products, and a decreased platelet count [<140,000/mL (mm^3)] confirms the diagnosis.

Chest radiographs may reveal pulmonary edema.

Clinical Therapy

Supportive treatment for the complications of ARF (fluid restriction and a high-calorie, high-carbohydrate diet low in protein, sodium, potassium, and phosphorus). Enteral nutrition may be needed.

Medications include calcium supplementation, aluminum hydroxide gel to bind to phosphorus, sodium polystyrene sulfonate to remove excess potassium, and antihypertensive agents. The use of antibiotics is controversial. Antimotility medications are contraindicated. Insulin may be needed for hyperglycemia.

Dialysis is necessary for approximately 40% of children (Trachtman, Cnaan, Christen, et al., 2003). CRF may develop.

Transfusions of fresh-packed red blood cells for severe anemia. Platelets are given if the child is bleeding or if surgery is needed. Transfusions are carefully administered to prevent hypertension.

Nursing Management

Assessment

Monitor vital signs, neurologic signs, electrolyte levels, and blood counts. Monitor daily weights, and assess intake and output. Observe for signs of progressive renal impairment. Monitor for petechia and ecchymosis. Monitor the child for abdominal discomfort from diarrhea or other gastrointestinal disturbances.

Assess the coping strategies of the child and family and their availability of support.

Implementation

Care is the same as for ARF (see Acute Renal Failure).

Avoid invasive procedures, when possible, to prevent unnecessary bleeding.

Provide enteral nutrition, as necessary, during acute illness phase. Give small portions of high-calorie, high-carbohydrate foods low in sodium, potassium, and phosphorus when oral foods are tolerated. Monitor bowel sounds, and observe for vomiting and diarrhea.

Encourage parents to participate in the child's care. Encourage parents to monitor siblings for signs of diarrhea or HUS.

Teach parents about medications, dietary and fluid restrictions, and reducing risk of consumption of contaminated beef.

Nephrotic Syndrome

An alteration in renal function of unknown cause in which the glomerular basement membrane has increased permeability to plasma protein. An upper respiratory infection often precedes the onset of edema by 2–3 days (Robinson, Nahata, Mahan, et al., 2003). Proteins and immunoglobulins are lost through the glomerular membrane. Decreased intravascular oncotic pressure causes edema. The liver increases synthesis of lipoprotein, resulting in hyperlipidemia. An increased platelet count increases the risk for thrombosis. Hypertension and renal failure may result. The large majority of children have minimal change nephrotic syndrome.

Clinical Manifestations
Edema develops over several weeks, noted with a gradual or rapid weight gain, snug-fitting clothing, and tight-fitting shoes. Periorbital edema on waking; pallor, shiny skin with prominent veins, brittle hair, skin breakdown also occur.

Malaise, irritable, fatigued, and weak; anorexia, abdominal pain, nausea and vomiting, diarrhea.

Decreased urine output and dark, frothy urine.

Hypertension, tachycardia; in severe edema, respiratory distress and pulmonary congestion may occur.

Thrombosis.

Diagnostic Testing
Serum creatinine, BUN, sodium, and other electrolytes are assessed. The albumin concentration is low, less than 2.5 g/dL.

Urinalysis with first morning specimen to detect proteinuria and measure the protein-to-creatinine ratio.

Renal ultrasound; renal biopsy.

Clinical Therapy
Corticosteroids are the primary treatment. Urine protein levels usually fall to trace or negative values within 2–3 weeks of the start of therapy, and remission generally occurs. See Table 22–6 for other medications. Albumin may be given to the child with severe edema who is resistant to diuretics (Robinson, et al., 2003).

A diet with no restriction or an increase in protein normal for the child's age. A *no added salt* diet during corticosteroid treatment.

A relapse may occur with a respiratory infection or live-virus immunization; however, relapses become less frequent or stop during puberty. Repeat therapy is administered to children who have a relapse after drug therapy is discontinued.

Nursing Management
Assessment
Assess the child for fluid volume excess, including weight gain, facial and periorbital edema, external genitalia edema, and ascites.

Table 22-6 Medications Used to Treat Nephrotic Syndrome

Medication	Action/Implication	Nursing Considerations
Corticosteroid therapy Prednisone or prednisolone	Stimulates remission Reduces the excretion of protein in the urine.	Children who respond successfully to therapy continue to take corticosteroids daily for 6 weeks followed by 6 weeks of alternate-day treatment. Monitor for infection, changes in blood pressure, and changes in growth and behavior. Observe for major side effects, such as weight gain and moon face, obesity, gastrointestinal bleeding, growth retardation, hyperglycemia, hypertension, adrenal suppression, and bone demineralization. Limit calorie intake to prevent excessive weight gain associated with the appetite stimulant effect of corticosteroids. Delay administration of live vaccines until child is no longer immunosuppressed.
Alkylating/cytotoxic agents Chlorambucil, cyclophosphamide	Stimulates remission and helps extend the interval between relapses Used when no response to corticosteroids or side effects are a problem.	Monitor WBC count. Assess for gastrointestinal bleeding, alopecia, and impaired growth. Serious long-term side effects include carcinogenesis and risk of sterility in males. Administer medications 1 hour before breakfast or 2 hours after evening meal. An antiemetic may be prescribed for nausea while taking medication. Encourage adequate hydration to reduce cystitis. Educate the family to report unusual bleeding, bruising, chills, fever, or other signs of infection.

(continued)

Table 22–6   Medications Used to Treat Nephrotic Syndrome (Continued)

Medication	Action/Implication	Nursing Considerations
Cyclosporine therapy (immunosuppressant)	Used in children with corticosteroid refractory nephrotic syndrome by decreasing immunologic responses, decreasing the glomerular filtration rate, and affecting the glomerular basement membrane permeability to albumin	Monitor blood pressure for hypertension and other side effects of nausea, vomiting, anemia, and abdominal discomfort. Monitor electrolytes, cyclosporine serum concentrations, creatinine clearance, and serum creatinine levels to assess renal status. Educate the family to administer medication with meals to reduce nausea, administer the medication at the same time each day, and use a glass rather than plastic container for mixing. May dilute with orange or apple juice. Do not use grapefruit juice.
Diuretics Loop diuretics	Used for severe edema	They may be administered orally or by IV.
Furosemide, bumetanide, torsemide	Prevents reabsorption of water, sodium, and potassium by the renal tubules, thereby reducing massive edema	Monitor for intravascular volume depletion (hypovolemia). Assess vital signs for tachycardia and hypotension. Monitor plasma concentration to identify child at risk for hearing loss. Monitor for other potential side effects, including hyponatremia, hypokalemia, and other electrolyte imbalances.
Thiazide diuretics	Blocks the sodium chloride transporter in the distal tubule, thereby reducing massive edema	
Angiotensin-converting enzyme inhibitor Enalapril maleate (Vasotec)	Antihypertensive agent Some renal protective effects	Monitor blood pressure. Assess for transient hypotension and lightheadedness. Monitor serum potassium for side effect of hyperkalemia. If given in combination with NSAIDs, educate the family to avoid salt substitutes because they are high in potassium.
Antibiotics	Administered for infection Routine prophylaxis in nephrotic syndrome not effective	Administered according to prescribed schedule. Monitor WBC count, and assess for signs and symptoms of infection.

(continued)

Table 22–6 Medications Used to Treat Nephrotic Syndrome (Continued)

Medication	Action/Implication	Nursing Considerations
Antithrombotic therapy Heparin, followed by oral anticoagulant therapy	Activates angiotensin III to reduce coagulation	Monitor clotting factors and platelet count. Assess for evidence of thrombosis. Assess for abnormal bleeding (oozing IV sites, nosebleeds).
NSAIDs	Promotes some decrease in protein excretion Analgesia	Establish a routine pain assessment schedule using a pain scale. Administer pain medications around the clock rather than prn.

NSAID, nonsteroidal anti-inflammatory drug; WBC, white blood cell.
Note: Data from R. F. Robinson, M. C. Nahata, J. D. Mahan, & D. L. Batisky. (2003). Management of nephrotic syndrome in children. Pharmacotherapy, 22(8), 1021–1036; and R. J. Hogg, R. J. Portman, D. Milliner, K. V. Lemley, A. Eddy, & J. Inglefinger. (2000). Evaluation and management of proteinuria and nephritic syndrome in children: Recommendations from a pediatric nephrology panel established at the National Kidney Foundation conference on proteinuria, albuminuria, risk, assessment, detection, and elimination (PARADE). Pediatrics, 105(6), 1242–1249.

Monitor intake and output and vital signs at least every 4 hours. Weigh the child daily using the same scale, and measure abdominal girth to monitor changes in edema and ascites.

Assess the child for signs of hypovolemia during periods of diuresis. Assess for skin breakdown.

Assess for respiratory distress associated with pulmonary congestion, pulmonary edema, and pleural effusion. Monitor for hypertension and signs of circulatory overload.

Test urine for proteinuria and specific gravity once each shift. Monitor electrolytes.

Assess for signs of infection. Assess the child's comfort level and activity tolerance.

Implementation

Administer medications, and monitor for adverse effects of corticosteroids. If the child is receiving IV albumin, monitor closely for hypertension or signs of volume overload.

Use standard precautions and good handwashing. Use strict aseptic technique during invasive procedures. Reduce exposure to individuals with respiratory infections and communicable diseases. Educate parents on signs of infection.

Prevent skin breakdown. Provide daily hygiene, and maintain dry skin. Avoid restrictive clothing.

Meet nutritional and fluid needs. Plan a diet high in calories and low in sodium, keeping the child's food preferences in mind. Provide calcium supplementation. Fluids are generally not restricted except during severe edema.

Promote rest with opportunities for quiet play.

Children may have a distorted body image related to sudden weight gain and edema. Encourage the child and parents to express their feelings and concerns.

Patient and Family Education

Explain the disease process, prognosis, medication administration, and the treatment plan.

Educate parents to monitor urine for protein daily and to maintain records. Encourage parents to monitor body weight and use a urine dipstick weekly during remission to identify early signs of a relapse.

Seek home tutoring until the child can return to school. Emphasize the importance of avoiding contact with individuals who have infectious diseases.

Polycystic Kidney Disease

An autosomal recessive and dominant genetic disorder in which cellular hyperplasia of the kidneys' collecting ducts causes dilation of the ducts. Fluid secreted into these ducts enables cyst sacs to form. The cysts become larger and fibrose, slowly replacing much of the kidney's mass and reducing renal function. Cysts can also form in the liver, leading to bile duct proliferation, hepatic fibrosis, portal hypertension, and biliary infection. Newborns with severe PKD die shortly after birth from pulmonary hypoplasia.

Clinical Manifestations

Potter facies (low-set ears, small jaw, and a flattened nose) in children with autosomal recessive PKD.

Hypertension in early infancy, often severe.

Expected urine output or oliguria may occur. Polyuria and polydipsia develop as the kidneys' ability to conserve sodium and concentrate the urine decreases.

Respiratory distress and feeding intolerance due to enlarged kidneys.

As uremia develops, children have progressive developmental delay, growth failure, and renal osteodystrophy.

Diagnostic Tests

Prenatal ultrasound may reveal fluid-filled cysts; enlarged kidneys may be palpated at birth.

Renal ultrasound detects enlarged kidneys with cysts.

Liver biopsy.

Clinical Therapy

Treatment is supportive. Ventilatory support for newborns with pulmonary hypoplasia.

Medications—diuretics for hypertension, antibiotics for UTIs, management of fluid and electrolyte abnormalities, growth hormones for some children.

Dialysis or kidney transplant, but liver problems complicate the child's health.

Other family members are screened for subclinical cases.

Nursing Management

Same as for the child with renal insufficiency and CRF. See Chronic Renal Failure.

Observe the child for signs of progressive renal impairment.

Establish a home management plan focusing on medications, diet adequate in protein and calories, and management of acute gastrointestinal illnesses.

Refer the family for genetic counseling.

Renal Replacement Therapy
Peritoneal Dialysis

The abdominal peritoneum is the membrane through which the body's waste products pass from the blood to the abdominal cavity. The dialysis solution that enters the abdomen through a catheter contains dextrose that pulls body wastes and extra fluid into the abdominal cavity. The wastes and extra fluid leave the body with the drained dialysate.

Continuous ambulatory peritoneal dialysis uses gravity to instill pre-filled bags of dialysis solution into the peritoneal cavity four or five times a day. The fluid remains in the cavity for 4–8 hours and is then drained by hanging the bag lower than the pelvis.

Automated peritoneal dialysis uses an automatic cycler to instill and drain the dialysate approximately five times over a 10-hour period, usually overnight. One additional exchange may be needed during the day.

Benefits include a continuous dialysis clearance that decreases the toxic effects of waste products, less severe dietary and fluid restrictions, and the child's ability to ambulate and interact with the environment. Treatment timing can minimize the interruption of school, play, or other social events. The primary complications are peritonitis and abdominal hernia.

Signs of peritonitis associated with peritoneal dialysis include cloudy dialysate, fever, vomiting, diarrhea, abdominal pain, and tenderness. Peritonitis is treated with antibiotics infused in the dialysate.

Nursing Management

Educate the child and family to perform peritoneal dialysis and catheter care using aseptic technique, washing the hands every time the catheter is touched, and using sterile gloves to perform exchanges.

Assist the family to develop home routines that minimize disruptions to attending school and daily family life. Reinforce the importance of adhering to the prescribed diet and daily exchanges.

Hemodialysis

Blood is pumped out of the body and through a dialyzer machine with a special filter, where waste products and extra fluids diffuse out across a semipermeable membrane.

- Continuous hemodialysis treatment 24 hours per day is used when the child has ARF, multiple organ failure, and hemodynamic instability.
- Outpatient hemodialysis is used for children with CRF when peritoneal dialysis is not possible, usually performed three times a week. Each session lasts approximately 3–4 hours.
- Vascular access is accomplished with an arteriovenous fistula, a synthetic graft between the arterial and venous circulation, or a double-lumen cannula inserted into a large vein. Two needles are inserted, one to carry blood to the dialyzer and one to return cleaned blood to the body.

Hemodialysis is more efficient than peritoneal dialysis but requires close monitoring for hypotension or rapid changes in fluid and electrolyte balance that may lead to shock. Disequilibrium syndrome—cerebral edema caused by a drop in plasma osmolality during dialysis is a complication. The child may complain of fatigue, nausea, vomiting, or tremors, and sometimes delirium, seizures, or coma may occur. Heparin is used to reduce the risk of thrombosis.

Nursing Management

Monitor vital signs, blood pressure, oral intake, and urinary output every half hour while the child is on the dialysis equipment. Weigh the child before and after the dialysis to determine any fluid imbalances that require adjustment during the next hemodialysis session.

Educate the child and family about the administration of heparin and the control of bleeding from minor trauma.

Reinforce dietary limitations, and review menu planning to assure that the child's daily nutritional needs are met.

Encourage daily care to the catheter site and showering rather than tub baths. Activities, such as swimming, may be discouraged.

Kidney Transplantation

A kidney transplant is the only alternative to long-term dialysis for children with ESRD. Blood type compatibility between the donor and recipient is required, and a human leukocyte antigen system match graft improves survival. A living-relative donor kidney has a higher survival rate than a cadaver kidney.

Screening performed before transplant identifies problems that could lead to rejection of the kidney or infection. The child should be fully immunized before transplant. Evaluation of family strengths, weaknesses, and coping skills important to adherence to the immune suppression treatment after transplant may be performed (Hillerman, Russell, Barry, et al., 2002).

After transplantation, the child receives immunosuppressive medications, such as corticosteroids, azathioprine, cyclosporine, and anti-lymphocyte antibodies, to suppress rejection.

Signs of rejection include fever, increased BUN and serum creatinine levels, pain and tenderness over the abdomen, irritability, and weight gain. Complications of immunosuppression therapy include opportunistic infection, lymphomas and skin cancer, and hypertension.

Nonadherence with therapy is the primary cause of transplanted kidney loss in 10–15% of all pediatric kidney transplant recipients. Some primary renal diseases, such as glomerulonephritis and HUS, can also recur in the transplanted kidney.

The child also needs ongoing monitoring and management of anemia, renal osteodystrophy, and short stature. The steroids used for immunosuppression cause bone resorption and growth hormone suppression. Growth hormone therapy is often prescribed.

Nursing Management

Educate the child and family about the transplantation process and protocols for immunosuppression. Emphasize that adherence with treatments is essential for the success of the transplant.

Educate the family about signs of acute rejection and infection and when to call the child's physician.

Evaluate the child and parents' understanding of and adherence to the prescribed regimen at all future visits, and reinforce education. Special family supports during periods of extra stress or family disruption may help them to maintain the daily immunosuppression regimen (Bell, 2000).

REPRODUCTIVE SYSTEM ANATOMIC AND PHYSIOLOGIC DIFFERENCES
Cryptorchidism (Undescended Testes)

In *cryptorchidism*, one or both testes fail to descend through the inguinal canal into the scrotum by the time of birth, but testes spontaneously descend in some infants by 3 months of age (Koo, 2001). Causes include a testosterone deficiency, an absent or defective testis, a narrow inguinal canal, short spermatic cord, or adhesions. The testes may be located in the inguinal canal, abdomen, perineum, or even the thigh. Testicular exposure to the higher abdominal temperature can lead to infertility, torsion of an undescended testis, atrophy, and psychological effects of *empty* scrotum. The risk of testicular cancer is 35–50 times greater in men with a history of cryptorchidism (Ferrer & McKenna, 2000).

Clinical Manifestations

Palpation of the scrotum fails to reveal one or both testes, and an inguinal hernia may also be present. The testes may retract into the inguinal canal but can sometimes be manipulated into the scrotum.

Diagnostic Tests

Ultrasound, CT scan, and MRI are used to determine the location of the testes. A diagnostic laparoscopy may also be required to locate the testes.

Hormonal and chromosomal evaluation may be performed to detect an intersex disorder.

Clinical Therapy

An orchiopexy is performed before 2 years of age. An incision made at the testicle's location allows blood vessels to be disentangled so the testis reaches the lower scrotum. The testis is stitched to the inside wall of the scrotum to keep it in place.

Nursing Management

Prepare the parents and infant for the outpatient surgical procedure, and address parents' concerns.

Postoperatively focus on maintaining comfort, monitoring urine output, and preventing infection. Administer prescribed analgesics.

Educate the parents to gently clean the incision site with each diaper change and to identify signs of infection. Provide guidelines for pain medication administration. Encourage loose clothing.

Avoid straddling the infant across the hip or on a riding toy for up to 2 weeks after surgery. Avoid vigorous activity and rough play.

Teach adolescents to perform monthly testicular examinations.

Inguinal Hernia and Hydrocele

An inguinal hernia is a painless inguinal or scrotal swelling that occurs when abdominal tissue, such as bowel, protrudes into the groin. A hydrocele is a fluid-filled mass in the scrotum that often resolves spontaneously by the second year of life. The major complication of an inguinal hernia is incarceration (intestinal strangulation and testicular ischemia).

Clinical Manifestations

An intermittent bulge in the groin or swelling in the scrotum appears with straining or crying. On palpation of the scrotum, a round, smooth, nontender mass is noted that may or may not reduce with manipulation. Transillumination may help determine whether the mass is a hernia or hydrocele.

Incarceration signs include an acute onset of pain, abdominal distention, vomiting, an irreducible mass, an edematous, erythematous scrotum, poor feeding, and bloody stools (Burd & Burd, 2002).

Clinical Therapy

Surgery for inguinal hernia repair during infancy. A regional nerve block may be used to reduce postoperative pain. In cases of incarceration, immediate manual reduction of the hernia is performed to prevent strangulation, necrosis, and perforation of the intestine. If unsuccessful, immediate surgical intervention is required. Surgical intervention for a hydrocele is rarely required.

Nursing Management

Before surgery, assess the newborn for signs of incarceration.

After surgery, assess the vital signs, pain level, peripheral circulation in the leg on the side of surgical repair, and the incision for swelling, bleeding, or drainage.

For an incarcerated hernia, postoperative care may include management of a nasogastric tube and IV antibiotics (Katz, 2001).

Educate the parents about incision site care, signs of infection, and the expected appearance of the scrotum (often bruised and edematous). Encourage provision of pain medication at home.

Phimosis

The foreskin over the glans penis cannot be retracted in infants and young males owing to natural adhesion; however, the foreskin usually separates from the glans during childhood and retracts. Narrowing of the preputial opening may obstruct urine flow and cause balanitis, inflammation, or infection of the glans penis. *Paraphimosis*, inability of the foreskin to return to its normal position over the glans, constricts the penis and is a medical emergency.

Circumcision, surgical removal of the foreskin, is commonly performed on newborns and sometimes on older children. Contraindications for circumcision include blood dyscrasias, hypospadias, epispadias, and chordee. Application of topical steroids (betamethasone cream) to treat phimosis is effective, safe, and economic (Ashfield, Nickel, Siemens, et al., 2003).

Nursing Management

Educate parents about care of the uncircumcised newborn male, and tell them to avoid forcibly retracting the foreskin. Educate the older child to return the foreskin to its normal position after cleaning to avoid constricting blood flow.

Discuss the risks, benefits, and potential complications of circumcision and pain relief for the infant during and after circumcision.

If topical steroids are prescribed, educate the parents about application of the medication.

Patient and Family Education

After circumcision, educate the parents to cover the head of the penis with a generous amount of petroleum jelly with each diaper change until the redness goes away. Use cotton balls moistened with tap water to gently clean the head of the penis. A pale yellow crust around the incision site and on the glans is normal for several days after surgery. Contact the healthcare provider if increased redness, bleeding, or swelling of the head of the penis is noted (Kaufman, Clark, & Castro, 2001).

Testicular Torsion

An emergency condition in which the testis suddenly rotates on its spermatic cord, obstructing its blood supply, leading to vascular engorgement and ischemia. The affected testis is positioned higher in the scrotum because of the shortened vascular pedicle. Testicular torsion may occur with trauma to the scrotum, but it may also occur during sporting activities, exercise, and sexual activity.

Clinical Manifestations

Severe pain and erythema in the scrotum, nausea and vomiting, abdominal pain, and scrotal swelling that is not relieved by rest or scrotal support

The testes are tender to palpation and become edematous; absent cremasteric reflex

Clinical Therapy

Diagnosis is based on signs and symptoms. A testicular scan or Doppler flow sonogram may be performed if immediately available. Torsion must be reduced within 4–6 hours to restore circulation and salvage the testis. Manual reduction with an analgesic is sometimes attempted. Emergency bilateral orchiopexy is performed to untwist the testis and stitch it to the side of the scrotum.

Nursing Management

Assess the child's symptoms, and recognize that pain and swelling in the scrotum is a true emergency. Provide analgesics, as ordered, and prepare the child for surgery. Educate the adolescent and family about the surgery and the need for rapid intervention. Reassure the child and family that fertility should not be affected because only one testis is affected.

Provide guidelines for home care of the incision, pain management, and avoidance of strenuous activity or lifting heavy objects for 2 weeks after surgery. Teach the adolescent to perform testicular self-examination.

SEXUALLY TRANSMITTED INFECTIONS
Common Sexually Transmitted Infections

Sexually transmitted infections (STIs) are caused by organisms of bacterial, parasitic, and viral origin. Children and adolescents can become infected through sexual experimentation, sexual play, molestation, and sexual abuse. When acquired after the neonatal period, infections almost always indicate sexual contact (Centers for Disease Control and Prevention, 2002). When a child younger than 10 years is infected, consider the possibility of sexual abuse.

See Table 22–7 for clinical manifestations and clinical therapy for STIs.

Table 22–7 Clinical Manifestations of Common Sexually Transmitted Infections

Sexually Transmitted Infection	Clinical Manifestations and Complications	Clinical Therapy
Chlamydia	Adolescent female: asymptomatic, or yellow mucopurulent endocervical discharge, dysuria, pelvic pain, mild abdominal pain, vaginal spotting, cervicitis, salpingitis, PID Adolescent male: asymptomatic, or urethritis, mucoid gray or clear discharge, dysuria, proctitis, epididymitis; 10% are asymptomatic	Recommended medication therapy includes doxycycline, erythromycin for 7 days, or single-dose azithromycin. HIV-positive persons receive the same treatment as those who are HIV negative. Evaluate, test, and treat all sexual partners. Abstain from sexual intercourse until they and their sex partners have completed treatment (approximately 7 days), otherwise reinfection is possible. Encourage use of condoms.
Genital herpes Herpes simplex virus 2	May not be aware of their infection when no symptoms are present. Dull pain, itching, and small lesions or pimples on genitalia, buttocks, or thighs. Lesions may be fluid-filled blisters on an erythematous base or, more commonly, painful papules and ulcers. Ulcers can appear between vaginal folds, in posterior cervix, on glans penis, or shaft of penis, in rectum, or in anus. Ulcers heal within 2–4 weeks. Lymph nodes closest to lesions are frequently enlarged. Disease frequently recurs four to five times a year with episodes lasting 5–10 days. Triggers include stress, menses, or trauma. Infection is lifelong. Individuals with immunosuppression may have systemic involvement.	No permanent cure. Recommended drug therapy to suppress the virus is an antiviral medication (acyclovir, valacyclovir, and famciclovir) given for 7–10 days. Treatment may also be used for recurrent episodes. Daily suppressive therapy for herpes can reduce or eliminate recurrences for the period of time taken. A cesarean delivery is usually performed for infected pregnant women with active lesions. Abstain from all types of sexual activity while lesions are present. Consistent and correct use of condoms may reduce the risk for transmission of genital herpes if the condom covers all lesions. Emphasize that the viral infection is lifelong. Transmission can occur when lesions are present and during asymptomatic periods. Sexual partners of infected persons should be advised about the potential of becoming infected.

(continued)

Table 22–7 Clinical Manifestations of Common Sexually Transmitted Infections (Continued)

Sexually Transmitted Infection	Clinical Manifestations and Complications	Clinical Therapy
Gonorrhea	Symptoms and severity vary from mild to severe and are different for males and females. Signs or symptoms often appear 2–5 days after infection; symptoms can take as long as 30 days to appear. Females: 80% are asymptomatic. The classic sign is purulent vaginal discharge, dysuria, and vulvovaginitis. Males: may be asymptomatic, yellow purulent urethral discharge, erythematous meatus, frequency, dysuria, and painful or swollen testicles. Symptoms of rectal infection in both genders include discharge, anal itching, soreness, bleeding, or painful bowel movements. Infections in the pharynx may cause a sore throat but are usually asymptomatic.	For uncomplicated gonorrhea, a single dose of cefixime, ciprofloxacin, ofloxacin, or levofloxacin PO, or a single dose of ceftriaxone IM. No follow-up is needed if symptoms resolve after treatment (Centers for Disease Control and Prevention, 2002). All sexual partners within the past 60 days should be notified and treated. Sexual activity should be avoided until therapy has had time to resolve all symptoms. Encourage proper and consistent use of condoms or abstinence. If any genital symptoms, such as discharge or burning during urination or unusual sore or rash, are experienced, discontinue having sex and seek medical attention immediately.
Human papillomavirus	Females: small, flat, flesh-colored warts clustered or alone on the vulva, perineal area, vagina, or cervix; itching, bleeding, burning, irritation. A subclinical infection may be detected through a Pap smear. Males: small, flat, flesh-colored warts on the penis, near base of penis on scrotal skin, or near anus.	No cure. Warts may resolve, remain unchanged, or increase in size and number if untreated. Treatment includes cryotherapy, topical podophyllin or imiquimod cream, laser ablation, intralesional interferon, or chemical cautery with trichloroacetic acid. Encourage abstinence or condom use. The disorder is transmissible even after treatment.

(continued)

Table 22–7   Clinical Manifestations of Common Sexually Transmitted Infections (Continued)

Sexually Transmitted Infection	Clinical Manifestations and Complications	Clinical Therapy
Trichomoniasis	Females: pale yellow to gray-green discharge that may be frothy or have a fishy odor, dysuria, vulvar pruritus, occasional abdominal pain; symptoms worsen during menses, more commonly have symptoms than males. Males: mucoid or purulent urethral discharge, pruritus, dysuria; usually asymptomatic.	A single dose of metronidazole PO or alternatively metronidazole PO for 7 days. No follow-up is needed if symptoms resolve after treatment. Treat both partners simultaneously to eliminate the parasite. Avoid sexual contact until both partners are cured. Do not drink alcoholic beverages during treatment and until symptoms resolve.
Syphilis	Appearance of classic signs and symptoms of syphilis depends on stage of disease. *Primary stage:* ulcer on labia, within vagina, on penis, in anus, or on lips or tongue that appears at invasion site approximately 2 weeks to 3 months after infection. Ulcer has an indurated border and smooth base (chancre), and it is painless. Lymphadenopathy is usually present. Ulcer spontaneously heals within 5 weeks. *Second stage:* appears up to 10 weeks after initial infection with fever, malaise, lymphadenopathy, patchy alopecia, and diffuse rash. Rash can be macular, papular, papulosquamous, or bullous, and appearance on the palms and soles is classic. Flat mucous patches called *condylomata lata* appear on genitals.	Recommended drug therapy includes a single dose of benzathine penicillin G IM. Alternative treatment for those with penicillin allergy is doxycycline or tetracycline PO for 14 days (Centers for Disease Control and Prevention, 2002). For children allergic to penicillin, use erythromycin PO for 15 days. Clinical examination and serology tests should be performed at 6 and 12 months after treatment to detect treatment failure or reinfection. Notify and treat all sexual contacts within the past 90 days to 1 year of diagnosis, depending on stage when diagnosed. During syphilis treatment, abstain from sexual contact with new partners until the syphilis sores are completely healed. Encourage abstinence or the correct and consistent use of condoms to prevent reinfection.

(continued)

Table 22–7 Clinical Manifestations of Common Sexually Transmitted Infections (Continued)

Sexually Transmitted Infection	Clinical Manifestations and Complications	Clinical Therapy
Syphilis (continued)	*Latent stage:* asymptomatic, follows the second stage by approximately 6 weeks. It can last for several years or be lifelong.	
	Tertiary stage: occurs more than 2 years after onset and manifests as neurosyphilis, cardiovascular disease, ophthalmic, or congenital syphilis.	

HIV, human immunodeficiency virus; PID, pelvic inflammatory disease.

Nursing Management

Assessment

Obtain a sexual history from the adolescent, identifying the number and gender of sexual partners and any protection used during sexual activity.

Identify signs and symptoms indicative of STIs during the physical examination. Routine screening of sexually active adolescents is recommended. When a child or adolescent is diagnosed with one STI, screen for the presence of others.

Assess the adolescent's anxiety or concern about an infection or fear that parents will be notified.

Implementation

Educate the adolescent about the specific infection diagnosed, its treatment, the need to complete all doses, potential adverse effects, and recommended follow-up. Reinforce the need to notify all sexual partners for treatment.

Provide psychological support, as the adolescent may be upset, ashamed, embarrassed, or angry about having the infection.

Encourage sexually active adolescents to receive hepatitis B immunization. Counsel the adolescent on ways to modify high-risk sexual behaviors.

When sexual assault is suspected, refer the child or adolescent to a healthcare provider specializing in collecting evidence and providing specialized care.

Patient and Family Education

Educate adolescents about the risk for STIs, potential complications, and methods to prevent an STI.

Abstinence is the best prevention.

Limit the number of sexual contacts; practice mutual monogamy.

Always use condoms and spermicidal gels or foams for vaginal and anal intercourse.

Refrain from oral sex if the partner has active sores in mouth, vagina, anus, or on the penis.

Reduce high-risk sexual behaviors. Use of recreational drugs and alcohol can increase sexual risk-taking.

Seek care as soon as symptoms are noticed, make sure the partner gets treatment, and avoid sexual intercourse until the STI is cured.

Seek annual screening as some STIs have no symptoms.

Pelvic Inflammatory Disease

An infection of the upper genital tract caused by the ascending spread of organisms from the cervix and vagina to the uterus and fallopian tubes. Usually caused by *Chlamydia trachomatis* or *Neisseria gonorrhea.*

Clinical Manifestations

Mild or dull bilateral lower abdominal pain or right upper quadrant pain.

Dysmenorrhea that is more severe or longer lasting than usual.

Dysuria, fever, mucopurulent vaginal discharge, pain with sexual activity, nausea and vomiting.

Diagnostic Tests

Clinical findings, such as uterine or adnexal tenderness or tenderness with cervical motion with pelvic examination.

Elevated erythrocyte sedimentation rate and C-reactive protein levels. Vaginal secretions contain WBCs. A pregnancy test, human immunodeficiency virus test, and cultures for STIs (particularly gonorrhea and *Chlamydia*) are performed.

A transvaginal sonogram may reveal thickened and fluid-filled fallopian tubes with or without free pelvic fluid.

Clinical Therapy

IV antibiotic therapy (cefotetan or cefoxitin plus doxycycline or clindamycin plus gentamicin) for the first 24 hours; oral antibiotics (ofloxacin, levofloxacin, and ceftriaxone or cefoxitin plus doxycycline) for the remaining 14 days of treatment.

Follow-up visit in 72 hours to monitor treatment adherence and condition improvement. If there is no improvement, IV antibiotics and hospitalization may be required. Male sexual partners should be examined and treated.

Nursing Management
Identify the risk for STIs and PID in all adolescent females. Administer first dose of medications by IV and make arrangements for her to return for a second dose 12 hours later. Educate the adolescent about the importance of taking all oral antibiotics on schedule for the full 14 days.

Assist the adolescent to discuss the health problem with the parents.

Provide counseling about methods to reduce the risk for reinfection. Provide information about the potential PID consequences, such as infertility, ectopic pregnancy, and chronic abdominal pain.

Encourage regular health visits with screening for STIs, as future *Chlamydia* and gonorrhea infections may be asymptomatic.

23. ALTERATIONS IN ENDOCRINE FUNCTION

ADRENAL FUNCTION DISORDERS
Adrenal Insufficiency (Addison Disease)

A rare disorder characterized by deficiency of glucocorticoids (cortisol) and mineralocorticoids (aldosterone) resulting from the body's lack of ability to handle stress (Gance-Cleveland, 2003). The primary cause is an autoimmune destruction of the adrenal gland acquired after trauma.

Clinical Manifestations

Adrenal insufficiency develops slowly as adrenal glands deteriorate.

Early signs: weakness with fatigue, lethargy, emotional lability, anorexia, salt craving, weight loss.

Additional signs: skin hyperpigmentation (at pressure points, lip borders, nipples, palms and soles, body creases), generalized skin bronzing, abdominal pain, nausea, vomiting, diarrhea, dehydration, tachycardia, dysrhythmias, postural hypotension.

Developmental delay and altered school performance if diagnosis is delayed.

Addisonian crisis: severe hypotension, weakness, fever, abdominal pain, hypoglycemia, seizures, dehydration, circulatory collapse, shock, and coma.

Diagnostic Tests

Serum cortisol (low) and urinary 17-hydroxycorticosteroid levels measured in early morning

Adrenocorticotropic hormone stimulation test of adrenal gland reserve

Serum electrolytes

Computed tomography scan of abdomen

Clinical Therapy

Replacement of deficient corticosteroids (hydrocortisone) and mineralocorticoids [fludrocortisone (Florinef)]. The dose of hydrocortisone is increased in the presence of any stressor.

Nursing Management
Assessment
Assess vital signs for changes in heart rate or blood pressure. Assess weight, skin turgor, and mucous membranes to determine presence of dehydration. Monitor laboratory values.

Stressful periods (illness, injury, cold, stress, burns, or surgery) can lead to acute adrenal insufficiency and addisonian crisis.

Implementation
Administer intravenous fluids as indicated, and encourage fluid intake as prescribed.

Monitor nutritional intake and intake and output.

Ensure the family recognizes symptoms that require reporting (bleeding, dizziness, lethargy, weakness, changes in blood pressure or heart rate, and weight gain).

If the child has vomiting within 1 hour of taking oral steroid dose, the dose is repeated. Increase dose of medication with illness.

Double or triple steroid medication is prescribed in anticipation of stressful events.

Injectable form of medication must be available at home and at school for emergencies.

Encourage a medical alert identification for the child.

Congenital Adrenal Hyperplasia
An autosomal recessive disorder causing deficiency of one of the enzymes necessary for the synthesis of cortisol and aldosterone. Increased secretion of adrenocorticotropic hormone occurs in response to low cortisol levels, leading to overproduction of adrenal androgens and virilization of female genitalia.

Seventy-five percent are salt-losing caused by aldosterone deficiency. Twenty-five percent are non–salt-losing with simple virilization.

Clinical Manifestations
Females: pseudohermaphroditism, masculinized genitalia at birth (enlarged clitoris, partial or complete labial fusion), normal uterus and fallopian tubes, vagina and urethra have a common opening (urogenital sinus).

Males: may appear normal at birth, may have slightly enlarged penis and hyperpigmented scrotum, may have an adult-size penis at school age, but testes are appropriately sized.

Precocious puberty, acne, tall stature, and excessive muscle development as the child grows.

Diagnostic Tests

Routine newborn screening for congenital adrenal hyperplasia (CAH) performed in 29 states (Lashley, 2002).

Diagnosis may be delayed until signs of adrenal insufficiency develop.

Adrenocorticotropic hormone with measurement of serum cortisol and 17-alpha-hydroxyprogesterone levels.

Karyotype to determine gender of the infant with ambiguous genitalia.

Serum testosterone level.

Electrolytes: hyponatremia, hyperkalemia, and high urinary sodium are present in salt-wasting varieties.

Ultrasonography to visualize internal pelvic structures.

Clinical Therapy

Lifelong replacement of deficient hormones with oral glucocorticoids.

If salt-wasting form, salt is added to the infant's formula.

Hormone replacement is doubled or tripled during acute illness and for surgery to replace the additional steroids that would be produced by the body during acute stress.

Reconstructive surgery for the enlarged clitoris before 1 year of age; vaginal reconstruction at a later age.

Adrenalectomy rarely performed.

Nursing Management

Assessment

Assess for signs of dehydration or shock. Frequently reassess the vital signs and peripheral perfusion.

Assess the parents' emotional response to a child with ambiguous genitalia and a chronic condition. Explore their values and beliefs with regard to gender roles and sexuality while awaiting karyotype results.

Implementation

Support parents having difficulty accepting that their infant, whose genitalia look male, is really female. With medication and surgery, the genitalia can assume a female appearance, and females have all of the organs necessary for future child bearing.

Assist parents in educating child's siblings and other family members about the condition.

Refer to infant as "your baby" not "your son" or "your daughter" until gender identity is confirmed.

Provide genetic counseling to parents and to the adolescent with CAH. Prenatal testing can detect congenital adrenal hyperplasia.

Educate family how to administer injectable hydrocortisone and the need for emergency treatment if hydrocortisone is not available. Carry an emergency kit with the child.

Inform parents of increased risk of rapid dehydration when child has salt-wasting form and develop an emergency plan for illness.

Encourage use of medical alert identification.

Cushing's Syndrome

Cushing's syndrome results from excess levels of glucocorticoids (especially cortisol) in the bloodstream, usually the result of adrenal cortex hyperfunction. Causes include adrenal or pituitary tumors or congenital adrenal hyperplasia.

Clinical Manifestations

Gradual excessive weight gain and growth retardation.

Often takes 5 years for the child to develop typical cushingoid appearance (moon face, buffalo hump).

Other signs include muscle weakness and wasting, bruising, hypertension, and striae on abdomen.

Diagnostic Tests

Serum sodium, calcium, potassium, and glucose levels; glycosylated hemoglobin concentration (hemoglobin A1C)

24-hour urine for free cortisol and 17-hydroxycorticosteroid

Adrenal (adrenocorticotropic hormone) suppression test

Computed tomography and magnetic resonance imaging to detect tumors in adrenal or pituitary gland

Clinical Therapy

Surgical resection for adrenal or pituitary tumors.

Lifelong hydrocortisone replacement when both adrenal glands are removed.

Prognosis for children with malignant adrenal tumors is poor.

Nursing Management
Assessment
Monitor the vital signs, weight, fluid status, and nutritional status.

Monitor serum electrolytes.

Implementation
Provide preoperative and postoperative teaching and care. Refer to Chapter 20 for care of the child with cancer. Postoperatively, elevate the head of the bed 30 degrees to promote effective breathing.

Patient and Family Education
Ensure that the patient and family understand this disorder and its treatment.

Explain that the child's cushingoid appearance is reversible with treatment.

Offer nutritional guidance for healthy food selections for weight management.

Encourage the child to discuss feelings about physical appearance.

Develop a schedule for administration of hydrocortisone replacement therapy, in the morning or every other day to mimic a diurnal pattern. Give oral preparations with meals to decrease gastric irritation.

Teach parents how to administer injectable hydrocortisone for times when the child cannot take oral medication. Steroid replacement is needed during illness to prevent severe illness or cardiovascular collapse.

Teach the signs of acute adrenal insufficiency: increased irritability, headache, confusion, restlessness, loss of appetite, lethargy, nausea and vomiting, diarrhea, abdominal pain, dehydration, and fever.

Encourage medical alert identification for the child.

GONADAL FUNCTION DISORDERS
Amenorrhea
Primary: Absence of menarche by 14.5 years with no growth or development of secondary sexual characteristics. Often caused by structural defects, chromosomal abnormalities, hypothalamic or pituitary tumors, thyroid dysfunction, or polycystic ovary disease. May be seen in competitive athletes.

Secondary: Absence of three or more consecutive menstrual periods after menstruation has begun. Most often due to pregnancy. May also occur in competitive athletes or in states of poor nutrition.

Diagnostic testing may include a pregnancy test, bone age, hormone levels (estrogen, luteinizing hormone, follicle-stimulating hormone, and prolactin), and a vaginal examination (to determine vaginal patency). Therapy is dependent on etiology. The most common approach is birth control pills containing estrogen and progesterone.

Nursing Management

Explain that irregular and variable duration cycles are common for 1–2 years after menarche.

Provide education about safe sexual practices to the adolescent who is or is considering being sexually active. Offer birth control.

Provide emotional support.

Encourage athletes to eat a well-balanced, high-calorie diet and to take calcium supplementation. Teach about medications prescribed.

Dysmenorrhea

Menstrual pain or cramping during the menstrual cycle due to an increased secretion of prostaglandins during the ovulatory cycle that causes uterine muscle contraction, leading to ischemia and pain. Endometriosis or pelvic inflammatory disease may cause secondary dysmenorrhea.

Pain usually occurs after the beginning of ovulation and ends on the second day of the menstrual cycle. Cramping in the lower abdomen and pelvic regions may radiate to the back. Other symptoms may include nausea, vomiting, headache, diarrhea, urinary frequency, or fatigue.

A gynecologic examination may detect tenderness and identify any abnormalities. Cultures are taken if a sexually transmitted infection (STI) is possible. Treatment includes nonsteroidal anti-inflammatory drugs and oral contraceptives. An increase in protein, magnesium, calcium, and vitamin B_6 may help relieve symptoms.

Nursing Management

Educate adolescents to begin taking nonsteroidal anti-inflammatory drugs 2–3 days before the onset of the menstrual cycle and to take with food to avoid gastrointestinal upset.

Suggest complementary therapies such as heating pad, guided imagery, massage, hypnosis, and meditation to manage symptoms.

Klinefelter Syndrome

A chromosomal disorder in which males have an extra X chromosome, usually 47,XXY causing hypogonadism and infertility in males.

Cardiac abnormalities, pulmonary disease, dental abnormalities, and scoliosis may be associated conditions.

Clinical Manifestations

Males appear normal at birth.

Disruptive behavior in school, emotional problems often occur due to auditory processing problems and speech delay.

Intelligent quotient (IQ) scores are often 10–15 points lower than unaffected siblings.

Tall and thin with disproportionately long legs, normal arm span for height.

Delayed onset of puberty with abnormal progression, decreased testicular size. Less facial and body hair may develop.

Gynecomastia.

Diagnostic Tests

Karyotyping, revealing one or more extra chromosomes

Clinical Therapy

Testosterone replacement, begun at puberty by injection of Depo-Testosterone (sustained-action preparation of testosterone cypionate) every 3–4 weeks, stimulates masculinization and development of secondary sexual characteristics.

Nursing Management

Assess secondary sexual characteristics, height, and weight.

Assess patient and family coping.

Support parents to work with the school to provide education tailored to needs.

Refer for speech therapy if needed.

Help parents identify child's strengths and promote success and self-esteem.

Turner Syndrome

The most common sex chromosome abnormality in females caused by a complete loss, partial absence, or other abnormality of one X chromosome has an incidence of 1 in 2,000–5,000 live births (Halec & Zimmerman, 2004).

Other associated conditions include congenital heart disease, hypertension, kidney abnormalities, hypothyroidism, chronic/recurrent otitis media, strabismus, ptosis, myopia, amblyopia, and inflammatory bowel disease.

Clinical Manifestations

Short stature (less than fifth percentile)

Short, webbed neck with low posterior hairline

Cubitus valgus (increased angle at the elbow), scoliosis, broad chest with widely spaced nipples

Lymphedema

Hyperconvex fingernails

Dark, pigmented nevi

Delayed puberty, amenorrhea, underdeveloped ovaries, infertility

Normal intelligence, risk for behavioral or social difficulties

Diagnostic Tests

Karyotype (reveals classic 45,XO or 46,XX pattern with one misshapen X chromosome)

Prenatal diagnosis with alpha-fetoprotein, estradiol, and human chorionic gonadotropin; maternal progesterone; inhibin A screening; and fetal ultrasound

Clinical Therapy

Growth hormone may be prescribed starting at age 2 years (Halec & Zimmerman, 2004).

Low dose estrogen is initiated at 15 years of age. Progesterone is added to the estrogen therapy to initiate menstrual periods.

Nursing Management

Assess for signs and symptoms of cardiac, renal, gastrointestinal, vision, hearing, musculoskeletal, or thyroid dysfunction.

Assess growth and plot on growth curve. A special growth curve is available from the Turner Syndrome Society.

Educate parents to administer growth hormone and to monitor for side effects.

Promote the girl's self-esteem.

INHERITED METABOLIC DISORDERS
Fatty Acid Oxidation Defects

Mitochondrial oxidation of fatty acids is an imperative energy-producing pathway during periods of starvation, when the body metabolizes fat for fuel. Autosomal recessive gene defects occur in almost every stage in the fatty acid oxidation pathway, leading to many subclasses of fatty acid oxidation defects.

Clinical Manifestations
Most commonly, acute life-threatening coma and hypoglycemia induced by a period of fasting.

May be asymptomatic except for times during illness or stress.

Other signs may include cardiomegaly, hepatomegaly, and muscle weakness.

Diagnostic Tests
Routine newborn screening may identify some disorders.

Most cases present with acute symptoms when the following diagnostic tests are performed: blood gases, electrolytes, hepatic profile, plasma lactate, plasma amino acids, urine organic acid, acylcarnitine profile, quantitative carnitine levels, and urine for ketones.

Skin biopsy often obtained for fibroblast analysis.

Clinical Therapy
Acute condition treated with 10% dextrose.

Frequent feedings and avoidance of fasting (no more than 10 hours without food).

Carnitine supplementation may be indicated in some disorders.

Nursing Management
Educate parents to feed the infant around the clock every 2–4 hours.

Do not let children or adolescents go longer than 8–12 hours without food. Encourage several low-fat and high-carbohydrate snacks throughout the day.

If the infant or child is unable to sustain oral intake during acute illness, refer to the hospital for intravenous dextrose supplementation. Simple infections can become life-threatening.

Refer family to genetic counseling. Test siblings even if asymptomatic.

Galactosemia
An autosomal recessive disorder of carbohydrate metabolism that results from a deficiency of the liver enzyme galactose 1-phosphate uridyltransferase, one of three enzymes needed to convert galactose to glucose. Galactose metabolites accumulate in the

eyes, liver, kidney, and brain, rapidly damaging the organs and causing life-threatening problems. Children become susceptible to gram-negative sepsis.

Clinical Manifestations

Early manifestations: poor suck and nutritional intake, failure to gain weight, vomiting, diarrhea, hypoglycemia, and enlarged liver.

Late signs: jaundice, ascites, sepsis, lethargy, seizures, hypotonia. cataracts, mental retardation, coma, and death.

Diagnostic Tests

Routine newborn screening in most states.

Physical examination, laboratory tests (elevated galactose, alanine aminotransferase, aspartate aminotransferase levels); urine specimens are checked for reducing substances.

Clinical Therapy

Elimination of galactose from diet, lactose-free formula (e.g., Nutramigen, meat-based, or soybean) *or*

Lifetime galactose-free diet (no milk, cheese products, foods with dry milk products)

Nursing Management

Educate the family about the disorder and required diet. Advise parents that several galactose-free cheeses are commercially sold.

Assess coping mechanisms and provide needed emotional support.

Teach families to screen foods for added milk solids and to avoid antibiotics with lactose fillers.

Calcium supplementation is often required.

Refer family for genetic counseling.

Maple Syrup Urine Disease

Maple syrup urine disease is a disorder of amino acid metabolism that has an autosomal recessive inheritance pattern.

A rare disorder (1 in 225,000 live births) with a high incidence in some Pennsylvania Mennonites at 1 in 380 live births (Robinson & Drumm, 2001).

Three essential amino acids (leucine, isoleucine, and valine) cannot be broken down because of absent or defective enzyme branched-chain alpha-ketoacid dehydrogenase, resulting in ketoacidosis.

All three amino acids are essential to form normal structures such as the hair, skin, and muscle. Leucine can accumulate in the brain and cause cerebral edema, progressive neurologic impairment, and death.

Clinical Manifestations

Within 3–7 days of life, the newborn develops poor appetite, lethargy, vomiting, variable muscle tone, irritability, seizures, high-pitched cry, severe ketoacidosis, and sweet smell.

Symptoms may quickly progress to coma and death if not treated (Larsson & Therrell, 2002).

Diagnostic Tests

Routine newborn screening; however, not performed in all states

Urine for ketones

Serum leucine, isoleucine, and valine

Clinical Therapy

Acute treatment: Remove branched-chain amino acids and their metabolites from tissues and body fluids by hydration or dialysis. Provide sufficient intravenous calories to reverse the infant's catabolic state.

Chronic treatment: Specially formulated medical formulas rich in amino acids, calories, vitamins, and minerals with the three amino acids removed; special low-protein foods for growth and adequate calories to support twice the child's basal metabolic rate; and daily urine testing for ketones to detect a catabolic state.

Nursing Management

Educate the family about the disorder and dietary requirements.

Ensure family understands how to mix the infant's formula.

Help parents develop a "sick day" plan that ensures food and formula when ill to prevent ketoacidosis.

Refer to nutritionist for diet counseling.

Permit moderate exercise only to prevent increase in leucine levels.

Help family identify support groups and sources of information.

Phenylketonuria

Phenylketonuria (PKU) is an autosomal recessive disorder of amino acid metabolism that affects the body's use of protein caused by a mutation of the phenylalanine hydroxylase gene. It results in phenylalanine accumulation in the blood or phenylalanine metabolites in the urine. Severe mental retardation, seizures, and death result if untreated.

Clinical Manifestations

Accumulation of phenylalanine causes a musty or mousy body and urine odor, irritability, hyperactivity, hypertonia, hyperreflexic deep tendon reflexes, seizures, and eczema-like rash (Rezvani, 2004).

Appears normal at birth, except for lighter complexion than siblings.

If untreated, develops microcephaly, prominent maxilla, widely spaced teeth, enamel hypoplasia, and growth retardation.

Diagnostic Tests

Routine newborn screening for PKU in all states after 48 hours of birth and repeated at 1–2 weeks of age

Serum phenylalanine measured in affected children periodically throughout life

Clinical Therapy

Special formulas and a diet low in phenylalanine (e.g., Lofenalac, Minafen, Albumaid XP).

Breastfeeding is possible if infant's serum phenylalanine levels are monitored.

Elemental medical foods with modified protein hydrolysates are substituted for high-protein foods (meats and dairy products).

Low-phenylalanine diet should be maintained for life and is especially important for adolescents and adult females before conception and during pregnancy to prevent congenital anomalies.

Nursing Management

Assess child for consequence of PKU (neurologic signs, atopic dermatitis, cognitive and behavioral problems).

Assess child's adherence to diet. If dietary control is lost before age 6 years, there is significant impact on IQ.

Teach patient/family to avoid high-protein foods (meats and dairy products) and aspartame because they contain large amounts of phenylalanine.

Support parents. Identify financial issues associated with purchase of elemental medical foods and assist with insurance coverage negotiations for those expenses.

PANCREATIC FUNCTION DISORDERS
Diabetic Ketoacidosis

Diabetic ketoacidosis (DKA) is a common and potentially life-threatening condition occurring in children with type 1 diabetes.

The body burns fat and protein stores for energy because no insulin is available to metabolize glucose, leading to hyperglycemia, dehydration, and metabolic acidosis.

Fatty acids are transformed by the liver into ketone bodies, leading to ketoacidosis.

Hyperglycemia causes an osmotic diuresis, resulting in dehydration, acidosis, and hyperosmolality.

Clinical Manifestations

Characteristic signs include dehydration, weight loss, tachycardia, and hypotension.

Kussmaul respirations (deep, rapid respirations) occur to rid the body of excess carbon dioxide and reduce acidosis.

Hyperglycemia, glycosuria, acidosis, and ketonuria.

Acetone breath (fruity smell).

Abdominal pain, chest pain, nausea, and vomiting.

Altered mental status (varies from lethargy to coma).

Headache, lethargy, change in mentation, tachycardia, or bradycardia may indicate development of cerebral edema, a life-threatening complication.

Diagnostic Tests

See Table 23–1 for laboratory findings.

Computed tomography of brain when cerebral edema develops.

Clinical Therapy

Intravenous fluids (child likely will require fluid resuscitation on presentation)

Insulin by continuous intravenous infusion to lower serum glucose at a rate no greater than 100 mg/dL/hour

Electrolyte supplementation

Mannitol if cerebral edema is suspected

Nursing Management
Assessment

Monitor vital signs, respiratory status, perfusion, and mental status continuously.

Table 23–1 Laboratory Findings in the Child with Diabetic Ketoacidosis

Laboratory Study	Results
Serum glucose	>300 mg/dL
Serum ketones	Positive
Arterial blood gas pH	Acidotic: pH 7.3 or below and bicarbonate < 15 mEq/L
Potassium	Elevated
Chloride	Elevated
Sodium	Decreased
Phosphate	Decreased
Calcium	Decreased
Magnesium	Decreased
Blood urea nitrogen and creatinine	Elevated due to dehydration
White blood cell count	Generally elevated due to presence of infection or dehydration
Serum osmolality	>350 mOsm/kg (normal is 275–295 mOsm/kg)
Urine	Positive for glucose and ketones

Connect the child to a cardiac monitor to detect arrhythmias associated with hypokalemia.

Monitor intake and output hourly.

Implementation
Monitor blood glucose, electrolytes, and acid–base balance. Monitor for signs of hypokalemia.

Manage intravenous fluid administration to reverse fluid deficit.

Initiate oral feeding when child is alert and glucose level is stabilized.

Provide support to the family.

Patient and Family Education
Signs that could indicate progression to DKA and should be reported to healthcare provider include the following (Boland & Grey, 2004):

- Vomiting more than two times in 6 hours
- More than five diarrhea stools in 1 day
- Has illness and is unable to eat
- Change in mental status
- Temperature higher than 102°F (38.9°C) for 12 hours
- Blood glucose level of more than 400 mg/dL on two separate readings or more than 200 mg/dL and moderate to large ketones
- Large ketones, acetone breath
- Difficulty breathing
- Decreased urine output
- Dysuria or other evidence of urinary tract infection

Test child's urine for ketones if three consecutive glucose readings are higher than 200 mg/dL, or if child is sick.

Teach family that extra insulin is required even when the child is not eating to counteract the hormones released in response to stressors.

Teach family to initiate extra insulin and fluids if urine has moderate or large ketone levels.

Diabetes Mellitus Type 1

Diabetes mellitus type 1, a disorder of carbohydrate, protein, and fat metabolism, is the most common metabolic disease in children, with prevalence among children of 1.7 per 1,000 (Centers for Disease Control and Prevention, 2004). Peak incidence is 7–15 years, but it presents at any age.

Destruction of pancreatic islet beta cells results in failure to secrete insulin. The body becomes dependent on exogenous sources of insulin. Type 1 has familial tendencies but no pattern of inheritance.

Insulin helps transport glucose into cells for use as an energy source. Without insulin, the serum glucose level rises and the glucose level inside the cells decreases.

When glucose is unavailable to cells for metabolism, free fatty acids are metabolized at an increased rate by the liver, producing acetyl coenzyme A and the by-product ketone bodies. Ketone bodies accumulate faster than they can be excreted, resulting in metabolic acidosis, or ketoacidosis.

Clinical Manifestations

Classic signs of polyuria, polydipsia, and polyphagia (excessive appetite) with significant weight loss.

Fatigue/lethargy.

Headaches.

Stomachaches.

Occasional enuresis in previously toilet-trained child.

Symptoms develop gradually over a month or shorter time period.

Diagnostic Tests

Fasting serum glucose at or above 126 mg/dL *or* random serum glucose of 200 mg/dL or higher.

Ketones may be found in the blood or urine.

Autoantibodies that can indicate an autoimmune dysfunction.

Hemoglobin A1c to measure glycemic control every 3 months.

Clinical Therapy

Multiple approaches to insulin therapy are available for children and adolescents:

- Basal-bolus therapy—basal insulin administered once or twice a day with boluses of rapid-acting insulin administered with meals and snacks matching carbohydrates consumed
- Conventional therapy—two or three insulin injections a day

Goal is to lower blood glucose levels, stabilize glucose levels (80–120 mg/dL before meals and 100–140 mg/dL at bedtime), and eliminate ketones.

See Table 23–2 for action times of different insulin types.

Insulin dose is adjusted according to frequent serum glucose monitoring, at least four times per day, and delivered by multiple subcutaneous injections or insulin pump.

Nutrition planning—counting carbohydrates, number of calories individualized to child for growth and activity.

Exercise program.

Pancreatic transplant for children receiving a kidney transplant.

Table 23–2 Action Times by Insulin Type Administered Subcutaneously

Type	Onset	Peak	Duration
Rapid-acting			
Insulin lispro (Humalog)	5–15 min	1 hr	2–4 hr
Insulin aspart	10–20 min	1–3 hr	3–5 hr
Short-acting			
Regular	0.5–1.0 hr	2–4 hr	4–6 hr
Intermediate-acting			
NPH	1–2 hr	6–12 hr	18–26 hr
Lente	1–2 hr	6–12 hr	24–26 hr
Long-acting			
Ultralente	4–8 hr	10–20 hr	16–24 hr
Lantos/insulin glargine	1–2 hr	None/slight	24 hr

Note: Intermediate-acting insulin mixed with short- or rapid-acting insulin (e.g., 70% NPH/30% regular, 50% NPH/50% regular, and 75% NPL/25% insulin lispro) is also available.

Nursing Management

Assessment

Assess physiologic status: vital signs, hydration, and level of consciousness.

Monitor growth and developmental milestones.

Monitor blood glucose, electrolytes, and blood gases as ordered.

Assess the adolescent's problem-solving skills.

Assess family strengths and coping for disease management.

- Do both parents or does the single parent work? Who else cares for the child?
- What is the child's daily schedule? Does it vary daily or on the weekend?
- Does the child have other chronic conditions, behavioral, cognitive, or visual problems?
- What other stressors exist in the family?
- Assess adolescent's willingness and challenges in adhering to treatment plan.

Implementation

Teach the family survival skills when child is newly diagnosed: blood glucose monitoring, drawing up and injecting insulin, urine testing for ketones, record keeping, survival food guidelines, and when to call the healthcare provider.

Coordinate care with diabetic nurse educator for disease management focusing on the following:

- Signs and symptoms of hypoglycemia and hyperglycemia
- Goals of insulin therapy, correct administration of insulin, rotation of sites
- Washing hands before pricking finger for blood
- Keeping a rapid acting source of sugar readily available
- Planning a balance of food intake, exercise, and insulin
- Healthy foot habits

Sick day guidelines to help prevent diabetic ketoacidosis:

- Monitor serum glucose levels more often than routine.
- Do not skip doses of insulin; insulin dose may need to be increased.
- Work to maintain food and fluid intake.
- Monitor urine for ketones.
- Call healthcare provider if fever or infection is present.

Coordinate with nutritionist to develop the food plan; use Food Guide Pyramid to identify correct portions of food, carbohydrate counting, and consistent intake of carbohydrates.

Encourage medical alert identification.

Provide emotional support and refer family to support groups and sources of information.

Assist family in coordinating with the school to develop an individualized health plan.

Diabetes Mellitus Type 2

Type 2 diabetes is associated with insulin resistance (alteration in the insulin receptor that signals the presence of insulin in the interior of cells).

It may be connected with an insulin secretory defect in the pancreas (causing a decrease in the beta cell weight or number) and insulin deficiency (Gungor & Arslanian, 2004).

Insulin fails to transfer glucose into the cells. The pancreas produces more insulin to facilitate glucose transfer and overcome insulin resistance, resulting in hyperinsulinemia. As insulin resistance worsens, the pancreas is unable to hypersecrete enough insulin.

Obesity is the most important risk factor. Other risk factors include sedentary lifestyle, diet high in fat, minority race, polycystic ovary syndrome, and type 2 diabetes in a first-degree relative (Alemzadeh & Wyatt, 2004).

Clinical Manifestations

Obesity, truncal adiposity.

Acanthosis nigricans, or color hyperpigmentation and thickening with velvety irregularities in skin folds of neck, axillae, elbows, knees, groin, and abdomen.

History of polyuria and polydipsia is rare.

Diagnostic Tests

Serum glucose level (fasting).

Urine test for glucose and ketones.

Hemoglobin A1c.

Lipid panel.

Autoantibodies and fasting C peptide are used to differentiate between type 1 and type 2 diabetes.

Clinical Therapy

Nutritional education for gradual sustained weight loss and metabolic control of blood glucose levels.

Exercise.

Emotional support.

Oral medication (e.g., metformin) if diet and exercise efforts are inadequate.

Insulin may be required at time of presentation and may ultimately be needed long term for glycemic control.

Nursing Management
Assessment

Assess child with body mass index above 85th percentile for signs of insulin resistance (acanthosis nigricans, hypertension, dyslipidemia).

Blood glucose monitoring.

Assess diet and activity patterns.

Consider evaluating siblings.

Implementation

Provide emotional support to child and family.

Teach the child and family about the disease and its management.

Help family plan strategies for daily management of condition, blood glucose monitoring, and medications.

Work with a nutritionist to help the family substitute high-calorie and high-fat foods for allowable foods matching the family's resources and ethnic preferences.

Encourage exercise and reduction of sedentary computer and television time.

Encourage annual evaluation for complications of diabetes.

Hypoglycemia

A sudden drop in blood glucose levels commonly occurs in children with type 1 diabetes because of an error of insulin dose or administration, inadequate caloric intake, or increased physical activity without increased caloric intake.

Signs occur with a serum glucose reading of approximately 70 mg/dL or less and include sudden onset of dizziness, tremulousness, anxiety, and confusion. Delirium, loss of consciousness, and seizures occur if not promptly managed with administration of glucose in a low-fat carbohydrate form such as sugar gel, glucose tablets, glucose paste, or a snack or drink. If the child loses consciousness, administer glucagon, intravenous dextrose, or sugar gel/paste onto the gums.

Nursing Management
Prompt recognition is essential to quickly manage symptoms and prevent further reduction in glucose level.

Patient and Family Education
Recognition of signs of hypoglycemia.

Test the blood glucose level.

If blood glucose level is 70 mg/dL or lower, give one of the following: $1/2$ cup of orange juice, $3/4$ cup of sugar-sweetened beverage, one small box of raisins, or three to four glucose tablets.

Wait 15 minutes to retest blood glucose level. Repeat the glucose drink or snack if still 70 mg/dL or below. Recheck the blood glucose level in 15 minutes.

Once the blood glucose level has returned to at least 80 mg/dL, give a more substantial snack such as cheese and crackers if it will be more than 30 minutes until the next meal or if an activity or exercise is planned.

Teach parents to administer intramuscular or subcutaneous glucagon.

PITUITARY FUNCTION DISORDERS
Diabetes Insipidus
A disorder in which the body is unable to concentrate urine, having both central (neurogenic) and nephrogenic forms. Both forms involve antidiuretic hormone (ADH).

In central diabetes insipidus, there is a deficiency or absence of production or release of ADH. In the absence of ADH, the kidneys are almost impermeable to water, leading to polyuria and dehydration.

In the less common nephrogenic diabetes insipidus, the kidney is unable to respond to ADH. The actual amount of ADH produced is adequate.

Clinical Manifestations
Both forms of diabetes insipidus have an abrupt onset and similar manifestations:

Central diabetes insipidus—polyuria, polydipsia, hypernatremia, dilute urine, nocturia, enuresis, irritable if fluids withheld, constipation, fever, and dehydration

Nephrogenic—polyuria, polydipsia, hypernatremia in neonatal period, dilute urine, vomiting, dehydration, and mental status changes

Diagnostic Tests

Serum electrolytes and osmolality: serum sodium (more than 145 mEq/L) and osmolality (more than 285 mOsm/L)

Urine osmolality (less than 200 mOsm/L)

Urine specific gravity (less than 1.005) (Trimarchi, 2001)

Plasma arginine vasopressin level before and after a water deprivation test

Clinical Therapy

Water replacement therapy is essential to prevent severe dehydration and hypotension.

Central (neurogenic) diabetes insipidus is treated primarily with intranasal, intravenous, or subcutaneous desmopressin acetate.

Nephrogenic diabetes insipidus is treated with thiazide diuretics, high fluid intake, and a low-sodium diet.

Nursing Management

Assessment

Assess for signs of fluid volume deficit, monitoring and documenting intake and output.

Frequently monitor electrolytes, osmolality, and urine specific gravity.

Monitor response to desmopressin acetate (i.e., expect significant decrease in urine output after administration).

Implementation

Administer replacement fluids, and keep fluids within child's reach at all times.

Notify healthcare team if there are signs of dehydration or no decrease in urine output after administration of desmopressin acetate.

Patient and Family Education

Ensure that parents understand and recognize signs of inadequate fluid intake and are able to appropriately adjust the child's fluid intake to prevent dehydration.

Encourage the family to obtain a medical alert identification for the child.

Notify the healthcare provider immediately when signs of acute illness occur, as increased metabolic activity from fever or illness can cause dehydration, hypernatremia, and increased risk for seizures.

Growth Hormone Deficiency

A disorder in which the pituitary gland fails to produce sufficient growth hormone. The cause may be idiopathic or related to a central nervous system disorder such as infection, infarction, tumor, trauma, and effects of chemotherapy or irradiation. Infants typically have normal birth weights and lengths and by 1 year of age are below the third percentile on the growth chart.

Clinical Manifestations

Primary characteristics include the following:

- Growth retardation, short stature, and delayed bone maturation.
- Growth rate is typically less than 5 cm (2 in.) per year.
- Higher-pitched voices, youthful facial features, and delayed dentition may also be noted as these children become older.

Other characteristics may include hypoglycemic seizures, hyponatremia, neonatal jaundice, pale optic disks, micropenis, and undescended testes.

Diagnostic Tests

Growth hormone levels, growth hormone stimulating tests, and insulin-like growth factor-1 levels are used to confirm the disorder.

Radiographic imaging of the hand or wrist is used to evaluate the bone age (stage of bone ossification). See Table 23–3 for diagnostic tests for short stature.

Clinical Therapy

Replacement growth hormone is administered by injection. Replacement therapy is continued until either the child achieves an acceptable height or growth velocity declines to less than 2 cm per year.

Nursing Management

Assessment

Carefully measure and document the child's height and weight on a growth chart, and monitor over time. Assess the child's psychosocial adaptation to short stature. Assess parents' ability to cope with child's short stature and treatment regimen.

Table 23–3   Diagnostic Tests for Short Stature

Test	Purpose Related to Short Stature
Insulin-like growth factor-1 and insulin-like growth factor binding protein-3	Excludes growth hormone deficiency if normal
Radiographic views of the sella turcica (site of the pituitary gland)	Demonstrates size of the sella turcica or a tumor
Karyotype (girls)	Detects Turner's syndrome
Thyroid function studies	Detects hypothyroidism
Urine creatinine, pH, specific gravity, urea nitrogen, electrolytes	Detects chronic renal failure
Bone age	Identifies other potential causes of delayed growth
Complete blood count and erythrocyte sedimentation rate	Screens for inflammatory bowel disease with anemia
Antigliadin antibodies	Screens for celiac disease

Note: Data from D'Ercole, A. J., & Underwood, L. (1996). Anterior pituitary gland and hypothalamus. In A. M. Rudolph, J. I. E. Hoffman, & C. D. Rudolph (Eds.). Rudolph's pediatrics (20th ed.) (p. 1692). Stamford, CT: Appleton & Lange. Modified.

Implementation

Provide instructions on site selections and injection administration.

Assist family with establishing techniques to minimize trauma of injections.

Discuss side effects of growth hormone with family (e.g., arthralgia, carpal tunnel syndrome, slipped capital femoral epiphysis, gynecomastia, scoliosis, hypothyroidism) and when to notify the healthcare provider (Miller & Zimmerman, 2004; Wilson, Rose, Cohen, et al., 2003).

Direct family to education resources such as The Magic Foundation (http://www.magicfoundation.org) or Human Growth Hormone Foundation (http://www.hgfound.org).

Hyperpituitarism

A rare condition associated with an excessive release of growth hormone and a pituitary adenoma, causing accelerated linear growth. Heights of 7–8 feet can be attained if oversecretion of growth hormone occurs before the closure of the epiphyseal plates. If oversecretion occurs after closure of the epiphyseal plates, acromegaly occurs.

Increased levels of insulin-like growth factors (insulin-like growth factor-1) establish the diagnosis. Radiographic testing is used to evaluate for presence of brain tumor. Treatment may include surgical removal of tumor, radiation therapy, radioactive implants, or administration of high doses of sex hormones to close the epiphyseal plates.

If the pituitary gland is removed, the child requires lifelong pituitary hormone replacement.

Nursing Management

Early identification is crucial. Monitor and document height on growth chart, and monitor trends. Early referral is necessary for children demonstrating growth rates exceeding expected development. Nursing care focuses on educating patients and families about the disorder, treatment, psychosocial support, and postoperative care (if surgical intervention is required).

Precocious Puberty

The appearance of any secondary sexual characteristics before 8 years of age in females and 9 years of age in males. Although not usually associated with abnormalities in females, a central nervous system disorder such as an intracranial tumor may be the cause in males (Traggiai & Stanhope, 2003).

Clinical Manifestations

Secondary sexual characteristics

Accelerated growth rate

Advanced bone age

Behavioral changes (e.g., mood swings, emotional lability)

Diagnostic Tests

Serum studies: luteinizing hormone, follicle-stimulating hormone, testosterone, estradiol

Provocative testing: gonadotropin-releasing hormone stimulation test

Radiologic imaging of head, hand or wrist for bone age, and pelvic ultrasound in females to assess uterus and ovaries

Clinical Therapy

Focused on arresting clinical signs of puberty, slowing growth velocity, retarding skeletal maturation, and returning ovarian function to prepubertal condition (Traggiai & Stanhope, 2003)

Administration of gonadotropin-releasing hormone analog via subcutaneous, intramuscular, or intranasal route

Nursing Management

Assessment

Assessment of secondary sexual characteristics and sexual maturity rating (see Chapter 3).

Document height and weight and plot on growth curve.

Assess child's psychosocial adaptation to changes in body image.

Assess for parental anxiety related to child's physical changes.

Implementation
Promote positive body image.

Ensure proper medication administration.

Reassure child that friends will experience the same stages of development eventually.

Patient and Family Education
Educate child and parents about treatment and condition.

Teach appropriate administration of gonadotropin-releasing hormone analog.

Advise parents of need to discuss issues of sexuality at an earlier age than normal.

Encourage parents to dress child to match child's chronologic age.

Syndrome of Inappropriate Antidiuretic Hormone

In syndrome of inappropriate antidiuretic hormone (SIADH), an excessive amount of ADH is secreted. It occurs in children with brain injury; diseases of the hypothalamus, pituitary stalk, or posterior pituitary; central nervous system infection; pneumonia; and positive pressure ventilation. SIADH results in water reabsorption by the kidneys despite low serum osmolality, hyponatremia, and euvolemia, increasing intravascular volume and decreasing urine output (Trimarchi, 2001). Often, this state reverses when the underlying etiology improves.

Clinical Manifestations

Signs are related to water intoxication and hyponatremia and include the following:

- Elevated blood pressure
- Crackles on lung examination
- Intake exceeding output; weight gain without edema; concentrated, amber-colored urine
- Nausea, anorexia, abdominal cramps, weakness
- Lethargy, confusion, seizures, and possible coma if significant hyponatremia

Diagnostic Tests

Serum sodium and blood urea nitrogen are low.

Serum osmolality is low, and urine osmolality is high.

Specific gravity is high.

Clinical Therapy

Fluid restriction to prevent further hemodilution.

Diuretics are considered to eliminate excess body weight.

Demeclocycline to block action of ADH.

Intravenous hypertonic saline to supplement sodium for severe hyponatremia.

Nursing Management

Assessment

Accurately document intake and output; weigh daily.

Monitor serum and urine electrolytes and urine specific gravity as ordered.

Monitor for altered mental status, headache, and seizures.

Implementation

If the patient is discharged with SIADH, teach the importance of daily weights and reporting weight gains to healthcare provider. Help family recognize hidden sources of water and fluids, such as popsicles, to prevent excessive fluid intake. Encourage child to wear medical alert identification.

THYROID FUNCTION DISORDERS
Hyperthyroidism

In hyperthyroidism, circulating thyroid hormone levels are increased, resulting in an increased basal metabolic rate, cardiovascular function, gastrointestinal function, and neuromuscular function, as well as weight loss and heat intolerance. It is rare in children and usually secondary to Graves' disease.

Clinical Manifestations

Signs vary based on amount of hypersecretion.

Enlarged, nontender thyroid gland (goiter)

Palpitations, tachycardia, heat intolerance

Nervousness, trembling hands, insomnia

Increased bowel movements, weight loss

Exophthalmus, staring gaze

Light menstrual periods

Diagnostic Tests

Thyroid-stimulating hormone (TSH) level is decreased; T_3 (triiodothyronine) and T_4 (thyroxine) levels are elevated.

Thyroid scan, radioactive iodine uptake scan.

Clinical Therapy

The excessive release of thyroid hormones is inhibited with antithyroid medication (methimazole or propylthiouracil), radiation therapy, or surgery (thyroidectomy). See Table 23–4 for medications used.

Nursing Management

Assessment

Assess vital signs and respiratory effort. Measure and monitor child's growth. Assess for goiter and exophthalmus. Observe behavior, activity, and level of fatigue. Assess elimination pattern, nutritional status, fluid balance, and sleep pattern.

Implementation

While the child is in hyperthyroid state, promote increased caloric intake, management of child's activity and rest periods, and cool environment. Protect the eyes.

After surgery, elevate the head of the bed to promote a patent airway, and keep emergency supplies immediately available. Monitor for life-threatening thyroid storm (elevated temperature, tachycardia, hypertension, diaphoresis, tremors, confusion, seizures, agitation, abdominal pain, nausea, vomiting, and diarrhea), and report immediately if noted.

Emphasize the need for lifelong thyroid hormone replacement if the child has undergone radiation or thyroidectomy.

Recommend medical alert identification.

Reinforce importance of follow-up to monitor thyroid levels and growth and development.

Hypothyroidism

Hypothyroidism is a disorder in which levels of active thyroid hormones are decreased.

Congenital hypothyroidism, occurring in 1 in 4,000 live births, may be caused by autosomal recessive gene mutation, hypoplasia of the

Table 23–4 Medications Used for the Management of Hyperthyroidism

Medication	Action or Indication	Nursing Considerations
Antithyroid medications Methimazole (Tapazole) Propylthiouracil (PTU)	Inhibits thyroid hormone secretion	Monitor for side effects, including rash, mild leukopenia, arthralgia; the more serious side effects include lupus-like syndrome, hepatitis, and glomerulonephritis. Emphasize the importance of taking medication as prescribed and to take it at the same time each day. Monitor for symptoms of hypothyroidism.
Propranolol (Inderal)	Beta-blocking agent Decreases beta-adrenergic activity to relieve tremors, tachycardia, anxiety, heat intolerance, and restlessness	Monitor for side effects, including hypotension. Emphasize the importance of taking the medication as prescribed.
Radioiodine (oral, in solution or capsule)	Produces radiation thyroiditis and fibrosis, resulting in euthyroid state	Assess for allergy to iodine. Antithyroid medications are discontinued 1 week before treatment. Liquid may be diluted in orange juice or other fluids to disguise taste. Ensure adolescent is not pregnant before beginning treatment. Teach family to avoid physical contact with secretions (urine, stool, saliva, sweat) for several days after the treatment. Emphasize the importance of monitoring thyroid function. Hypothyroidism is a potential complication.

thyroid gland, failure of the thyroid feedback mechanism to develop, and iodine deficiency (Palma Sisto, 2004).

Acquired hypothyroidism can be idiopathic or result from autoimmune thyroiditis (Hashimoto's thyroiditis), late-onset thyroid dysfunction due to pituitary or hypothalamic dysfunction, or exposure to certain medications.

Clinical Manifestations

Congenital hypothyroidism has few clinical symptoms in the first weeks of life. When untreated, characteristic features—thickened protuberant tongue, thick lips, dull appearance—appear in the first few months of life. Other signs include prolonged neonatal jaundice, hypotonia, macroglossia, respiratory distress, bradycardia, hypothermia, cool extremities, posterior fontanel larger than 1 cm in diameter, lethargy, difficulty feeding, and swollen eyelids. Mental retardation is irreversible if the disorder is not treated.

Acquired hypothyroidism: decreased height velocity, delayed bone and dental age, delayed or precocious puberty, decreased appetite, cool skin, thinning hair, hair loss, depressed deep tendon reflexes, bradycardia, constipation, sensitivity to cool temperatures, abnormal menses, and goiter.

Diagnostic Tests

Congenital hypothyroidism: usually detected during newborn screening of T_4 and TSH. A thyroid scan or ultrasound of thyroid to confirm presence and position of thyroid gland. See Table 23–5.

Acquired hypothyroidism: T_4, TSH, and antithyroid antibody measurement.

Clinical Therapy

Lifetime thyroid replacement hormone: levothyroxine (Synthroid)

Nursing Management

Assessment

Perform routine newborn screening when child is discharged from newborn nursery and at first health visit.

Periodic monitoring of T_4 and TSH and bone age in affected children.

Measure and record height and weight on growth curve.

Table 23–5   Diagnostic Laboratory Values for Testing Thyroid Function

Diagnostic Study	Hypothyroidism	Hyperthyroidism
Serum T_4	Decreased	Markedly elevated
Serum T_3	Normal	Markedly elevated
Serum thyroid-stimulating hormone	Elevated	Decreased

Note: Normal values vary based on infant/child age.

Implementation

Educate patient and family about lifelong need for hormone replacement therapy.

Teach side effects of hypothyroidism to patient and family and instruct them to promptly report any of these changes to their health-care provider.

Reinforce importance of follow-up to monitor growth and thyroid levels.

24. ALTERATIONS IN NEUROLOGIC FUNCTION

SIGNIFICANT MEDICAL CONDITIONS
Altered States of Consciousness

An altered level of consciousness (LOC) is an important indicator of neurologic dysfunction. *Consciousness* is the brain's responsiveness to sensory stimuli and involves alertness and cognitive power. *Unconsciousness* is depressed cerebral function, or the inability of the brain to respond to stimuli. Categories of altered LOC are confusion, delirium, obtunded, stupor, and coma. Causes of altered LOC include hypoxia, trauma, infection, poisoning, seizures, metabolic disturbance, and congenital structural defect.

Clinical Manifestations

Signs of progressive alteration in LOC:

- Slight disorientation to time, place, and person
- Restless or irritable
- Drowsy but responds to loud verbal commands, withdraws from painful stimuli
- Response to pain progresses from purposeful to nonpurposeful
- Decorticate or decerebrate posturing

Some children may have signs of increased intracranial pressure (ICP). See Table 24–1.

Newborns may have lethargy, irritability, or hyperalertness.

Diagnostic Testing

Performed to identify potential cause of altered LOC:

- Complete blood cell count, blood chemistry, clotting factors
- Culture of blood, urine, cerebrospinal fluid (CSF)
- Toxicology assessments of blood and urine
- Electroencephalogram
- Radiologic studies [computed tomography (CT), magnetic resonance imaging (MRI), skull radiographs]
- ICP monitoring

Clinical Therapy

Oxygen and assisted ventilation (when gas exchange is inadequate)

Metabolic, acid–base, or electrolyte imbalance correction

Table 24–1 Signs of Increased Intracranial Pressure

Timing of Signs	Signs
Early signs	Headache
	Visual disturbance, diplopia
	Nausea and vomiting
	Dizziness or vertigo
	Slight change in vital signs
	Pupils not as reactive or equal
	Sunsetting eyes
	Seizures
	Slight change in level of consciousness
Additional signs in infants	Bulging fontanel
	Wide sutures, increased head circumference
	Dilated scalp veins
	High-pitched, cat-like cry
Late signs	Significant decrease in level of consciousness
	Cushing's triad
	Increased systolic blood pressure
	Bradycardia
	Irregular respirations
	Fixed and dilated pupils

Antibiotics

Cerebral perfusion pressure (CPP) maintained

Intravenous (IV) fluids for hypovolemia

ICP reduced or controlled

Nursing Management
Assessment
Identify a potential cause of altered LOC from history.

Assess the child's physiologic status: responsiveness, ability to maintain the airway, vital signs, head circumference, breathing patterns, air exchange, cranial nerves, pupil size and reactivity, eye movements, motor function, pulse oximetry, and arterial blood gases.

A modification of the Glasgow Coma Scale may be used at specific intervals to monitor changes in LOC in infants and young children (Table 24–2).

To rapidly assess responsiveness in infants, the acronym AVPU helps:

*A*lert, responsive to parents, cuddles, coos or babbles, smiles

Table 24–2   Glasgow Coma Scale for Infants and Young Children

Category	Score*	Criteria
Eye opening	4	Spontaneous opening
	3	To loud noise
	2	To pain
	1	No response
Verbal response	5	Smiles, coos, cries to appropriate stimuli
	4	Irritable; cries
	3	Inappropriate crying
	2	Grunts, moans
	1	No response
Motor response	6	Spontaneous movement
	5	Withdraws to touch
	4	Withdraws to pain
	3	Abnormal flexion (decorticate)
	2	Abnormal extension (decerebrate)
	1	No response

*Add the score from each category to get the total. The maximum score is 15, indicating the best level of neurologic functioning. The minimum is 3, indicating total neurologic unresponsiveness.

Note: From James, H. E. (1986). Neurologic evaluation and support in the child with acute brain insult. Pediatric Annals, 15(1), 17, with permission.

*V*erbal, responsive to verbal stimulation
*P*ain, responsive to painful stimulation only
*U*nresponsive to painful stimulation

Implementation

Maintain airway patency, oxygen, assisted ventilation, endotracheal tube or tracheostomy management, suctioning.

Monitor neurologic status, prepare for seizures, and protect child from injury.

Perform routine care and oral care; protect eyes.

Provide nutrition.

Provide sensory stimulation, talk, or play music or tapes of stories; stroke and touch the child in a soothing manner; orient child to time, place, and person.

Provide emotional support to parents, involve them in care, encourage them to express feelings.

Plan for transition to long-term care or home.

Bacterial Meningitis

An inflammation of the meninges often caused by *Haemophilus influenzae* type b, *Neisseria meningitidis*, *Streptococcus pneumoniae*, or group B streptococcus in the newborn (Prober, 2004). Inflammation causes the brain to swell, causing headache and increased ICP. Inflammation of the spinal nerves and roots causes a stiff neck. Potential complications include hearing loss, seizures, subdural effusion, hydrocephalus, septicemia, and septic arthritis.

Clinical Manifestations

In infants: fever, change in feeding pattern, vomiting, or diarrhea; bulging or flat fontanel; alert, restless, lethargic, or irritable.

Older children: fever, upper respiratory or gastrointestinal illness, increasing irritability and alteration in LOC; vomiting; complaint of muscle or joint pain.

Petechiae progressing to purpura is seen in meningococcal meningitis.

Signs of meningeal irritation: headache, photophobia, esotropia, and nuchal rigidity (resistance to neck flexion); positive Kernig or Brudzinski sign.

Symptoms can progress to include seizures, apnea, cerebral edema, photophobia, altered mental status, subdural effusion, hydrocephalus, disseminated intravascular coagulation, and shock.

Diagnostic Testing

Complete blood count, serum electrolytes and osmolality, and clotting factors

Blood and CSF culture

CT scanning when increased ICP or brain abscess is suspected

Clinical Therapy

IV antibiotics administered as soon as diagnostic tests are obtained, often changed once culture and sensitivity results are known.

Corticosteroids (dexamethasone) for children older than 6 weeks of age to reduce the risk of severe neurologic sequelae such as sensorineural hearing loss. In some cases, anticonvulsants and antipyretics are given (American Academy of Pediatrics, 2003).

Initial IV fluid restriction while monitoring for increased ICP and syndrome of inappropriate antidiuretic hormone. Nothing by mouth initially.

Aggressive fluid resuscitation if child is in shock to maintain CPP.

Intensive care monitoring.

Nursing Management

Assessment

Assess the child's physiologic status, including vital signs and LOC. Monitor for increased ICP.

Measure the infant's head circumference frequently and compare to previous measurements.

Be alert for signs of a change in the child's condition and response to treatment.

Monitor the child's ability to control secretions and to drink sufficient fluids. Monitor intake and output. Monitor the serum sodium concentration and urine specific gravity.

Assess for sensory deficits.

Implementation

Maintain hydration.

Administer medications and monitor the child's response to antibiotics. Monitor for gastrointestinal distress and blood in the stool associated with corticosteroids.

Promote comfort with reduced stimulation (dim lights, quiet room) and a side-lying position. Assess pain management.

Use standard and droplet precaution isolation until effective treatment is under way.

Provide support to the family. Help the parents comfort the child and participate in daily care.

Encourage infants and children to be fully immunized to prevent potential meningitis.

Refer infants and toddlers with neurologic sequelae to an early-intervention program.

Cerebral Palsy

Cerebral palsy (CP) is a disorder of movement and posture from an intrauterine insult to the brain or structural abnormality of the central nervous system (CNS). Intrauterine infection (chorioamnionitis) increases the risk for CP (Van Eerden & Bernstein, 2003). CNS infection and brain trauma are the major sources of acquired brain injury and subsequent CP in young children. Four types of motor dysfunction seen include spastic, dyskinetic, ataxic, and mixed. The prognosis for infants and children with CP depends on the level of physical involvement and on the presence of intellectual, visual, or hearing deficits.

Clinical Manifestations

Delay in meeting developmental milestones

Visual defects such as strabismus, nystagmus, or refractory errors; hearing loss; language delay; speech impediment; seizures; or mental retardation

Difficulty feeding because of oral motor involvement

Behavior problems such as attention deficit hyperactivity disorder and self-injurious behavior

Wide variability in symptoms depending on the area of the brain involved and the degree of anoxia

Spastic (Cerebral Cortex or Pyramidal Tract Injury)

Persistent hypertonia, rigidity, leads to contractures and abnormal curvature of the spine

Exaggerated deep tendon reflexes

Persistent primitive reflexes

Dyskinetic (Extrapyramidal, Basal Ganglia)

Impairment of voluntary muscle control; bizarre twisting movements; tremors, difficulty with fine and purposeful motor movements

Exaggerated posturing

Inconsistent muscle tone that may change hour to hour or day to day; rigid muscle tone when awake and normal or decreased muscle tone when asleep

Ataxic (Cerebellar, Extrapyramidal)

Abnormalities of voluntary movement involving balance and position of the trunk and limbs; difficulty controlling hand and arm movements during reaching

Increased or decreased muscle tone; muscle instability and wide-based unsteady gait

Hypotonia in infancy

Mixed (Multiple Areas)

No dominant motor pattern

Unique compensatory movements and posture to maintain control over specific neuromotor deficits

Combination of characteristics from other types

Diagnostic Testing

Ultrasonography to detect fetal and neonatal brain abnormalities, such as intraventricular hemorrhage

Neuromotor tests of movement patterns, tone, and primitive reflexes

CT scans and MRI to view anatomic structures and positron emission tomography to evaluate brain metabolic functioning

Clinical Therapy

Braces and splints to prevent contractures or to manage scoliosis

Tone reducing casts to keep spastic muscles in stretched position

Static positioning devices

Surgery to lengthen tendons, reduce spasticity, balance muscle power, and stabilize uncontrollable joints

Nerve blocks; diazepam, baclofen, dantrolene to control spasticity; botulinum toxin injections into specific muscle groups (Buck, 2003). See Meds 24–1.

Physical and occupational therapy to promote improved muscle tone and better motor control for function; speech therapy

Assistive devices, technology, mobility options (tricycle, walker, wheelchair)

Nursing Management

Assessment

Assess for developmental delays and orthopedic, visual, auditory, and intellectual deficits.

Assess for abnormal muscle tone or abnormal posture, persistence of primitive reflexes beyond the expected age (see Chapter 3).

Identify asymmetric or abnormal crawling by using two or three extremities; identify hand dominance before the preschool years.

Implementation

Provide adequate nutrition—high-calorie diets or supplements needed due to chewing and swallowing difficulties. Give small amounts of soft foods at a time. Use feeding utensils with large, padded handles.

Meds 24–1 Medications Used to Treat Cerebral Palsy

Medication	Nursing Considerations
Diazepam, lorazepam, or clonazepam *Oral*	Can cause drowsiness and excessive drooling. May interfere with feeding and speech. Physiologic dependence can develop, so taper drug when discontinued.
Dantrolene *Oral*	Can cause drowsiness, muscle weakness, and increased drooling. May cause liver damage, so liver function testing should be performed periodically.
Baclofen *Intrathecal* *Oral*	Adjustable dosing is possible. May cause hypotonia, increased seizures in children with known epilepsy, sleepiness, and nausea and vomiting. Monitor for pump failure and signs of infection.
Botulinum toxin type A *Injection*	Used to improve walking in children with equinus gait, may be used in hip adductors and hamstrings to improve positioning. May have stumbling, leg cramps, leg weakness, and calf atrophy. Repeated injections needed to continue effect.

Maintain skin integrity—protect the skin over bony prominences, under splints and braces.

Maintain proper body alignment—in the bed or in a chair. Use splints and braces to support the child and reduce the risk for contractures.

Promote physical mobility—range of motion exercises to maintain joint flexibility and to prevent contractures. Position the child to foster flexion to enhance interaction with the environment. Encourage use of child's adaptive appliances during hospitalization. Refer parents to get help with the acquisition of adaptive devices, such as customized wheelchair.

Promote safety—use safety belts in strollers and wheelchairs. Determine if an adaptive car safety seat is needed.

Promote growth and development—child may not be intellectually disabled; refer to early intervention programs.

Promote communication—if hearing impaired, refer to learn sign language or other communication methods; computer may help communication.

Provide emotional support—listen to parents' concerns, encourage them to ask questions and share feelings. Refer to support group.

Provide referral to social services for financial resources for adaptive equipment or for special transitions in the child's life, such as plans for adult living.

Patient and Family Education

Educate about the disorder and the child's special needs.

Teach administration, desired effects, and side effects of medications prescribed for CP and seizures.

Encourage regular dental care, as enamel defects and malocclusion are common, along with hyperplasia when anticonvulsants are prescribed.

Prepare parents for possible seizure when pertussis and measles-mumps-rubella vaccines are given, when child has coexisting seizure disorder.

Prepare parents to become the child's case manager when appropriate.

Provide guidance for development of an individualized education plan (IEP) to address mobility and educational support for behavior problems, perceptual problems, and speech difficulties. Explore vocational training options during adolescence.

Encephalitis

An inflammation of the brain and often the meninges, usually caused by a viral infection.

Clinical Manifestations

Severe headache, fever, signs of an upper respiratory infection, malaise, and nausea or vomiting.

Disorientation or confusion may progress to stupor and coma. Behavioral or personality changes, hallucinations, periods of screaming.

Hemiparesis, ataxia, or weakness; cranial nerve deficits; or alterations in reflex response; focal or generalized seizures.

Diagnostic Testing

Analysis of CSF, blood serology tests, and nasopharyngeal and stool specimens for viral pathogens. Virus-specific immunoglobulin M antibodies.

CT scan, MRI, and electroencephalogram may also be performed.

Clinical Therapy

Supportive care in the pediatric intensive care unit (PICU). Treated with antibiotics until bacterial pathogens have been ruled out. Acyclovir may be used for herpes viral infections.

Nursing Management
Monitor the child's airway and ability to handle secretions. Monitor vital signs, color, pulse oximetry readings, capillary refill time, arterial blood gas values, LOC, and urine output.

Anticipate seizures, have appropriate equipment for managing seizures at bedside.

Prevent complications with skin care, proper positioning and turning, chest physiotherapy, and passive range of motion exercises.

Orient child to environment as LOC improves. Offer therapeutic play, age-appropriate toys, and diversional activities.

Keep parents informed about the child's condition, treatment, and prognosis.

Refer parents to home care, social services, family counseling, and support groups.

Headaches
Headaches have both benign (migraine, inflammatory, and tension) and structural causes (tumors and increased ICP).

Clinical Manifestations
Migraines
Triggered by stress; foods containing nitrates, glutamate, caffeine, tyramine, and salt; menses; oral contraceptives; stress; fatigue; and hunger

Aura (auditory, visual, or taste sensation)

Unilateral or bilateral pulsatile throbbing pain lasting for hours or days, pain often in retro-orbital frontal and temporal region

Nausea and vomiting

Photophobia and phonophobia

Tension Headaches
May be associated with stresses associated with school, insecurity, or conflict in the family.

Dull, achy pain in band around head, in temporal or occipital areas, in neck and shoulders that may last for days; intermittent or constant pain with fluctuations in severity.

Dizziness and fatigue may be present.

Sensitive to light or sound.

Pain may be aggravated with increased physical activity.

Medication-Overuse Headaches

Associated with the frequent use of medications for headaches, more than two to three times a week (Reimschisel, 2003)

Dull, bilateral or unilateral pain in frontal area

Occur at least two to four times a week or almost daily

Can vary in character, location, and severity from time to time

Usually increase in frequency and severity over time, paralleling the increase in medication use

Recur when the abortive therapy or medication wears off

Diagnostic Testing

Usually based on detailed history and physical examination

Radiologic studies (CT scan or MRI) only if a structural problem is suspected

A lumbar puncture if an infection or inflammatory process is suspected

Clinical Therapy

Migraines

Food elimination trial to identify food triggers

Caffeine avoidance

Noise and light avoidance

Medications to abort migraine (ergot, isometheptene, sumatriptan); cyproheptadine, beta-blockers, tricyclic antidepressants, and anticonvulsants (valproic acid, topiramate, and gabapentin) may be used prophylactically if headaches significantly interfere with usual activities (Lewis, Scott, & Rendin, 2002)

Analgesic medication (ibuprofen, acetaminophen)

Relaxation techniques and biofeedback

Tension Headaches

Relaxation techniques

Analgesic and anti-inflammatory medications

Ice pack

Rest

Medication-Overuse Headaches

Discontinuation of all medications for headaches (caffeine, acetaminophen, nonsteroidal anti-inflammatory drugs, and triptans).

Clonidine may be used to treat withdrawal symptoms.

Nursing Management

Assess the child for potential neurologic signs associated with headaches.

Encourage the child to keep a calendar or diary of headaches, including the events and stresses occurring at the time. Analyze diary for patterns of triggers or stress. Identify and discuss strategies that may help reduce triggers or stress.

If a food elimination trial is implemented, educate the child and family about foods to eat and not eat and how to gradually add foods to identify offending chemical triggers.

Educate child and family when to take analgesics and other prescribed medications appropriately. Teach child and parents that medications should not be used for more than 2–3 days a week.

Hydrocephalus

An imbalance between the production and absorption of CSF that leads to an increase in the volume of CSF. The condition may be congenital, associated with CNS malformations such as myelomeningocele, or develop as a complication of an injury, an acute illness, or intraventricular hemorrhage in the premature newborn.

Communicating hydrocephalus—the CSF flows freely between normal channels and pathways, but absorption of CSF in the subarachnoid space and the arachnoid villi is impaired.

Noncommunicating hydrocephalus—an obstruction in the channels or pathways impedes the flow of CSF and prevents it from entering the subarachnoid space.

When a Chiari II malformation associated with myelomeningocele is present, hydrocephalus causes displacement of the cerebellum, brainstem, and fourth ventricle leading to herniation. Sudden death, respiratory difficulty, swallowing difficulties, and the need for assisted ventilation may occur at any time.

Clinical Manifestations

Infants

Rapidly increasing head circumference, tense, full or bulging fontanel, split sutures, Macewen's sign (cracked-pot sound).

Bossing (protrusion) of frontal area, face is disproportionate to the skull size.

Sunsetting eyes (sclera visible above iris), sixth cranial nerve palsy.

Prominent, distended scalp veins, translucent scalp skin.

Increased tone or hyperreflexia, brisk deep tendon reflexes, Babinski sign, difficulty holding head up.

Irritability or lethargy, decline in LOC, poor feeding.

Late signs include apnea, a shrill, high-pitched cry, difficulty swallowing or feeding, and vomiting.

Older Children with Acquired Hydrocephalus
No head enlargement

Irritability, lethargy, altered LOC, poor appetite

Fussiness, sleepiness, confusion, or apathy

Personality change, loss of interest in daily activities; poor judgment or verbal incoherence, worsening school performance, memory loss

Ataxia, spasticity, or other alterations in motor development

Visual defects due to pressure on second, third, and sixth cranial nerves; papilledema

Signs of increased ICP, headache on arising with vomiting

Signs of Shunt Failure
Low-grade fever, malaise, headache, nausea

Changes in LOC, irritability after fever is controlled

Diagnostic Testing
Head circumference measurement.

CT scanning and MRI may reveal the anatomic cause of hydrocephalus.

Ultrasonography or echoencephalography in infants with open fontanels.

Shunt failure is evaluated with CT scanning; MRI; lateral radiographs of the skull, neck, chest and abdomen; a radionucleotide CSF study; and a culture of the CSF obtained by tapping the shunt.

Clinical Therapy
Medications (furosemide and acetazolamide) to reduce the rate of CSF production until surgery is performed.

A ventricular access device to withdraw CSF may be inserted before shunt placement.

Surgery to remove the obstruction such as a tumor or to create a new CSF pathway.

Placement of a catheter or shunt in the ventricle to divert CSF to the peritoneal cavity, atrium of the heart, or the pleural spaces. Mechanical complications may include catheter blockage, kinking of the tubing, or valve breakdown.

Antibiotics, shunt removal, and placement of an external ventricular drainage system when a shunt infection occurs. A new shunt is inserted when the CSF cultures are sterile.

Some children with shunt drainage to the heart receive endocarditis antibiotic prophylaxis to reduce the risk of shunt infections (see Chapter 17).

Nursing Management
Assessment
Routinely measure the head circumference of all infants and plot on a growth curve to detect unexpected head enlargement.

After shunt placement surgery, monitor the vital signs, respiratory status, irritability, and LOC to detect increased ICP. Assess pain. Monitor intake and output.

Inspect surgical sites for drainage and signs of infection; redness and swelling of the shunt tract; leakage of CSF; nuchal rigidity; neck or back pain; headache; and photophobia (Ditmyer, 2004).

Measure head circumference daily and compare to previous measurements.

Assess the child for shunt failure and infection at all healthcare visits. Monitor for signs of visual problems as well as cognitive, speech, and motor developmental delays.

Implementation
Postoperatively, the child is initially in a flat position to prevent rapid CSF drainage, and the head of the bed is elevated gradually.

Keep body in alignment with splints or towel rolls. Do not stretch or strain the neck muscles that must support the large head.

Passive range of motion exercises three to four times per day as ordered.

Maintain skin integrity:
- Change position every 2 hours, inspect for areas of redness, keep skin clean and dry, massage gently using lotion.

- Place child on pressure-reducing surface.
- Place transparent dressing over surfaces exposed to frequent friction.

Provide frequent, small feedings with frequent burping, as the infant is prone to vomiting.

Provide emotional support, and keep the parents informed about the child's condition and all procedures to be performed. Assure parents that most children with shunts lead normal lives.

Refer to early intervention program to promote development. School children may need IEP or individualized health plan (IHP).

Patient and Family Education
Important signs and symptoms of shunt failure (signs of increased ICP) and infection (changes in LOC, irritability, personality change, malaise, headache, diplopia, nausea, loss of developmental milestones or loss of coordination and balance, and low-grade fever).

When and how to contact the healthcare provider. Assist with development of an emergency care plan in case of shunt failure.

Infants with poor head control should not be placed in forward-facing car safety seats, regardless of age. This position increases the risk of cervical spine injury and death to these children in the event of a car crash.

Use a helmet for bicycle riding and skateboarding. Do not participate in sports with high risk for head or abdominal impact.

Myelodysplasia or Spina Bifida
Myelodysplasia is a malformation of the spinal cord and spinal canal or neural tube defect. Types of neural tube defects include the following:

- Anencephaly—no development of the brain above the brainstem.
- Encephalocele—protrusion of meningeal tissue or meningeal-covered brain through a defect in the skull.
- Spina bifida occulta—a vertebral defect without visible protrusion of the meninges or spinal cord tissue. An abnormal growth of hair, a dimple or sinus tract, a lipoma, or a vascular skin lesion may be over the defect.
- Meningocele—a spinal fluid–filled meningeal sac protruding through a vertebral defect, associated with no abnormalities of the spinal cord.

- Meningomyelocele (spina bifida)—a spinal fluid–filled meningeal sac that contains a portion of the spinal cord and nerves protruding through a vertebral defect.

Spina bifida can occur at any location along the vertebral column. The cause is unknown, but genetics, maternal use of seizure or acne medications, excessive use of alcohol, and folic acid deficiency before and during pregnancy are implicated.

Clinical Manifestations

A sac-like protrusion on the infant's back indicates meningocele or myelomeningocele. The higher the defect on the vertebral column, the greater the neurologic dysfunction:

- Thoracic or lumbar 1–2 level: paralysis of the legs, weakness and sensory loss in the trunk and lower body region
- Lumbar 3: can flex hips and extend the knees, ankles and toes paralyzed
- Lumbar 4–5 level: can flex hips and extend knees, weak or absent ankle extension, toe flexion, and hip extension
- Sacral level: mild weakness in ankles and toes, bladder and bowel function may be affected

Hip abnormalities such as hip dysplasia; clubfoot; scoliosis or kyphosis.

Sensory loss. Bowel and bladder sphincters may be affected. Renal involvement may result from neurologic impairment and urinary retention.

Hydrocephalus due to the Chiari II malformation when defect is above the sacral level.

- Signs of Chiari II complication in infants: difficulty swallowing, apnea, respiratory difficulty, inspiratory stridor, weak or poor cry, sustained backward arching of the head (opisthotonus).
- Signs of Chiari II complication in older children: choking, hoarseness, vocal cord paralysis, disordered breathing during sleep, stiffness or spasticity of arms and hands, loss of feeling or sensation.

Other disabilities: mobility problems, cognitive impairment, seizures, and visual impairment such as strabismus.

Potential complications: spinal curvatures, musculoskeletal and joint abnormalities, skin sores, urinary dysfunction, and sexual dysfunction.

Diagnostic Testing

Before birth: prenatal maternal serum tests for alpha-fetoprotein and a high-resolution fetal ultrasound

After birth: ultrasonography, radiologic imaging by CT scan, MRI, and flat films of the spinal column

Evaluation of bladder and bowel function, neurologic and motor function, and cognitive function

Clinical Therapy

Surgery to close and repair the lesion within 48 hours of birth to reduce infection.

Braces to support joint position and mobility. Assistive devices such as walkers, crutches, and wheelchairs to enhance mobility. Encourage weight bearing.

A diet with adequate calcium and vitamin D to minimize risk for osteoporosis.

Use of nonlatex equipment and supplies, as child is at risk for latex allergy.

Surgery or an orthotic jacket to correct spinal deformities.

Bowel and bladder interventions: clean intermittent catheterization, stool softeners, glycerin or bisacodyl suppositories.

Multiple surgeries and invasive procedures for orthopedic and urologic problems.

Comprehensive healthcare planning with a team of physicians, nurses, and therapists from neurosurgery, orthopedics, urology, and physical therapy.

Nursing Management

Assessment

Newborn

Monitor for integrity of the sac and leakage of CSF. Inspect area for wound healing after surgery. Note any signs of infection.

Assess the extremities for deformities and motor defects.

Assess the vital signs, monitor intake and output, and assess for bladder and bowel involvement.

Measure the head circumference daily to assess for hydrocephalus.

Assess family's financial status, health insurance, and need for social services.

Child
Assess the child's vital signs, growth, and head circumference.

Assess neurologic status for any deterioration in function that could be associated with shunt failure or problem with the spinal cord. Assess the range of motion of joints and mobility status.

After surgery to correct deformities, assess vital signs, responsiveness, and level of pain. Assess dressing sites for bleeding and draining. Monitor the distal extremities for swelling and circulation. Assess intake and output.

Implementation
Newborn before Surgery
Cover the sac with a sterile saline dressing and protect it from pressure, infection, and trauma. Prone position with hips slightly flexed and legs abducted to minimize tension on the sac.

Feed the newborn with the head turned to one side until surgery has been performed. Comfort the neonate before surgery with tactile stimulation such as touching, patting, and cuddling.

Postsurgical Care
Observe for infection, especially meningitis. Keep the diaper away from incision site.

If a ventriculoperitoneal shunt is placed, see Hydrocephalus for care information.

Keep in prone position until healed, and then convert to supine position for sleeping. Splints may help maintain extremity alignment.

Promote mobility—gentle range of motion exercises.

Provide emotional support to parents and involve them in the care.

Encourage use of local healthcare provider for primary care and episodic illnesses with care coordination by a multidisciplinary team of health professionals.

Obtain special devices such as splints, wedges, and rolls for care in the home.

Make home health nursing referral and identify a case manager until parents assume that role.

Refer parents to resource groups such as the Spina Bifida Association of America.

Patient Education

Instruct parents how to position, handle, feed, and perform range of motion exercises.

Teach parents the signs and symptoms of increased ICP, hydrocephalus, shunt infection or malfunction, and urinary tract infection.

Teach skill of intermittent catheterization.

Educate the child and families about the proper use of braces, walkers, crutches, canes, custom-designed wheelchairs, and car safety seats. Encourage independent mobility.

Discuss nutritional needs to promote growth, reduce osteoporosis, and reduce constipation. Emphasize importance of preventing excessive weight gain.

Teach bowel training to control evacuation of bowel with diet and a glycerin or bisacodyl suppository in either the morning or evening.

Inspect daily all skin areas under braces and splints, pressure areas on buttocks when in wheelchair; and provide skin care.

Identify and use latex-free products. See Chapter 18.

Begin teaching children to assume responsibility for self-care as their intellectual ability and fine motor skills develop.

Provide guidance on coordination of educational services, development of an IEP, and individualized transition plan.

Neonatal Abstinence Syndrome

Illicit substances used during pregnancy that may cause neonatal abstinence syndrome include opiates (heroine, meperidine, methadone), CNS stimulants (cocaine, propoxyphene, amphetamines), and CNS depressants (barbiturates, alcohol, and marijuana). Children with prenatal cocaine exposure may have difficulties with language development, attention span, memory, and motor skills (Campbell, 2003).

Clinical Manifestations

Withdrawal symptoms for opiates within 24–48 hours after birth; for barbiturates within 4–14 days after birth, for cocaine or amphetamines within 7 days after birth.

Prematurity, intrauterine growth retardation, microcephaly, and low birth weight are common results of prenatal cocaine exposure.

Jitteriness, seizures, hyperexcitability, and poor feeding may be related to the effects of cocaine on developing CNS rather than signs of drug withdrawal (Kuehne & Reilly, 2004).

Hypertonia, tremors, and extensor leg posture; poor sucking and feeding difficulties; less time in quiet sleep; more stressed behaviors such as mouthing and clenched fists; and difficulty regulating their behaviors.

Excoriated skin due to continuous movement on crib sheets.

Sneezing, stuffy nose, sweating, tachycardia, and tachypnea.

Diarrhea, vomiting, and poor feeding.

Diagnostic Testing
Maternal and infant urine toxicology screening.

Toxicologic screening of meconium or infant hair reveals mother's drug use for the last half of the pregnancy.

Chain of custody for specimens may be needed.

Brazelton Neonatal Behavioral Assessment Scale evaluates infants on habituation general arousal level, orientation, quality of movement and tone, autonomic stability, reflexes, and responsiveness when aroused (Campbell, 2003).

Clinical Therapy
Supportive treatment: reduced environmental stimuli and swaddling.

Medications such as phenobarbital, diazepam, methadone, clonidine, and paregoric may be prescribed to alleviate symptoms of drug withdrawal.

Breastfeeding is discouraged, as the drugs cross over into breast milk.

Nursing Management
Assessment
Observe for poor sucking, seizures, vomiting and diarrhea, dehydration, and an increased metabolic rate. Consider if the newborn could have both neonatal abstinence syndrome and another condition such as infection, bowel obstruction, electrolyte disorder, hydrocephalus, and intracranial anomaly with similar signs.

Monitor the skin for abrasions.

Assess the strengths, safety, and competence of the mother and other potential caregivers. Determine if the mother is still using illicit drugs and identify other family supports that may help provide the care and safety needed by the newborn.

Implementation

Provide frequent, small, high-calorie feedings (24 calories per ounce formula). Be patient when feeding infants with poor coordination of sucking and swallowing. Teach parents to use a calm approach and soothing voice when feeding. Newborns may initially feed better in side-lying position while swaddled.

Administer prescribed medications if ordered for drug withdrawal and monitor the infant's response.

Use techniques to calm and soothe the newborn:

- Quiet environment with subdued lighting to minimize stimulation and promote sleep.
- Comfort and pacify the infant with swaddling, rocking, and a pacifier for sucking needs. Infant massage may be beneficial.
- Hold the infant with the spine flexed to decrease extensor tone.

Promote parent–infant interaction, minimizing stimulation, and promoting feeding.

Refer for careful long-term follow-up (social services, physicians, and nurses) to ensure the infant's safety and to assess growth and development.

Support from social services or child protective services may be needed to manage complex family situations.

Neurofibromatosis 1

An autosomal dominant disorder in which tumors grow along nerves leading to skin changes and bone deformities. Most children and adults with mild symptoms can live a normal, productive life.

Clinical Manifestations

Six or more café au lait spots or dark macules 5 mm or larger seen at birth or by 2 years of age. The spots grow to 15 mm or larger in diameter by adulthood.

Multiple neurofibromas or benign tumors begin to grow on or under the skin during puberty.

Plexiform neurofibromas—freckling in the axillary or inguinal areas.

Pain when tumors grow around and compress a nerve or grow in the spinal cord.

Scoliosis, thinning of tibia, and fractures that do not heal well.

Vision deficits when tumors develop in the optic nerve (optic glioma).

Precocious puberty or delayed puberty with delayed menarche (Virdis, Street, Bandello, et al., 2003).

Diagnostic Testing
Diagnosis is based on physical examination. Prenatal diagnosis using amniocentesis or chorionic villus sampling procedures is possible. Genetic testing may be useful in some cases.

Clinical Therapy
Monitor for signs of developing problems (growth and development, blood pressure, scoliosis, timing of sexual development, and neurofibromas).

Radiologic imaging (MRI of the brain and radiographs of the spine and other bones) performed when problems are detected.

Annual ophthalmic examinations to detect optic gliomas and vision deficits and to monitor Lisch nodules.

Genetic counseling is offered.

Surgery when neurofibromas are disfiguring, cause pain, or are life-threatening.

Nursing Management
Assess for café au lait spots, axillary and inguinal freckling, and small tumors on the body. Note growth of any mass or pain caused by a mass. Monitor for hypertension. Monitor growth and pubertal development. Perform vision and scoliosis screening on a frequent basis. Note any evidence of tibial bowing or thinning.

Monitor school performance for learning disabilities and hyperactivity.

Provide psychological support to the child and family, as tumor development causes self-image and self-esteem problems. Identify peers or refer the adolescent to support groups. Focus on the child's strengths.

Seizure Disorders
Seizures result from abnormal excessive electrical discharges of the cortical neuronal network of cells on the surface of the brain. Common causes include CNS infection, hypoxia, brain injury, and a sudden rise in temperature. Other causes include hypoglycemia, toxins, and tumors.

Clinical Manifestations

Partial seizures—often start with an aura (sensory warning of impending seizure) or abrupt unprovoked alteration in behavior. May progress to generalized seizure.

Generalized seizures—often begin with a tonic phase (unconsciousness, continuous muscular contraction, and sustained stiffness), followed by the clonic phase (alternating muscular contraction and relaxation as a rhythmic repetitive jerking). The postictal period follows with decreased LOC.

Febrile seizures—generalized seizures in association with a rapid temperature rise above 39°C (102°F).

Newborn seizures are subtle [horizontal deviation of eye, repetitive blinking, sucking or lip smacking/tongue thrusting, rhythmic repetitive movement of an extremity (like bicycling of the legs)].

Status epilepticus—a generalized seizure lasting longer than 10 minutes or a series of seizures during which consciousness is not regained.

Diagnostic Testing

Testing varies with potential cause of seizures

Complete blood cell count, blood chemistry

Cultures of urine, blood, CSF

Serum drug level if the child is taking any anticonvulsants

Electroencephalogram

Toxicology screening, lead level, tests for inborn errors of metabolism

Radiologic tests (CT, MRI)

Clinical Therapy

Anticonvulsant therapy—a single medication for seizure control is preferred. Monitor therapeutic drug levels and regular blood testing to identify hematologic or liver problems (Meds 24–2).

Surgery to remove a tumor, lesion, or even a portion of the brain causing the seizures when the seizures are not responsive to medication.

A vagal nerve stimulator for children who are unable to tolerate several antiepileptic medications but are not candidates for surgery (Blair & Selekman, 2004).

A ketogenic diet may be used for myoclonic and absence seizures. The diet with very high fat, adequate protein, and low carbohydrates produces ketosis and has anticonvulsant effects (Freeman, 2003).

Meds 24–2 Commonly Used Medications for the Treatment of Seizures

Medication	Nursing Considerations
Diazepam IV	IV push medication is administered very slowly as close to vein as possible. Monitor vital signs for hypotension, tachycardia, and respiratory depression.
Phenobarbital PO, IV, IM	IV medication must be administered slowly. Monitor child's vital signs frequently when given intravenously. May crush tablets and mix with food or fluid.
Phenytoin PO, IV	Educate family to ensure adequate intake of vitamin D, folic acid, and calcium. Promote frequent dental care for gingival hyperplasia. Ginkgo may decrease anticonvulsant effectiveness.
Carbamazepine PO	Give with food to enhance absorption. Do not administer suspension simultaneously with another liquid medication to prevent formation of a precipitate. Causes photosensitivity reactions.
Valproic acid PO	Do not use carbonated beverage to dilute syrup. Tablets and capsules should not be chewed. Give with food to decrease irritation. Monitor platelet count and bleeding times. Drug should not be used in combination with aspirin, sedatives, and allergy medications.
Ethosuximide PO	Monitor for weight loss or anorexia. Give with food if gastrointestinal upset occurs.
Primidone PO	Tablet may be crushed and given with fluid; may be given with food. Do not combine with over-the-counter medications unless approved by healthcare provider. Educate family to ensure adequate intake of vitamin D, folic acid, calcium, and vitamin B_{12}.
Clonazepam PO	Monitor for signs of overdose (confusion, irritability, sleepiness, sweating, muscle cramps, diminished reflexes). Do not combine with over-the-counter medications unless approved by healthcare provider.
Felbamate PO	Monitor weight for gain or loss. Child needs regular monitoring for hematologic and liver problems. Careful dosing is needed when combined with other anticonvulsants.
Gabapentin PO	Vision, concentration, and coordination may be impaired by the medication. Do not take medication within 2 hours of an antacid.

(continued)

**Meds 24–2   Commonly Used Medications for
                the Treatment of Seizures (Continued)**

Medication	Nursing Considerations
Lamotrigine PO	Drug increases photosensitivity. Monitor for adverse effects if used with valproic acid.
Tiagabine PO	Give with food. Monitor for signs of central nervous system depression. Avoid using with over-the-counter medications that cause drowsiness.
Topiramate PO	Increase fluid intake to reduce risk of kidney stones. Psychomotor slowing as well as speech and language problems may develop with use of medication.

Note: Data from Wilson, B. A., Shannon, M. T., & Stang, C. L. (2005). Nurse's drug guide 2005. Upper Saddle River, NJ: Prentice Hall.

Clinical Therapy for Status Epilepticus
Emergency assessment and interventions (see Chapter 12).

Monitor electrolytes, glucose, blood gases, increasing fever, and abnormal blood pressure.

Anticonvulsants such as diazepam are given intravenously or rectally.

A nasogastric tube is inserted to reduce risk of aspiration.

Manage thermoregulation.

Monitor for adverse effects of cumulative doses of anticonvulsants (apnea, need for airway control and assisted ventilation).

Nursing Management
Assessment
Observe the specific seizure activity, LOC, vital signs, and signs of hypoxia. The child's lack of response may be the result of the postictal state.

Collect and analyze historical information about the seizure activity, clustering, aura, description of motor activity or changes in muscle tone, automatisms, and any changes in development or school performance.

Assess the family's adaptation. Identify how well the child copes when a seizure happens at school.

Implementation
Maintain airway patency; place nothing in child's mouth during a seizure.

Monitor oxygenation.

Protect the child from self-harm during seizures.

Administer IV medications for acute management of seizures slowly to minimize risk of respiratory or circulatory collapse.

Provide emotional support to family, permit them to express fears and frustrations.

Patient and Family Education

Teach about potential causes of seizures and home management (medication administration, ketogenic diet, protecting from injury).

Develop emergency care plan and IHP.

Educate adolescents about potential teratogenicity of some anticonvulsants, and encourage contraception for sexually active adolescent females.

Provide child and family with safety guidelines:

- Do not leave the child alone in the bathtub. Children who bathe alone should use the shower.
- Have a buddy and lifeguard present when the child swims.
- Wear a life vest when boating.
- Use a helmet when the child has frequent seizures to protect the head during a fall.
- Keep child away from open flames or outdoor grills.
- Avoid activities where fall risks are increased (e.g., rock climbing).
- Wear medical alert identification.

INJURIES OF THE NEUROLOGIC SYSTEM
Concussion

A transient impairment of consciousness often resulting from blunt head trauma. Nerve fibers are stretched, compressed, or sheared by the impact injury to the head, but no gross structural damage or focal injury results. Sports such as hockey, football, and soccer place the child at a high risk for concussion.

Athletes who sustain a concussion are nearly three times as likely to have a second concussion in the same season (Guskiewicz, Weaver, Padua, et al., 2000). Second-impact syndrome (a second concussion before complete recovery from the first) results in acute brain swelling, neurologic or cognitive deficits, and sometimes death.

Clinical Manifestations

Clinical manifestations are the same as those of a mild brain injury (see Traumatic Brain Injury). Severity is graded by three levels, as follows:

Grade 1—transient confusion, no loss of consciousness, mental status abnormalities last less than 15 minutes

Grade 2—transient confusion, no loss of consciousness, and a duration of mental status abnormalities of 15 minutes or longer

Grade 3—Loss of consciousness, either brief (seconds) or prolonged (minutes or longer)
(Quality Standards Subcommittee, American Academy of Neurology, 1997)

Pediatric Concussive Syndrome
Occurs in children younger than age 3 years.

Toddlers are stunned at time of injury, with no loss of consciousness.

Later become pale, clammy, lethargic, and may vomit.

Postconcussive Syndrome
Headache, dizziness, vertigo, fatigue, photophobia, ataxia.

Subtle changes in personality, irritability, poor concentration, poor memory.

Symptoms may last several weeks, and in cases up to 6 months.

Clinical Therapy
Supportive treatment. Monitored over several hours for decreased LOC.

May be admitted if unconscious for more than 5 minutes or amnesia of event.

Postconcussive syndrome: supportive treatment, prepare parents and teachers to expect child's altered behavior during weeks to months of recovery.

Removal from sports participation according to guidelines for severity of concussion and number of concussions.

Nursing Management
See guidelines for child with a mild brain injury in Traumatic Brain Injury.

Hypoxic–Ischemic Brain Injury (Drowning and Near Drowning)
Drowning is defined as death within 24 hours of a submersion incident. *Near drowning* is survival for at least 24 hours after submersion. Children at high risk include toddlers because of inability to

escape from the water, adolescent boys because of risk-taking behavior, and children with seizure disorders. More than 90% of drowning incidents occur in fresh water such as ponds and residential swimming pools (Zuckerman & Conway, 2000).

The immersion injury causes hypoxemia, and irreversible CNS damage within 4–6 minutes. Water in the airway inactivates surfactant and damages the alveoli, leading to pulmonary edema and acute respiratory distress syndrome. Pneumonia may develop. Secondary damage from cerebral edema and increasing ICP compound the injury. Near drowning may result in complete recovery, severe brain injury, or variable neurologic deficits. Predictors of good outcome are submersion for less than 5 minutes and cardiopulmonary resuscitation (CPR) for less than 10 minutes (Zuckerman & Conway, 2000).

Clinical Manifestations
Submersion and resuscitated—the child has few symptoms and recovers without complication.

Longer submersion—decreased LOC, seizures, irregular respirations, apnea, gastric distention, cerebral edema, increased ICP, respiratory acidosis.

Clinical Therapy
Upon rescue, assess for spontaneous breathing, heart rate, and responsiveness. Clear mouth of foreign matter and perform CPR.

Cardiorespiratory monitoring equipment, arterial blood gases, chest radiograph.

Oxygen (100%) by nonrebreather face mask and rewarming. Airway secured with an endotracheal tube. Assisted ventilation with positive end-expiratory pressure to keep the alveoli open.

IV fluids if hypovolemic. Once hypovolemia is corrected, fluids are often restricted to reduce the risk of cerebral edema.

Potential medications used include diuretics to reduce cerebral edema, vasopressors to maintain a normal blood pressure, and antibiotics if signs of pneumonia develop.

Hospital admission for at least 24 hours even when asymptomatic, as respiratory distress and cerebral edema may take 12 hours to develop.

Nursing Management
Assessment
Assess LOC, spontaneous respiratory efforts, and pulse.

Attach a cardiorespiratory monitor and pulse oximeter. Monitor the child's respiratory status, oxygenation, cardiopulmonary function, neurologic status (Glasgow Coma Scale, pupil checks), and vital signs. Assess intake and output.

Assess frequently for respiratory distress and decreasing LOC, indicating potential cerebral edema.

Assess response of family members and need for support associated with the child's life-threatening injury.

Implementation

The child with seriously compromised respiratory and neurologic status is cared for in the PICU.

Administer oxygen and positive end-expiratory pressure or mechanical ventilation if acute respiratory distress develops.

Position the child properly to promote respiratory function.

Note any change in respiratory status, blood gases, and notify the physician promptly.

Implement nursing interventions for the child with altered LOC as described in Altered States of Consciousness.

If cerebral edema develops, implement nursing interventions as described in Traumatic Brain Injury.

Provide emotional support to the family. Encourage parents to seek assistance from social workers, clergy, close friends, and relatives. Arrange for appropriate referrals.

If the child's prognosis is poor, an ethical consult may be offered to educate the family about options for decision making regarding sustaining or terminating life support.

When the child has significant neurologic disabilities, identify a case manager to work with the family for long-term care and rehabilitation options.

Become involved in community efforts to prevent drowning through education and enactment/enforcement of regulations such as fencing around all four sides of swimming pools.

Patient and Family Education

Teach ways to prevent drowning episodes, such as empty buckets, fencing and controlled access around swimming pools, and close supervision of children in and near the water, including the bathtub.

Encourage parents with private pools to get CPR training and to keep a phone at poolside.

Educate adolescents about the dangers of mixing alcohol and swimming.

Traumatic Brain Injury

Traumatic brain injury (TBI) is an injury to the brain caused by blunt force or penetration that causes a change in LOC and/or an anatomic abnormality of the brain. Secondary effects of trauma may include diffuse cerebral edema, malignant brain edema, and increased ICP. TBI leads to nearly a third of all injury-related deaths (Adekoya, Thurman, White, et al., 2002).

TBI is the most common injury in childhood, often caused by falls in young children. Highest risk for TBI occurs in children younger than age 5 years or during adolescence. A permanent disability may result from a moderate or severe injury such as epilepsy, cognitive impairment, learning problems, and behavioral or emotional problems.

Primary injury (initial cellular damage) occurs at the time of the insult (direct impact to the head or inertial forces). Scalp injuries, skull fractures, contusions, and hematomas of brain tissue may occur at the time of impact. The inertial forces tear nerves, fibers, and blood vessels.

Secondary injury results from the biochemical and cellular response to the initial insult. Hypoxia, hypotension, edema, change in the blood–brain barrier, or hemorrhage result and cause increased arterial pressure and ICP.

Clinical Manifestations
Mild Brain Injury
No loss or very brief loss of consciousness

Low-grade headache that will not go away

Slowness in thinking, acting, speaking, reading

Amnesia or memory problems

Loss of balance, unsteady walking

Difficulty paying attention or concentrating, change in performance at school; lack of motivation or interest in favorite toys

Feeling tired all the time, change in sleeping pattern

Change in eating patterns

Increased sensitivity to lights, sounds, distractions; easily irritated

Moderate Brain Injury

Decreased responsiveness; Glasgow Coma Scale score of 9–12

Post-traumatic amnesia for 1–24 hours

Loss of consciousness for 5–10 minutes

Severe Brain Injury

Glasgow Coma Scale score of 8 or less

Post-traumatic amnesia for more than 24 hours

Coma

Increased ICP

Other Potential Clinical Manifestations

Post-traumatic seizures.

Retinal hemorrhages in many children with inflicted TBI.

Cushing's triad is characterized by hypertension, increased systolic pressure with wide pulse pressure, bradycardia, and irregular respirations.

Reflexes may be hyporesponsive, hyperresponsive, or areflexic. Child may assume a decorticate, decerebrate, or flaccid posture.

Diagnostic Testing

Glasgow Coma Scale to monitor changes in responsiveness.

Cranial nerve assessment.

Complete blood cell count, blood chemistry, toxicology screening, and urinalysis.

Radiologic testing includes skull and cervical spine radiographs, CT, MRI, and positron emission tomography scanning.

ICP monitoring.

Clinical Therapy

Emergency care—ensure that the airway is clear and stable, intubating if necessary. Administer oxygen and assist ventilation to prevent hypoxemia and hypercarbia.

Maintain CPP to ensure brain has adequate oxygen and nutrients and to promote removal of accumulated neurotoxins. Treat shock aggressively with IV fluid, and inotropic medications if needed to maintain the blood pressure. Restrict fluids only after the child is hemodynamically stable.

Depressed, compound, and basilar fractures: irrigation, surgical débridement, and elevation of bone; tetanus prophylaxis; and antibiotics.

Surgical débridement of any penetrating injury tracts, evacuation of hematomas, and removal of accessible bone or bullet particles.

Manage increased ICP. Brain swelling leads to worsening cerebral ischemia and more swelling. Hypoxia and hypercapnia can cause vasodilation and increased ICP. If unrelieved, brain shifting begins in the cranium as a precursor of herniation.

- Mechanical ventilation with 100% oxygen at the child's normal respiratory rate is used in the first 24 hours after injury to maintain oxygenation levels.
- Medications to decrease the ICP and promote comfort. See Meds 24–3.
- Invasive procedures such as bur holes, a ventriculostomy catheter, or decompressive craniectomy may be used.
- Head of the bed elevated up to 30 degrees, head maintained at midline to promote venous drainage. Avoid hip flexion.
- Environment kept as quiet as possible. Body temperature kept within normal limits.

Provide total parenteral nutrition or enteral nutrition within 72 hours.

Meds 24–3 Medications Used for Increased Intracranial Pressure (ICP)

Medication	Action
Analgesics and sedatives	Neuromuscular blockade causes muscular paralysis that helps with ventilatory control, prevents increases in arterial blood pressure, and minimizes anxiety and pain.
Mannitol	Osmotic agent that reduces blood viscosity and lowers ICP as fluid is moved out of brain tissue into the circulation. Cerebral blood volume is maintained as less viscous blood reduces resistance to blood flow.
Furosemide	A diuretic that works to reduce cerebrospinal fluid production and reduces sodium transport to the brain. It also causes a reduction in total body fluids.
Hypertonic saline (3%) infusion	Osmotic agent that moves fluid out of the brain tissue into the circulation to lower ICP.
Barbiturates (pentobarbital)	In high doses, barbiturate coma is induced to lower the resting cerebral metabolic rate for oxygen. Used when other therapies have not been successful.
Anticonvulsants	Used to treat status epilepticus or prevent breakthrough seizures that can cause spikes in ICP.

Prevent complications from immobilization, disuse, and neurologic dysfunction.

Rehabilitation care.

Nursing Management
Assessment
Assess the child's ability to maintain an open airway, regulate breathing, and circulation.

Assess the neurologic status frequently with the pediatric Glasgow Coma Scale (see Table 24–2), pupil size and reactivity, and cranial nerves. Note decerebrate or decorticate posturing.

Carefully inspect any area of the skull with swelling or a hematoma for a possible fracture.

Monitor vital signs closely, watching for changes indicating increased hypoxia, ICP, or Cushing's triad.

Observe for physiologic and behavioral signs of pain.

Assess the family's coping with the child's life-threatening injury and their support systems.

Implementation
Minimize increases in ICP by maintaining oxygenation and ventilation, keeping the airway clear, suctioning the airway only when excessive secretions are present, and providing careful thermoregulation.

Administer IV fluids at the rate that maintains hydration and blood pressure. Monitor the effects of medications on hydration status.

Stabilize and protect the intraventricular catheter or bolt from becoming displaced.

Position the child with head at midline supine on a flat surface or side-lying with neck and head straight to prevent compression of the neck blood vessels. Turn child by logrolling. Head of bed may be elevated only when CPP is maintained.

Minimize unpleasant stimuli and pain from procedures and increased ICP.

Promote nutrition to promote wound healing.

Provide oral care and good skin care. Pad and cushion bony prominences and change the child's position frequently.

Protect the eyes from corneal irritation with ophthalmic ointment and patching.

Prevent constipation with stool softeners and suppositories as needed.

Perform passive range of motion exercises to prevent contractures. Coordinate initiation of physical, occupational, and speech therapy. Use splints to position extremities in functional positions. Encourage parents to learn techniques.

Provide stimulation based on the child's age and ability using toys, books, music, or games. Encourage parents to bring in the child's favorite music.

When the child may die or have a new disability, provide emotional support to parents in collaboration with social services, mental health providers, or clergy members.

Rehabilitation

Mild Brain Injury

Prepare parents for altered behavior during 6 weeks of brain healing. Behaviors may include tiring easily, memory loss or forgetfulness, easy distractibility, difficulty concentrating and following directions, irritability or short temper, and needing help starting and finishing tasks. An educational assessment should be initiated if recovery takes longer than 6 weeks.

Moderate and Severe Brain Injury

Children often have behavior problems that include inattention, increased or decreased activity, impulsivity, irritability, lowered frustration tolerance, emotional lability, apathy, aggression, and social withdrawal (Michaud, Semes-Concepcion, Duhaime, et al., 2002). Children may also have long-term problems with attention, problem solving, and speed of information processing that compromise their school performance. Encourage neuropsychological testing to identify the subtle learning disabilities and appropriate educational accommodations.

Severe Brain Injury

Coordinate rehabilitation services to help the child regain self-care skills and improve functioning. Determine what adaptations and assistive technology are needed to care for the child at home. Refer families to home health services to help care for the child and to develop case management skills.

25. ALTERATIONS IN MENTAL HEALTH AND COGNITION

DEVELOPMENTAL AND BEHAVIORAL DISORDERS

Pervasive Developmental Disorders—Autism

Description/Etiology

Pervasive developmental disorders (PDDs) begin in early childhood and are characterized by impaired social interactions and communication, with restricted interests, activities, and behaviors (Baird, Charman, Cox, et al., 2001); they are also called "autistic spectrum disorders."

There are five types of PDDs: autistic disorder, Asperger's syndrome, Rett disorder, child disintegrative disorder, and PDD not otherwise specified.

The etiology of autistic spectrum disorders is unclear, but several theories have been proposed; genetic transmission, immune responses, and neuroanatomy are being investigated as causes (Williams, Dalrymple, & Neal, 2000).

Neurotransmitters such as dopamine, serotonin, and opioids are abnormal in some children and a focus of present research (Cade & Tidwell, 2001).

Congenital rubella syndrome, fragile X syndrome, phenylketonuria, Down syndrome, and tuberous sclerosis are all associated with a higher than normal incidence (American Academy of Pediatrics, 2001; Hudson & Dixon, 2003).

Clinical Manifestations

The essential features typically become apparent by the time a child is 3 years of age and involve impairment in social reciprocity, communication, and behavior (Towbin, Mauk, & Batshaw, 2002).

The child may be unable to converse normally, fail to initiate conversations, and have impaired observations of nonverbal behavior.

Stereotypy or rigid, obsessive, repetitive behavior may occur.

Responses to sensory stimuli are frequently abnormal and include an extreme aversion to touch, loud noises, and bright lights.

Emotional lability is common.

Communication difficulties or delays in speech and language are common and are often the first symptoms that lead to diagnosis.

Absence of babbling and other communication by 1 year, absence of two-word phrases by 2 years, and deterioration of previous language skills are characteristic; abnormal communication patterns include both verbal and nonverbal communication.

They often have rituals and become upset if normal routines are disrupted.

Autistic children may manifest disturbances in the rate or sequence of development; they are frequently cognitively impaired but can demonstrate a wide range of intellectual ability and functioning.

See further clinical manifestations of particular types in Table 25–1.

Diagnostic Tests

Diagnosis is based on the presence of specific criteria, as described in the American Psychiatric Association's *Diagnostic and Statistical Manual of Mental Disorders*, 4th edition (DSM-IV-TR).

Diagnosis includes developmental testing, neuroimaging (computed tomography scan or magnetic resonance imaging), lead screening, metabolic studies, DNA analysis, and electroencephalogram.

Clinical Therapy

Early intervention assists in maximizing the child's potential and establishing helpful support for parents.

Treatment focuses on behavior management to reward appropriate behaviors, foster positive or adaptive coping skills, and facilitate effective communication.

Some goals of treatment are to reduce rigidity or stereotypy (repetitive, obsessive, machinelike movements) and other maladaptive behaviors.

Some parents choose to use complementary therapies such as vitamin supplements and dimethylglycine.

Medications are used with some children to treat associated disorders but are not effective in treatment of these disorders; they may include stimulants, selective serotonin reuptake inhibitors (SSRIs), and mood stabilizers.

Further therapy is listed in Table 25–1.

Table 25–1   Clinical Manifestations of Autistic Spectrum Disorders (Pervasive Developmental Disorders)

Disorder	Clinical Manifestations	Clinical Therapy
Autistic disorder	Impaired social, communicative, and behavioral development, usually noted in first year of life.	Early intervention is key to maximal performance. Interventions focus on improving behaviors and communication skills, providing physical and occupational therapy, structuring play interactions with other children, and educating parents about the child's needs.
Asperger's syndrome	Impaired social interactions with normal language development for age; pitch, tone and other speech characteristics may be abnormal. Verbal skills involving spelling and vocabulary are high, with concept formation, language flexibility, and comprehension low.	Social interactions are focus of therapy.
Rett disorder	Early development appears normal and symptoms emerge at 6–18 mo. Ataxia, hand-wringing, intermittent hyperventilation, dementia, and growth retardation show progressive increase. Appears only in females as an X-linked dominant disorder; mutations occur in the gene MeCP2, affecting methyl-CpG-binding protein 2, which is important in brain development.	Early intervention in areas of abnormal behaviors.
Childhood disintegrative disorder	First 2–5 years of development appear normal followed by deterioration in many areas of functioning. Behaviors finally stabilize at some point without further deterioration.	Focus on areas of developmental function that show abnormality. Individualized education plans are needed in school to deal with communication, play, physical therapy, and teaching management skills to parents. Regression in toileting and other skills may occur.
Pervasive developmental disorder not otherwise specified	Severe social impairment without meeting DSM criteria for other types of autistic spectrum disorder.	Behavioral therapy focuses on building social skills.

Nursing Management

Carefully evaluate the child for history of developmental milestones; perform developmental screening that considers several areas of development, including motor activity, social skills, and language.

Perform hearing and vision screening if possible to rule out sensory problems.

The child needs to be oriented to new settings such as a classroom or the hospital room; ask parents about the child's usual routines and maintain these routines as much as possible.

Adjust communication techniques and teaching to the child's developmental level.

Schedule daily care and routine procedures at consistent times to maintain predictability.

Evaluate methods of communication and adapt to the child's needs.

Maintain a safe environment.

Partner with parents to promote the child's development through behavior modification and specialized educational programs.

Families of autistic children need a great deal of support to cope with the challenges of caring for the autistic child; help them to identify resources for childcare, such as special toddler programs and preschools; assist them to work with schools to establish an individualized education plan.

The parent or primary caretaker often has difficulty obtaining respite care and may need assistance to find suitable resources.

Siblings of the autistic child may need help to explain the disorder to their friends or teachers.

Attention Deficit Disorder and Attention Deficit Hyperactivity Disorder
Description and Etiology

Attention deficit disorder is a variation in central nervous system (CNS) processing characterized by developmentally inappropriate behaviors involving inattention; when hyperactivity and impulsivity accompany inattention, the disorder is called *attention deficit hyperactivity disorder.*

Attention deficit hyperactivity disorder is most commonly manifested and affects from 4% to 12% of all school-age children, boys almost four times more commonly than girls (National Initiative for Children's Healthcare Quality, 2003).

Some prenatal and environmental exposures are associated with higher incidence of the disorder; examples of known associations include exposure to high levels of lead or mercury in childhood, prenatal exposure to alcohol or tobacco smoke, preterm labor, impaired placenta functioning, and impaired oxygenation in the perinatal period; seizures and serious head injury are other potential associations.

Genetic factors may be important, as well as family dynamics and environmental characteristics.

The pathophysiology of attention deficit disorder/attention deficit hyperactivity disorder is unclear, but there may be a deficit in the catecholamines dopamine and norepinephrine in some children, lowering the threshold for stimuli input.

Clinical Manifestations

Children with attention deficit disorder and attention deficit hyperactivity disorder have problems related to decreased attention span, impulsiveness, and/or increased motor activity.

Diagnostic Tests

Obtaining an accurate diagnosis by a pediatric mental health specialist is vital; specific diagnostic criteria must be applied to all children with the potential diagnosis (see DSM criteria in American Psychiatric Association, 2000).

Behaviors both at home and school or childcare must be evaluated because abnormal patterns in two settings are needed for diagnosis.

A variety of tests are available for use by the trained professional in establishing the diagnosis.

Diagnosis begins with a careful history of the child, including family history, birth history, growth and developmental milestones, behaviors such as sleep and eating patterns, progression and patterns in school, social and environmental conditions, and reports from parents and teachers.

A physical examination should be performed to rule out neurologic diseases and other health problems.

A mental health specialist performs testing of the child and administers questionnaires to the parent and teacher to identify the disorder and to rule out other conditions that may mimic or occur concurrently, such as depression, anxiety, learning disorder, conduct disorder, or oppositional defiant disorder (Adesman, 2003).

Clinical Therapy

Treatment is established to meet the desired behavioral outcomes and includes a combination of approaches, such as environmental changes, behavior therapy, and pharmacotherapy (American Academy of Pediatrics Committee on Quality Improvement, 2001).

See Table 25–2 for a listing of common pharmacologic treatments.

Table 25–2 Medications Used to Treat Attention Deficit Hyperactivity Disorder

Medication	Action and Indication	Nursing Implications
Methylphenidate	A derivative of piperidine that acts like an amphetamine. May work in attention deficit hyperactivity disorder treatment by enhancing catecholamine effects in the nervous system, improving attention span and task performance. Schedule II drug in Schedule of Controlled Substances.	Available in short-acting forms of 5-, 10-, and 20-mg as Ritalin and Methylin and in 2.5-, 5-, and 10-mg forms as Focalin. Also in intermediate-acting forms of 20 mg (Ritalin SR), 10 and 20 mg (Metadate ER and Methylin ER). Available in long-acting forms of 18, 27, 36, and 54 mg (Concerta); 20 mg (Metadate CD); and 20, 30, and 40 mg (Ritalin LA). The variety of available forms makes it important to read labels carefully and inform families about proper administration of the child's specific type of drug. Periodic growth measurements are needed. Behavior and school performance are monitored.
Amphetamine preparations	Synthetic sympathomimetic amine with stimulant effect on central nervous system. Increases release of norepinephrine and dopamine by blocking their reuptake. Schedule II drug in Schedule of Controlled Substances.	Available in short-acting forms of 5 mg (Dexedrine), 5 and 10 mg (DextroStat), and 5 and 7.5 mg (Adderall). Intermediate-acting forms include 10-, 12.5-, 15-, 20-, and 30-mg Adderall and 5-, 10-, and 15-mg Dexedrine Spansules. A long-acting form is 5-, 10-, 15-, 20-, 25-, or 30-mg Adderall-XR. Read labels and instruct in proper administration. Monitor vital signs and growth measurements periodically.

(continued)

Alterations in Mental Health and Cognition **541**

Medication	Action and Indication	Nursing Implications
Atomoxetine	This is the first nonstimulant drug for treatment of attention deficit hyperactivity disorder. It inhibits norepinephrine reuptake. Decreases hyperactivity and impulsivity of attention deficit hyperactivity disorder and may assist with improving mood and decreasing anxiety.	Available in 10-, 18-, 25-, 40-, and 60-mg capsules. Recommended starting dose for children is 0.5 mg/kg/day. Has been shown to have long-lasting effect of 1 day or longer. Side effects are uncommon and transient, with dyspepsia or vomiting, fatigue, decreased appetite, and dizziness most common. Have the child change position slowly if dizziness occurs; caution teen not to drive until effects of drug are clear. Perform periodic growth measurements.

Note: Data adapted from Buck, M. L. (2003). Atomoxetine: A new alternative for the treatment of attention-deficit/hyperactivity disorder. Pediatric Pharmacotherapy, 9(2). http://www.medscape.com/viewarticle/452714. Accessed September 24, 2005; and Stein, J. A., & Baren, M. (2003). Welcome progress in the diagnosis and treatment of ADHD in adolescence. Contemporary Pediatrics, 20(8), 83–107.

Nursing Management

Assess the child's development, and observe interactions and activity level.

Refer to mental health specialist for diagnosis.

When medications are used for treatment, be alert for side effects; careful periodic monitoring of weight, height, and blood pressure is necessary.

Promote the child's self-esteem by emphasizing the positive aspects of behavior and treating instances of negative behavior as learning opportunities; help the child to develop ego strengths.

Behavior modification programs can help to reduce specific impulsive behaviors.

Parents must cope simultaneously with managing the difficult needs and demands of a hard-to-handle child, obtaining appropriate evaluation and treatment, and understanding and accepting the diagnosis, even when the child exhibits different behaviors with different people; family support is essential.

Provide information on behavioral techniques, including need for daily exercise and quiet places for homework; work closely with the school and healthcare provider; and provide information about medication effects, safe storage, and administration.

MOOD DISORDERS
Depression
Description and Etiology
Depression is psychological distress that can range from mild to severe.

The incidence of major depression is estimated to be approximately 2% in prepubertal children and approximately 4% to 8% in adolescents; males and females are equally affected until adolescence, when the incidence in girls rapidly increases until they are twice as commonly afflicted (Castiglia, 2000a; Castiglia, 2000b; Shugart & Lopez, 2002).

Many theories have been proposed to explain the cause of depression in children and adolescents; depression may be biologic in origin (decrease in monoamines needed for neurotransmission) or a result of learned helplessness, cognitive distortion, social skills deficit, or family dysfunction; other mental health disorders commonly accompany depression.

Clinical Manifestations
Characteristic findings of major depression in children and adolescents include declining school performance, withdrawal from social activities, sleep disturbance (either too much or too little), appetite disturbance (too much or too little), multiple somatic complaints, especially headaches and stomachaches, decreased energy, difficulty concentrating and making decisions, low self-esteem, and feelings of hopelessness.

Symptoms of depression in children vary according to their developmental levels.

- Infants may fail to eat and grow.
- Toddlers can show regressive behaviors in toileting and other activities.
- School children may show a decrease in academic performance, increased or decreased activity, somatic complaints, and loss of friends; they may be irritable and manifest frequent death themes in their play.
- Adolescents can have a wide array of symptoms such as anxiety, decreased social contact, poor school performance, lack of prior involvement in activities, poor self-care, difficulty with parents and teachers, and focus on violence.

Diagnostic Tests

Initial assessment is performed by a child psychologist or child psychiatrist; a variety of scales and techniques are used, such as the following:

- Children's Depression Inventory
- Revised Children's Manifest Anxiety Scale
- Beck Depression Inventory
- Reynolds Child Depression Scale
- Reynolds Adolescent Depression Scale
- Center for Epidemiologic Studies Depression Scale of Children

Clinical Therapy

Treatment may include psychotherapy in combination with psychotropic medication.

Often a combination of individual, family, and group therapy provides the greatest benefits for young children and adolescents.

Involving parents and other family members in the treatment plan is essential.

Group therapy is an effective treatment measure for adolescents because of the importance of peer group relationships during the teenage years.

Cognitive therapy may be used with adolescents, and play therapy with younger children.

Antidepressant medications, most commonly the SSRIs, tricyclic antidepressants such as imipramine (Tofranil) and desipramine (Norpramin), and amitriptyline (Elavil), may be prescribed (see Table 25–3 for medications commonly used in treatment of depression).

Nursing Management

Nursing assessment includes a thorough history, physical examination, and screening for risk factors of depression (Table 25–4).

Monitor vital signs of youth receiving antidepressant medications.

Watch for common side effects of the agent(s) used, and carefully monitor for serious side effects of tricyclic antidepressants or SSRIs.

Monitor cardiovascular status, including hypertension and tachycardia; observe motor movement; and record dietary intake.

Help parents to evaluate inpatient settings if the child needs hospitalization to be certain the care provided best meets the needs of the child or adolescent.

Table 25–3 Selective Serotonin Reuptake Inhibitor Drugs Used to Treat Depression and Anxiety Disorders

Medication	Pediatric Dose	Adolescent Dose	Selected Side Effects
Fluoxetine (Prozac)	2.5–40 mg qd or 0.5–1 mg/kg/day	10–60 mg qd	Restlessness, headaches, akathisia
Sertraline (Zoloft)	25–125 mg qd or 1.5–3 mg/kg/day	50–200 mg qd	Dry mouth, gastric upset
Paroxetine (Paxil)	5–40 mg qd or 0.25–0.7 mg/kg/day	20–40 mg qd	Dry mouth, weight gain
Fluvoxamine (Luvox)	50–100 mg bid or 1.5–4.5 mg/kg/day	50–300 mg qd	Dry mouth, gastric upset
Citalopram (Celexa)	Little data available	10–40 mg qd	Dry mouth, nausea, sleep disturbance

Although a variety of selective serotonin reuptake inhibitors are used in treatment of children and adolescents, the only approved U.S. Food and Drug Administration medication for major depressive disorder in this age group is Prozac, and the only approved Food and Drug Administration medications for obsessive-compulsive disorder in the pediatric age group are Prozac, Zoloft, Luvox, and clomipramine (Anafranil).
Note: Data from Shugart, M. A., & Lopez, E. M. (2002). Depression in children and adults. Postgraduate Medicine, 112,53–61; Walsh, K. H. (2002). Welcome advances in treating youth anxiety disorders. Contemporary Pediatrics, 19(9),66–82.

Teach parents and school personnel to recognize signs and symptoms of worsening depression and to report these symptoms promptly.

Parents should be taught dosages and side effects of any prescribed medications.

Table 25–4 Risk Factors for Child and Adolescent Depression

Child	Family	School and Social Situations
Frequent feelings of sadness, sleep problems, loss of interest in activities	Parental neglect, abuse, or loss	Academic pressures and underachievement
Increase in risk taking and impulsivity	Dysfunctional family relationships	Stressful social relationships
Previous suicide attempt	Family history of depression, suicide, substance abuse, alcoholism, other psychopathology	Declining participation in social events
Alcohol or substance abuse		
Diagnosed psychotic disorder		
Chronic illness and frequent hospitalization		

Refer the family to appropriate healthcare professionals and to support groups for family members dealing with depression.

Bipolar Disorder (Manic Depression)

Bipolar disorder is a mental illness in which extreme changes in affect and energy are manifested. Moods most often alter between mania and depression. Children often present with irritability or hyperactivity.

The average age for children to demonstrate bipolar disorder is 11 years, but a first manic episode at 5 years is not uncommon; children may show mainly depressive symptoms and then develop mania in adolescence or may have episodes of both mania and depression in the same day.

The manic phase of bipolar illness is characterized by hyperactivity and high energy, irritability, aggression, and sometimes hallucinations.

In the depressive phase, the child is sad, has alterations in sleep and eating patterns, and is socially withdrawn, similar to any depressive illness.

Diagnosis and treatment of bipolar disorder should be performed by mental health specialists; there are not specific criteria for diagnosis of bipolar disease in children.

The treatment of bipolar disease involves a variety of drugs used to stabilize mood. Lithium, valproate (Depakote), and carbamazepine (Tegretol) are most frequently used (Weller, Calvert, & Weller, 2003).

Individual and family education and therapy can be helpful.

The child with bipolar disorder needs ongoing care to ensure implementation of therapy and return to function.

The nurse administers medications in some settings and instructs parents, the child, and other family members in other settings; observe for side effects to the specific drug regimen used.

Assist parents to find resources for healthcare because medications and other treatments may be costly; parents and children need information about the disorder because it may recur several times during life; assist the child to find social events and groups that build a sense of self-esteem.

ANXIETY AND RELATED DISORDERS

Anxiety is a subjective feeling of uncertainty, worry, and helplessness, usually accompanied by CNS signs, including restlessness, trembling, perspiration, and rapid pulse.

Generalized anxiety disorder is often manifested in children by restlessness, excessive fatigue, poor concentration, irritability, muscle tension, and sleep disturbance (American Psychiatric Association, 2000).

Separation anxiety disorder is a particular type of anxiety character-ized by an extreme state of uneasiness when in unfamiliar surroundings and often by refusal to visit friends' homes or attend school for at least 2 weeks; children with separation anxiety disorder tend to be perfectionis-tic, overly compliant, and eager to please; they often cling to the parent or caretaker; they may use physical complaints such as headaches, ab-dominal pain, nausea, and vomiting in an attempt to avoid being away from the parent, and depression frequently accompanies separation anx-iety disorder.

Another type of anxiety disorder is *panic disorder*, the presence of recurrent, unexpected panic attacks; these attacks are periods of in-tense fear and discomfort in the absence of real danger; physical symptoms experienced are palpitations, sweating, chills, hot flashes, shaking, shortness of breath, choking, chest pain, nausea, and dizzi-ness; the person describes feelings of danger or doom.

Another disorder is *obsessive-compulsive disorder*, in which children have recurrent ritualistic thoughts or actions that interfere with daily life; examples of behaviors and concerns are obsessions about dirt or germs, worries about harm, and sexual thoughts; common behaviors are exces-sive handwashing, counting objects, and hoarding substances.

School phobia (also called "school avoidance" or "school refusal") is another anxiety disorder described as persistent, irrational, or exces-sive fear of attending school.

Posttraumatic stress disorder victims have experienced or witnessed a life-threatening event with death or severe injury (Meltzer-Brody, Hidalgo, Connor, et al., 2000); the event is persistently reexperienced through thoughts, dreams, or memories, leading to feelings of fear, terror, and helplessness; the child with posttraumatic stress disorder is often irritable and has sleep problems and inattentiveness; there is a state of hypervigilance and exaggerated startle response, such as to touch or loud noises; the child feels detached from others and alone.

The diagnosis for anxiety and related disorders is made by a mental health specialist.

Counseling by a mental health specialist is the main therapy for anx-iety disorders; techniques such as play therapy and group techniques are frequently used with children.

A variety of antidepressants and SSRIs can be used for pharmaco-logic treatment (see Table 25–3).

The nurse gathers information about family history, the events that have occurred in the child's life, behavioral descriptions and recent changes, developmental progression, and social interactions.

Nursing care for anxiety disorders focuses on behavioral and cognitive therapies to enhance coping skills—for example, mental health nurses may conduct group therapy sessions both in inpatient and community settings.

Children can learn relaxation techniques, and nurses may teach such techniques or recommend that the child consider participation in yoga or guided-imagery classes.

Parents or other significant people should be included in the treatment program; nurses often teach them basic information about the child's diagnosis and therapy, provide resources that they need to get relief from worry about the child, and help them identify financial resources to cover cost of treatment.

Nurses often administer medications to children being treated for anxiety; be alert for and promptly report side effects; ensure that the family knows how to safely administer the drugs; drugs should be kept locked securely; the child should wear a medical alert tag with the medications noted.

Have the child return for follow up as needed because some medications may take several weeks to achieve effects, and close monitoring is essential.

School personnel may need to know about the child's treatment, so partner with the families to provide needed information.

Some schools have counselors who can be instrumental in carrying out treatment plans at school and acting as a resource in that setting; school personnel may be asked to provide feedback about the child's attendance, performance, and social skills as a measure of the success of therapy, and the community or school nurse can relay this information to the mental health therapist.

SUICIDE

Suicide is the third leading cause of death in adolescents between 15 and 19 years of age and has grown in incidence in the last decade (Fish, 2000; National Strategy for Suicide Prevention, 2001).

The most common precursor to adolescent suicide is depression; common signs or symptoms of an underlying depression that could lead to suicide include boredom, restlessness, problems with concentration, irritability, lethargy, intentional misbehavior, preoccupation with one's own body or health, and excessive dependence on or isolation from others (especially adults or caregivers); the depression may be exacerbated by a recent psychosocial stress such as loss or perceived rejection or ridicule.

Many risk factors for suicide exist in children and adolescents, and there are also known protective factors (Table 25–5).

The child or adolescent found to be at high risk for suicide may be admitted to a psychiatric unit for care or cared for in a community mental health facility; it is important to provide crisis intervention at the time of the suicide attempt to minimize the opportunity for repeat attempts and begin a therapeutic treatment plan.

Treatment may include individual, group, or family therapy.

Table 25–5 Risk and Protective Factors for Suicide in Children and Adolescents

Risk Factors	Protective Factors
History of previous attempted suicide	Emotional well-being
	Satisfactory school performance
Suicide or attempt by friend	Participation in sports or other group events
School problems or changes in grades	Weight satisfaction
Pregnancy	Parent/family connectedness
Drug use or abuse	Discuss issues with family frequently
Problems with a romantic relationship	School connectedness
Minority sexual practice	Safe school
Loneliness, withdrawal	Safe neighborhood
Feelings of anxiety	Caring adult presence at school or elsewhere
History of chronic family problems	Availability of school counseling
Chronic illness	School policies against fighting, bullying
Physical, emotional, or sexual abuse	
History of suicide in a family member	
History of depression	
Chronic low self-esteem	
Change in behavior	
Change in weight	
Giving away special possessions	
Access to firearms and ammunition	

Alterations in Mental Health and Cognition 549

Negotiating a no-suicide contract is an important first step in therapy; in the contract, the child agrees not to attempt suicide during a specified time period; the presence of a contract is not a guarantee of child safety, so vigilant monitoring of the youth's condition continues.

Comorbidities such as depression or substance abuse must also be addressed for treatment to be successful.

Nursing Management

The major nursing role is in prevention of suicide; all children and adolescents in health promotion visits and emergency rooms should be evaluated for risk.

During health promotion visits, be alert for children with depression, substance abuse, recent stresses, and changes in behavior.

Gather a family history of mental health disorders, suicide attempts, and stresses.

Ask about how often the youth talks with or has meals and other activities with the family.

Most suicides are committed with firearms present in the home, so ask at each healthcare visit if the family has firearms; encourage families to keep firearms unloaded, with ammunition and firearms locked in separate locations; be sure that children and adolescents do not have access to the keys for the locked firearms.

Nursing care of the child or teen hospitalized after a suicide attempt centers on taking appropriate precautions to ensure the safety of a child or adolescent at risk of suicide.

- The child and the environment of the hospital or other setting are monitored for any object that could be used for self-harm.
- All potentially harmful objects, such as shoestrings, belts, pantyhose, and hair ribbons, are removed.
- All personal care items (including toothbrush and shampoo) are kept locked at the nursing station and monitored constantly when used by the child.
- Children or adolescents who are considered at high risk for suicidal behaviors are attended by a nursing staff member at all times, including while using the bathroom and sleeping.

When the child is receiving care in the community, encourage parents to keep follow-up clinic appointments, to watch for self-destructive behaviors, and to administer any prescribed medications according to the treatment schedule; arrange home visits and other community resources for families.

Education in all school settings is appropriate to assist children in knowing about resources of help when needed and in identifying peers at risk.

- Teach students to report to teachers, nurses, or counselors about friends who have threatened suicide or seem depressed or display behaviors different than usual.
- Nurses often plan with mental health specialists to implement suicide prevention programs in schools and communities.

Provide supportive grief-counseling services to family and friends when suicide occurs.

SUBSTANCE ABUSE
Tobacco Use

Tobacco use is the most preventable cause of adult death in the United States, Canada, and most other developed nations.

Major health problems linked to tobacco use include cardiovascular disease, cancer, chronic lung disease, low birth weight, and other maternal problems; even passive smoking or environmental tobacco smoke is linked to increased heart disease, blood pressure, and respiratory problems (Leone, 2003).

Cigarettes are most common; however, chewing tobacco, snuff, cigars, and bidis may also be used and also pose significant health hazards.

Characteristics that contribute to the likelihood of tobacco use include increasing age, male gender, ethnic group, ease of obtaining tobacco products, and smoking among family members; low socioeconomic group membership, access to tobacco products, low price of products, advertising, and lack of parental involvement in the youths' lives are also associated with tobacco use (U.S. Department of Health and Human Services, 2000).

Cigarette use may be associated with use of alcohol and marijuana, suicidal thoughts, and younger age at first sexual intercourse (Busen, Modeland, & Kouzekanani, 2001).

Educational programs have been developed to encourage youth to avoid tobacco use, and smoking cessation programs are available to assist youth who are already regular smokers to lead to cessation or decrease in tobacco use.

Questions about tobacco use should be inserted by nurses into all well-child visits, beginning at approximately 9–10 years of age; inquire about whether family members (especially parents and siblings) smoke or chew, and ask if some of the child's friends have tried smoking.

Determine the child's knowledge and beliefs about the benefits and risks of tobacco use.

Assess for associated risk behaviors such as alcohol and drug use, sexual behavior, and suicidal thoughts.

The roles of nurses in preventing and intervening in youth smoking are to inform youth, identify smokers, and implement programs.

Offer information on available prevention and cessation programs to youth and families in clinics, outpatient surgery centers, community activities, and hospitals.

Use opportunities such as adolescent pregnancy and presence of illness to reinforce the hazardous effects of tobacco on the individual and on those nearby.

Speak to young athletes about the effects of tobacco on athletic performance.

Show youth the ways in which this product can interfere with their meeting of life goals.

Role-play how to tell other youth no when tobacco is offered.

Establish programs that increase the sense of self-esteem without tobacco use.

Be sure to include parents in the programs so that they see and acknowledge their role in setting an example about tobacco use and in providing guidelines for the child; influence of environmental tobacco (secondhand smoke) should be acknowledged.

Work with the schools and school districts to help establish preventive and cessation programs.

Alcohol and Drug Abuse

Abuse of many substances—particularly marijuana, alcohol, cocaine, crack, and heroin—remains high among youth.

Substance abuse represents a maladaptive coping response to the stressors of childhood and adolescence.

Children in families with a history of substance abuse are at higher risk of abusing drugs and alcohol; other risk factors include rebelliousness, aggressiveness, low self-esteem, dysfunctional parental relationships, lack of adequate support systems, academic underachievement, poor judgment, and poor impulse control.

Substance abuse in children and adolescents is commonly overlooked and underdiagnosed by healthcare providers.

Common physical manifestations include alterations in vital signs, weight loss, chronic fatigue, chronic cough, respiratory congestion, red eyes, and general apathy and malaise; the mental status examination may reveal alterations in level of consciousness, impaired attention and concentration, impaired thought processes, delusions, and hallucinations; low self-esteem, feelings of guilt or worthlessness, and suicidal or homicidal thoughts are also common; poor school performance and changes in mood, sleep habits, appetite, dress, and social relationships are nonspecific characteristics of the substance-abusing child (see Table 25–6 for further information on clinical manifestations).

The primary goal of treatment is to teach the child and other family members to develop and sustain positive coping patterns and to support them during this process.

Table 25–6   Clinical Manifestations of Commonly Abused Drugs

Drug	Potential for Dependence	Clinical Manifestations
Depressants Alcohol, barbiturates (amobarbital, pentobarbital, secobarbital)	Physical and psychological: high; varies somewhat among drugs	Physical: decreased muscle tone and coordination, tremors Psychological: impaired speech, memory, and judgment; confusion; decreased attention span; emotional lability
Stimulants Amphetamines (e.g., Benzedrine), caffeine, cocaine	Physical: low to moderate Psychological: high; withdrawal from amphetamines and cocaine can lead to severe depression	Physical: dilated pupils, increased pulse and blood pressure, flushing, nausea, loss of appetite, tremors Psychological: euphoria; increased alertness, agitation, or irritability; hallucinations; insomnia

(continued)

Table 25–6   Clinical Manifestations of Commonly Abused Drugs (Continued)

Drug	Potential for Dependence	Clinical Manifestations
Opiates		
Codeine, heroin, meperidine (Demerol), methadone, morphine, opium, oxycodone (Percodan, OxyContin)	Physical and psychological: high; varies somewhat among drugs; withdrawal effects are uncomfortable but rarely life-threatening	Physical: analgesia, depressed respirations and muscle tone (may lead to coma or death), nausea, constricted pupils Psychological: changes in mood (usually euphoria), drowsiness, impaired attention or memory, sense of tranquillity
Hallucinogens		
Lysergic acid diethylamide (LSD), mescaline, phencyclidine (PCP)	Physical: none Psychological: unknown	Physical: lack of coordination, dilated pupils, hypertension, elevated temperature; severe PCP intoxication can result in seizures, respiratory depression, coma, and death Psychological: visual illusions and hallucinations, altered perceptions of time and space, emotional lability, psychosis
Volatile inhalants		
Glues, typing correction fluid, acrylic paints, spot removers, lighter fluid, gasoline, butane	Physical and psychological: varies with drug used	Physical: impaired coordination, liver damage (in some cases) Psychological: impaired judgment, delirium
Marijuana	Physical: low Psychological: usually low; occasionally moderate to high	Physical: tachycardia, reddened conjunctiva, dry mouth, increased appetite Psychological: initial anxiety followed by euphoria; giddiness; impaired attention, judgment, and memory

Most treatment programs offer inpatient and outpatient services, as well as aftercare programs; they usually consist of peer support focusing on the development of a lifestyle free of drugs or alcohol, healthy family relationships, and positive coping skills; family involvement is strongly encouraged.

Hospitalization is required if the physical dependence is significant and withdrawal places the child at risk for complications such as seizures, depression, or suicidal behavior.

Nursing management focuses on prevention of substance abuse, early identification of users, and referral to treatment options.

Assessment tools provide useful information for the healthcare provider; an example is the PACES tool:

- P = parents, peers
- A = accidents, alcohol/drug use
- C = cigarettes
- E = emotional problems
- S = school, sexuality
  (Knight, 1997)

CHILD ABUSE

Child abuse includes physical abuse, physical neglect, emotional abuse and neglect, verbal abuse, and sexual abuse.

Abuse generally involves an act of commission—that is, actively doing something to a child physically, emotionally, or sexually, such as hitting, belittling, or molesting; neglect more often involves an act of omission, such as not providing adequate nutrition, emotional contact, or necessary physical care.

Physical abuse is the deliberate maltreatment of another individual that inflicts pain or injury and may result in permanent or temporary disfigurement or even death.

Physical neglect is the deliberate withholding of or failure to provide the necessary and available resources to the child.

Emotional abuse involves shaming, ridiculing, embarrassing, or insulting the child or the destruction of a child's personal property.

Emotional neglect is characterized by the caretaker's emotional unavailability to the child.

Child sexual abuse is the exploitation of a child for the sexual gratification of an adult.

The most common abuser is the child's parent or guardian or the male friend of the child's mother.

Risk factors associated with abusive behavior in adults include the following:

- Psychopathology, such as drug addiction or alcoholism, low self-esteem, poor impulse control, and other personality disorders
- Poor parenting experiences, such as abuse in the abuser's own childhood, rejection by the abuser's own parent(s), lack of knowledge of alternative methods of discipline, strong belief in or family tradition of harsh discipline, and lack of parental affection
- Marital stressors and problems with partners, such as hostile-dependent, abusive, or nonsupportive relationships and one-sided decision making
- Environmental stressors, such as legal, financial, medical, or housing problems
- Social isolation, such as few friends and limited use of sitters, family, or other resources
- Inappropriate expectations for the developmental level of the child

See Tables 25–7 and 25–8 for some common clinical manifestations of abuse.

Diagnosis of abuse is made on the basis of a careful history and thorough physical examination; radiologic, computed tomography, and magnetic resonance imaging studies may be ordered to identify signs of recurrent abuse such as healed fractures and other damaged tissues; laboratory studies may involve urine culture for signs of infection or screening for sexually transmitted diseases; genitourinary examination may be performed if sexual abuse is suspected.

Neglect, which is more difficult to define and identify, frequently requires hospitalization with a comprehensive medical, social, and psychiatric evaluation.

Table 25–7   Clinical Manifestations of Child Abuse

Multiple bruises in various stages of healing

Scald burns with clear lines of demarcation and in a glove or stocking distribution

Rope, belt, or cord marks, usually seen on the mouth, buttocks, back, legs, and arms

Burn scars in various stages of healing

Multiple fractures in various stages of healing

Shortness of breath and distress on being moved, indicating chest contusions and possible rib fractures

Sedation from overmedication

Exacerbation of chronic illness (such as diabetes or asthma) because of withholding of medication

Table 25–8 Clinical Manifestations of Sexual Abuse in Children and Adolescents

Vaginal discharge
Blood-stained underpants or diaper
Genital redness, pain, itching, or bruising
Difficulty walking or sitting
Urinary tract infection
Sexually transmitted disease
Somatic complaints, such as headaches or stomachaches
Excessively seductive behavior
Sleeping problems, such as nightmares or night terrors
Bedwetting
Unwillingness to go to babysitter, family member, neighbor, or other person
Fear of strangers
New or excessive sexual curiosity or play
Constant masturbation
Curling into fetal position
Phobias about particular places, people, or things
Abrupt changes in school performance and attendance
Changes in eating habits
Abrupt changes in behavior (especially withdrawal)
Child or adolescent female acts like a wife or mother

Initial therapy focuses on providing safety; physical injuries are treated, and the child is removed from the abusive situation.

Children who have been physically, emotionally, or sexually abused are at risk for major mental health problems, such as depression and posttraumatic stress disorder; they require skilled care by mental health professionals who are specially trained in this area.

Initially, the treatment goals include prevention of self-destructive or other dangerous acts.

Children are encouraged to express their fears and feelings in a safe and supportive environment.

The child is assisted to build coping skills and self-esteem.

The child must be reassured and convinced that he or she is in no way responsible or to blame for what happened.

Nursing assessment in instances of suspected child abuse or neglect requires a comprehensive history and physical examination, with documentation of findings.

Be alert for discrepancies between the history and physical assessment data.

Work with social services and community agencies to assess the child's home environment, individuals living in the home, and the actions surrounding the abuse.

Assist in removing the child from the home to temporary custody of the court or foster care of another relative, if indicated.

Counsel family members about abuse and refer for appropriate therapy.

Protect and treat the child's injuries.

Work within schools to inform all children about where they may turn in abusive situations, and help establish information sessions for teens about date rape and safety precautions.

FEEDING AND EATING DISORDERS
Feeding Disorder of Infancy and Early Childhood (Failure to Thrive)

Feeding disorder of infancy and early childhood, or failure to thrive (FTT), describes a syndrome in which infants or young children fail to eat enough food to be adequately nourished.

The cause of FTT can be organic, as in congenital acquired immunodeficiency syndrome, inborn errors of metabolism, neurologic disease, and esophageal reflux; however, most cases of FTT are nonorganic in origin; FTT resulting from nonorganic causes is called *feeding disorder of infancy or early childhood.*

Infants and children whose parents or caretakers experience depression, substance abuse, mental retardation, or psychosis are at risk for this disorder; parents may be socially and emotionally isolated or may lack knowledge of infant nutritional and nurturing needs.

A reciprocal interaction pattern may exist whereby the parent does not offer enough food or is not responsive to the infant's hunger cues, and the infant is irritable, not soothed, and does not give clear cues about hunger (Corrales & Utter, 1999).

The characteristics of this feeding disorder are persistent failure to eat adequately with no weight gain or with weight loss in a child 6 years of age or younger that is not associated with other medical conditions or mental disorders and is not caused by lack of or unavailability of food (American Psychiatric Association Working Group on Eating Disorders, 2000).

Infants with feeding disorders refuse food, may have erratic sleep patterns, are irritable and difficult to soothe, and are often developmentally delayed.

A thorough history and physical examination are needed to rule out any chronic physical illness; the infant or child may be hospitalized so that healthcare providers can establish a routine for feeding and sleeping.

The goals of treatment are to provide adequate caloric and nutritional intake, promote normal growth and development, and assist parents in developing feeding routines and responding to the infant's cues of physical and psychologic hunger.

Nurses perform accurate measurement of weight and height each time any child is seen for healthcare to provide a record of growth patterns over time.

The child's activity level, developmental milestones, and interaction patterns provide important information.

When feeding the child, the nurse observes how the child indicates hunger or satiety; the ability of the child to be soothed; and general interaction patterns such as eye contact, touch, and cuddliness.

Nursing care centers on performing a thorough history and physical assessment, observing parent–child interactions during feeding times, and providing necessary teaching to enable parents to respond appropriately to their child's needs.

Observations of feeding and continued careful physical assessments are needed; the child's intake is carefully recorded at each meal or feeding.

Parents are taught how to understand and respond to the child's cues of hunger and satiety; they are taught to hold, rock, and touch the infant during feedings and to establish eye contact with infants and children during feeding situations.

Refer the family to an agency that can continue monitoring of the home situation; this provides an opportunity to observe feeding during a home visit and evaluate stresses and behavior patterns among family members.

Frequent growth measurement and development must be ensured so the child is adequately nourished.

Parents may need referral to community resources to help them manage stressful situations in their lives and to enhance their parenting skills.

Finding a nurturing relationship for the parent may provide the support needed to enhance parenting.

Anorexia Nervosa

Anorexia nervosa is a potentially life-threatening eating disorder that occurs primarily in teenage girls and young women.

Anorectic adolescents are characterized by extreme weight loss accompanied by a preoccupation with weight and food, excessive compulsive exercising, peculiar patterns of eating and handling food, and distorted body image.

Cultural overemphasis on thinness may contribute to the overconcern with dieting, body image, and fear of becoming fat that is experienced by many adolescents; chemical changes have been found in the brain and blood of anorectic patients, leading to theories about a biologic cause; often a significant life stress, loss, or change precedes the onset of anorexia. Stress hormones are commonly elevated in anorectics, and immune system function may be disturbed (Brambilla, 2001; White, 2000).

The adolescent may engage in lengthy and vigorous exercise (up to 4 hours daily) to prevent weight gain; laxatives or diuretics may be used to induce weight loss.

Leukopenia, electrolyte imbalance, and hypoglycemia develop as a result of protein–energy malnutrition; once the body mass decreases below a critical level, menstruation ceases.

Accompanying signs and symptoms of depression, crying spells, feelings of isolation and loneliness, and suicidal thoughts and feelings are common; the disorder is often associated with mental illness such as obsessive-compulsive disorder, anxiety disorders, and history of abuse (Herpertz-Dahlmann, Muller, Herpertz, et al., 2001).

Physical findings include cold intolerance, dizziness, constipation, abdominal discomfort, bloating, irregular menses, and malnutrition; hypothalamic suppression can lead to disturbances of gynecologic function, osteoporosis, decreased bone density, and fractures (Seidenfeld & Rickert, 2001); lanugo (fine, downy body hair) may be present.

Fluid and electrolyte imbalances, especially potassium imbalances, are common; extreme weight loss often leads to cardiac arrhythmias (bradycardia).

Diagnosis is based on a comprehensive history, physical examination revealing characteristic clinical manifestations, and the DSM-IV criteria.

Diagnostic tests commonly include hematocrit and hemoglobin, serum electrolytes, and serum vitamins and vitamin precursors.

The goal of treatment is to address the physiologic problems associated with malnutrition, as well as the behavioral and cognitive components of the disorder.

A firm focus is placed on reaching a targeted weight, with a gradual weight gain of 0.1–0.2 kg/day (0.25–0.5 lb/day); enteral feedings or total parenteral nutrition may be necessary to replace lost fluid, protein, and nutrients.

Individual treatment and family therapy are used to address any individual and family patterns that may contribute to the disorder.

Nursing care centers on meeting nutritional and fluid needs, preventing complications, administering medications, and providing referral to appropriate resources.

Monitor nutritional and fluid intake, encourage consumption of food, and observe eating behaviors at mealtime; elimination patterns may be altered as a result of increased intake during hospitalization, so monitor for abdominal distention, constipation, or diarrhea. Daily monitoring of serum electrolytes is necessary during acute hospitalizations with electrolyte imbalance.

If total parenteral nutrition is administered, watch for complications such as circulatory overload, hyperglycemia, or hypoglycemia; use strict aseptic technique when changing tubing or dressings.

Monitor vital signs if the adolescent is receiving antidepressants; watch for signs of hypertension and tachycardia, as well as changes in mood and behavior.

Refer parents and other family members to the American Anorexia and Bulimia Association, National Anorectic Aid Society, and National Association of Anorexia Nervosa and Associated Disorders for further information about the disorder and a list of support groups in their area.

Bulimia Nervosa

Bulimia nervosa is an eating disorder characterized by binge eating (a compulsion to consume large quantities of food in a short period of time); usually the episodes of bingeing are followed by various methods of weight control (purging), such as self-induced vomiting, large doses of laxatives or diuretics, or a combination of methods.

Causes of bulimia nervosa are similar to those of anorexia nervosa: sensitivity to social pressure for thinness, body image difficulties, and long-standing dysfunctional family patterns; depression is commonly associated with the disorder.

Bulimic adolescents, like anorectics, are preoccupied with body shape, size, and weight; they may appear overweight or thin and usually report a wide range of average body weight over the years.

Physical findings depend on the degree of purging, starvation, dehydration, and electrolyte disturbance; erosion of tooth enamel, increased dental caries, and gum recession, which result from vomiting of gastric acids, are common findings; the back of a hand can have calluses from inducing vomiting; abdominal distention is often seen; esophageal tears and esophagitis may also occur.

Treatment includes management of physiologic problems, behavior modification, and psychotherapy.

During hospitalization, the patient should keep a food diary.

Be alert to the adolescent who hides, gives away, or discards food from the tray or who exits to use the bathroom after meals; the adolescent should be monitored for at least 30 minutes after meals by remaining in a central area in the company of the nurse or other responsible individuals.

Withdrawal from laxatives and diuretics is managed with careful observation for alterations in fluid and electrolyte status.

Cardiac monitoring may be necessary if potassium levels are seriously altered.

Esophageal tearing or esophagitis is treated to promote mucosal healing.

Medications such as antidepressants may be administered.

Encourage continuation of group and other therapy sessions.

COGNITIVE DISORDERS
Learning Disabilities

Learning disabilities affect approximately 5% of school children.

The brain is unable to receive or process information in the normal manner.

Common types of learning disorders are listed in Table 25–9.

Table 25–9 Clinical Manifestations of Various Learning Disabilities

Disorder	Clinical Manifestations
Dyslexia	Difficulty with writing, reading, and spelling
Dyscalculia	Mathematics and computation problems
Dysgraphia	Difficulty with writing, spelling, and composition
Dyspraxia	Problems with manual dexterity and coordination

Children may have difficulty in processing visual information, which may be manifested in reading, writing, and mathematics performance; others may have more difficulty with oral information, leading to problems in language development and reading (National Center for Learning Disabilities, 2004).

The causes of learning disorders are complex. Sometimes they are related to low birth weight or problems during the perinatal period; there may be a genetic component because their occurrence is more common when other family members are affected.

Treatments involve learning how to compensate for the difficulties by using capabilities that are intact.

Children with learning disabilities should have individualized education plans established with realistic goals for school performance.

Nurses play a major role in identification of children with learning disabilities; assess the child for the following developmental milestones that can indicate learning disability:
- Lack of ability to phrase sentences together by 2.5 years
- Inability to use speech that is understandable at least 50% of the time by 3 years
- Unable to tie shoes, button, hop, or cut by kindergarten
- Inability to sit for a short story by 3–5 years
  (American Academy of Pediatrics, 2000)

When a child may have a learning disability, refer the family to the school or other testing resource.

Partner with the family to plan for the child's learning needs.

Help the family to work closely with the child, provide a setting at home to maximize potential for learning, and build healthy self-esteem in the child.

Assist the family to work with the school to establish annual goals for the child.

Mental Retardation
Description and Etiology

Mental retardation is defined as significant limitation in intellectual functioning and adaptive behavior. It is manifested in differences in conceptual, social, and practical life skills and begins before the age of 18 years (American Association of Mental Retardation, 2004).

Intellectual functioning is generally characterized by an IQ below 70–75, and there are significant impairments in adaptive functioning (the ability of an individual to meet the standards expected for his or her cultural group); the child with mental retardation has adaptive deficits in at least two areas such as communication, self-care, home living, social/interpersonal skills, use of community resources, self-direction, functional academic skills, work, leisure, health, or safety.

The causes of mental retardation can be grouped into three general categories: prenatal errors in the development of the CNS, prenatal or postnatal changes in the biologic environment of the person, and external forces leading to CNS damage; in each instance, the precipitating factor causes a change in the form, function, and adaptation of the CNS (Table 25–10).

Three common conditions associated with mental retardation from prenatal conditions are Down syndrome, fragile X syndrome, and fetal alcohol syndrome; see Table 25–11 for physical characteristics of children with each of these conditions.

In the United States, approximately 1 in 1,000 infants, or 4,000 infants each year, are born with Down syndrome (Roizen, 2002); the

Table 25–10 Common Conditions Associated with Mental Retardation

Prenatal Conditions	Biologic Environment	External Forces
Down syndrome	Inborn errors of metabolism (e.g., phenylketonuria, hypothyroidism)	Traumatic brain injury (e.g., accident)
Fragile X syndrome		Poison ingestion (acute or chronic)
Fetal alcohol syndrome		Hypoxia/anoxic insult
Maternal infection (e.g., rubella, cytomegalovirus)		Infection (e.g., meningitis)
		Environmental deprivation

Table 25–11 Characteristics of Three Common Conditions Associated with Mental Retardation

Down Syndrome	Fragile X Syndrome	Fetal Alcohol Syndrome
Small head (microcephaly)	Long face	Flat midface
Flattened forehead	Prominent jaw	Low nasal bridge
Wide, short neck	Large ears	Long philtrum with narrow upper lip
Epicanthal eye folds	Frequent otitis media	
White spots on eye iris (Brushfield spots)	Large testicles	Short, upturned nose
	Epicanthal eye folds	Poor coordination
Congenital cataracts	Strabismus	Failure to thrive
Flat nose	High-arched palate	Skeletal and joint abnormalities
Small, low-set ears	Scoliosis	
Protruding tongue	Pliable joints	Hearing loss
Short, broad hands		
Simian line on palm		
Wide space between first and second toes		
Hearing loss		
Increased incidence of diabetes, congenital heart defect, and leukemia		
Hypotonia		

condition is caused by an extra chromosome, so the child has 47 rather than 46 chromosomes.

Fragile X syndrome is caused by a single recessive gene abnormality on the X chromosome.

Fetal alcohol syndrome is caused by the effect of ethyl alcohol on the developing fetus; alcohol ingestion by the pregnant woman can influence development of many body organs and effects can range from mild to severe.

Clinical Manifestations

Children who are mentally retarded manifest delays in all areas of development, including motor movement, language, and adaptive behavior.

Children achieve developmental milestones more slowly than the average child.

Mental retardation is sometimes accompanied by sensory impairment, speech problems, motor and orthopedic disabilities, and seizure disorders.

Diagnostic Tests

Mental retardation is diagnosed and initial treatment is planned in a multistep process and by involving a multidisciplinary team; members of the team are commonly a developmental specialist, physician, geneticist, nurse, teacher, language therapist, occupational therapist, and physical rehabilitation specialist.

A comprehensive history and evaluation of the child's physical characteristics, developmental level, and intellectual and adaptive functioning are carried out.

Laboratory tests such as chromosome analysis, blood enzyme levels, and lead levels and cranial imaging provide valuable information in some circumstances.

Tests of intellectual and adaptive functioning are performed when mental retardation is suspected.

A neurologic examination may indicate asymmetry of movement or strength, irritability or lethargy, or abnormal pitch to an infant's cry.

Because mental retardation may be accompanied by physical abnormalities, it is important to observe the child for facial symmetry, distance between the eyes, level of the ears, hair growth, and palmar creases.

Clinical Therapy

Based on the results of the evaluation, a multidisciplinary team plans the support needed to maximize the child's potential for development.

Management focuses on early intervention to improve the degree of adaptive functioning.

Simultaneous treatment of associated physical, emotional, and behavioral problems is provided.

Depending on the child's condition, special education programs and physical or occupational therapy may be necessary.

Nursing Management

Assessment

Nurses can help to identify children with mental retardation through history taking, observation, and developmental screening during early childhood.

The history should provide information about the mental and adaptive functioning of birth parents and other family members, as mental retardation may cluster in some families and conditions such as fragile X syndrome are genetic in origin.

The pregnancy and birth history can provide important information relating to alcohol and drug use by the mother during pregnancy; be alert for a history of difficult pregnancy and problems.

During home visits, during clinic appointments, in childcare centers, and during hospitalization, be alert for signs of developmental delays, multiple (more than three) physical anomalies associated with a specific condition, or neurologic alterations.

Developmental assessment should be part of each health promotion/health maintenance visit to aid in early identification.

Once the diagnosis of mental retardation has been made, assess the adaptive functioning of the child and family.

A functional assessment of the child should be performed, including toileting, dressing, and feeding skills.

Assess the child's language, sensory, and psychomotor functioning.

Assess the home and community for safety hazards.

Observe how the family is managing with the child.

To determine the impact of the child with mental retardation on the family, ask parents to describe (1) family activities that include the child; (2) strategies that parents and siblings use to deal with community attitudes about the child; and (3) the case of a child with other disabilities, methods of managing the child's care, and planning for future care needs.

Assess the availability of services such as support groups for parents and special education opportunities for children.

Intervention

Family members need empathy and support both at the time of diagnosis and in the ensuing years.

Parents and other family members may be in an acute or chronic state of grief over the loss of the perfect child.

Encourage the family members to verbalize their feelings.

Introduce the parents to parents of other mentally retarded children to provide assistance and support as they learn how to manage the child's needs.

Discuss the availability of respite care to provide parents with a break from caretaking.

Parents need honest information and answers to their questions about the child's condition.

Reinforce information provided by genetic counselors and other healthcare professionals.

Inform parents about community resources designed to assist children with mental retardation, including the Zero to Three Project, special education preschools and schools, county health services, and respite care.

Assist with plans for education and services such as physical or speech therapy; children need an individualized education plan designed to meet their specific learning needs.

Children with mental retardation require close supervision because they may lack an understanding of common hazards; ensure safety in the hospital environment, and assist parents to provide safety at home and school and to teach their child necessary skills such as pedestrian safety; consider both physical and emotional safety because the child with mental retardation may be trusting of others and sometimes is at risk for physical or sexual abuse.

Encourage parents' efforts to maximize the child's areas of strength and identify needs related to adaptive behaviors.

Assist parents as necessary to acquire the skills required to coordinate the child's plan of care.

Continue to evaluate the child's needs regularly, and assist parents with the treatment plan revision as necessary.

26. ALTERATIONS IN MUSCULOSKELETAL FUNCTION

DISORDERS OF FEET AND LEGS
Metatarsus Adductus
Most common congenital foot deformity

Characterized by an inward turning of the forefoot at the tarsometatarsal joints

Caused by both intrauterine positioning and genetic factors

Foot radiographs and physical assessment performed for diagnosis

Clinical Therapy
Simple exercises may correct the problem by approximately 3 months of age.

Serial casting is the treatment of choice for curvature angles of more than 15 degrees, or in cases that do not improve.

Braces and orthopedic shoes may also be used to maintain correction after casting.

Nursing Management
Reassure parents that the child's condition can be corrected.

Teach parents simple stretching exercises that can be performed at each diaper change:
- Hold the infant's foot securely by the heel. Maintain the heel in this position.
- Move the forefoot outward away from the body with the other hand.
- Hold the foot in this position for 5 seconds.
- Repeat five times during each diaper change.

If casting is necessary, provide cast care, and teach parents how to care for the child in a cast at home.

Clubfoot
Clinical Manifestations
Occurs in approximately 1 in 1,000 births, affects boys nearly twice as often as girls, and is bilateral in approximately half of affected infants.

Involves three areas of deformity: The midfoot is directed downward (equinus), the hindfoot turns inward (varus), and the forefoot curls toward the heel (adduction) and turns upward in partial supination.

Muscles, tendons, and bones are all involved in the abnormality, and clubfoot cannot be corrected by exercise.

The foot is small, with a shortened Achilles tendon; muscles in the lower leg are atrophied, but leg lengths are generally normal.

Diagnostic Tests
Visual inspection, examination, and radiographs confirm the diagnosis and extent of involvement.

Clinical Therapy
Serial casting beginning as soon as possible after birth is the first therapy; the foot is manipulated to achieve maximum correction first of the varus deformity and then of the equinus deformity.

A long leg cast is applied to hold the foot in the desired position and is changed every 1–2 weeks; the regimen of manipulation and casting continues for approximately 8–12 weeks until maximum correction is achieved.

If the deformity has been corrected, the child may then wear a splint with a crossbar between shoes (most commonly called a *Denis Browne splint*) or reverse last corrective shoes (shoes with the toes pointing outward rather than inward) to maintain the correction (Gilmore & Thompson, 2003; Morcuende, Dolan, Dietz, et al., 2004).

If the deformity has not been corrected, surgical intervention using posteromedial release is required at approximately 3–12 months of age.

Surgery is followed by casting for 6–12 weeks, followed by a physical rehabilitation program and, commonly, use of a brace and corrective shoes.

Nursing Management
The goals of nursing care for the child with a clubfoot are to provide necessary information to parents and ensure safety and adequate healing during the treatment process.

Assessment
Perform a physical examination, including position and appearance of the foot.

Assess the child's motor development.

Evaluate the family's coping mechanisms and access to transportation to healthcare agency for serial casting visits.

Intervention

Explain the treatment to parents and involve them in the child's care.

Provide cast care to ensure skin and neurovascular integrity (Box 26–1).

Box 26–1 Nursing Care of the Child in a Cast

- A plaster cast takes anywhere from 24 to 48 hours to dry. When handling the cast, be gentle and use the palms of your hands, as fingertips can indent plaster and create pressure areas.
- After the cast is applied, elevate the extremity on a pillow above the level of the heart. Elevation helps to reduce swelling and increases venous return.
- If the cast is applied after surgery, there may be drainage or bleeding through the cast material. Circle the stain, and note the date and time on the cast to provide a means of assessing the amount of fluid lost. Once a cast is dry, a "window," or opening, is sometimes cut so that a wound can be viewed or to allow the stomach to expand more comfortably.
- Assess the distal pulses, and check the fingers and toes for color, warmth, capillary refill, and edema. Assess sensation as well as movement. Any deviation from normal may indicate nerve damage or decreased blood supply.
- During the first 24 hours, the casted extremity should be checked every 15–30 minutes for 2 hours, then every 1–2 hours thereafter. The skin should be warm. It should blanch when slight pressure is applied and then return to its normal color within 3 seconds. For the next 2 days, the casted extremity should be assessed at least every 4 hours.
- Check the edges of the cast for roughness or crumbling. If necessary, pull the inner stockinette over the edge of the cast and tape.
- The rough edges of the cast may also be alleviated by "petaling." This is done by securing adhesive tape to the inside of the cast and pulling it over the edge, covering the jagged or broken pieces of plaster, and securing it to the outer surface of the cast. Moleskin may be used on the cast as well. Petal the opening around a window in the cast if one is present.
- Keep the cast as clean and dry as possible. Cover the cast with a plastic bag or plastic wrap when the child bathes or showers.
- The skin under the cast may itch; however, do not use powders or lotions near the edges or under the cast, as they can cause skin irritation.
- Be sure that children do not put small objects between the casts and their extremities; these actions can cause skin irritation as well as neurovascular compromise.

Routine postoperative care after surgical correction includes neurovascular status checks every 2 hours for the first 24 hours and observing for any swelling around the cast edges, application of ice bags to the foot, and keeping the ankle and foot elevated on a pillow for 24 hours to promote healing and help with venous return.

Keep new casts open to air to facilitate drying; monitor, record, and report drainage or bleeding.

Administer pain medication routinely for 24–48 hours after surgery; popliteal or epidural blocks may be placed during surgery and used in the immediate postsurgical period for pain control; monitor these blocks for effectiveness and any undesired effects.

Patient and Family Education

Parents should be given written instructions for care of the child with a cast.

Skin care:

- Check the skin around the cast edges for irritation, rubbing, or blistering. The skin should be clean and dry.
- Cleanse the skin just under the cast edges and between the toes or fingers with a cotton-tipped applicator and rubbing alcohol. Avoid using lotions, oils, and powders near the cast, as they may cause caking.
- Avoid poking sharp objects down inside the cast, as this may result in sores.

Cast care:

- Keep the cast dry. Protect plaster with a cast shoe, thick sock, or sling.
- Allow a new, wet cast to air dry for 24 hours.
- Begin walking on a leg cast only when the physician gives permission.

Be alert for possible complications:

- Toes or fingers should be pink, not blue or white.
- Skin should be warm and the tips of the toes should blanch when pinched.
- Raise the casted arm or leg above heart level, and rest it on pillows to prevent or reduce any swelling.

Notify the healthcare provider if any of the following occur:

- Unusual odor beneath the cast
- Tingling

- Burning or numbness in the casted arm or leg
- Drainage through the cast
- Swelling or inability to move the fingers or toes
- Slippage of the cast
- Cast cracked, soft, or loose
- Sudden, unexplained fever
- Unusual fussiness or irritability in an infant or child
- Fingers or toes that are blue or white
- Pain that is not relieved by any comfort measures (e.g., repositioning or pain medication)

General care:
- Demonstrate the use of a sponge bath to protect the cast from water breakdown.
- Discuss several options for clothing that accommodate a cast, for example, one-piece snap suits or sweatpants.
- Discuss potential safety hazards that may result from awkward positioning. Be sure the child is properly situated in a car safety seat for the trip home.
- Suggest that parents make an effort to place toys within the child's reach because movements of a child in a cast may be slowed.
- Have parents avoid use of "umbrella" strollers and infant swings because they do not provide adequate support for the casted leg.

Adapted from and courtesy of Shriners Hospital for Children-Spokane (Washington).

Parents should be given written instructions for care of the child with a brace:
- Braces should be as comfortable as possible and the child should have adequate mobility while wearing the brace.
- Begin wearing the brace for periods of 1–2 hours and then progress to 2–4 hours.
- Check the skin at 1- to 2-hour intervals initially, then lengthening to every 4 hours once skin has been clear for several days. If redness is apparent, leave the brace off and allow the skin to clear. If breakdown has occurred, the brace cannot be replaced until healing is complete.
- Always have the child wear a clean white sock, T-shirt, or other thin white liner beneath the brace. Be sure the liner is wrinkle-free under the brace. Avoid using powders or lotions that can

cause skin to break down. Toughen any sensitive areas using alcohol wipes.

- Reapply the brace when the skin returns to its normal color.
- Return to the physician or orthotic specialist if discomfort or red areas persist or if the brace needs adjustment or repair or is outgrown.
- Check the brace daily for rough edges.

Genu Varum and Genu Valgum

Genu varum (bowlegs) is a deformity in which the knees are widely separated while the ankles are close together and the lower legs are turned inward (varus).

In genu valgum (knock-knees), the knees are close together while the ankles are widely spaced so that the lower legs are directed outward (valgus).

At certain stages of a child's development, the appearance of bowlegs or knock-knees is normal. Until 2–3 years, the knees are normally bowed, showing varus alignment, and by 4–5 years, some knock-knee or valgus alignment commonly emerges.

Blount's disease and rickets are two pathologic causes of bowlegs and should be ruled out if the condition is severe or has not improved by 2 years of age.

Excessive or continued knock-knees should also be evaluated by an orthopedist, although unlike genu varum, the condition has no pathologic causes.

Physical measurements, radiographic studies, arthrography (joint radiograph), magnetic resonance imaging (MRI), and computed tomography imaging may be used for accurate diagnosis of varus and valgus conditions.

Treatment may include braces, supplementation with calcium and vitamin D if rickets is a cause, and occasional surgery.

Nursing care centers on instruction on brace wear or dietary supplementation as needed, along with postsurgical care for that intervention.

DISORDERS OF THE HIP
Developmental Dysplasia of the Hip
Clinical Manifestations
Limited abduction of the affected hip.

Asymmetry of the gluteal and thigh fat folds.

Telescoping or pistoning of the thigh.

The older child with untreated developmental dysplasia of the hip walks with a significant limp.

Diagnostic Tests
Physical examination, including Allis' sign (one knee lower than the other when the knees are flexed) and positive Ortolani-Barlow maneuver.

Sonogram may be used until 4 months of age and radiographs after that time.

Clinical Therapy
Pavlik harness, a dynamic splint that allows movement but ensures hip flexion and abduction while not allowing hip extension or adduction.

External or skin traction is sometimes used.

Surgery and application of spica cast may be needed.

Nursing Management
Encourage families to make regular healthcare visits so assessment of hips can occur throughout the infancy period.

Provide care for the child in traction or who has surgery and has spica cast application (see Box 26–1). If permitted by physician's orders, release the child from traction for meals and daily care. The time out of traction should not exceed 1 hour per day. Encourage parents to hold and cuddle the child at this time to promote comfort and bonding.

Special care after surgery for developmental dysplasia of the hip includes the following:
- Use adequate padding and skin wrapping to avoid placing pressure on the popliteal space. Such pressure could lead to nerve damage.
- Change the casted child's position every 2–3 hours while awake to help avoid areas of pressure and promote increased circulation. The child can be placed either prone or supine or positioned on the floor and supported with pillows.
- Help prevent skin irritation and breakdown in the child with a cast. Use moleskin to provide protection from rough edges. Place tape around the perineal opening of the cast to prevent soiling.

- Increase fluids and fiber in the child's diet, as a change in bowel or bladder status is commonly associated with immobility.
- Assess respiratory system carefully, and plan games to encourage deep breathing by the young child.

Patient and Family Education

Instruct families on proper use of the Pavlik harness when it is prescribed:

- Position the chest halter at nipple line and fasten with Velcro.
- Position the legs and feet in the stirrups, being sure the hips are flexed and abducted. Fasten with Velcro.
- Connect the chest halter and leg straps in front.
- Connect the chest halter and leg straps in back.
- All the straps are marked at the first fitting with indelible ink so they can be reattached easily after the harness is rinsed and dried.

Instruct parents on care of the child in a spica cast, including safe transport home in a car (see Box 25–1).

Emphasize importance of neurovascular checks and reporting promptly any signs of circulatory impairment.

Consider safety because the child cannot move away from dangers such as heat and may easily fall from high places.

Instruct about ways to encourage normal growth and development while the child is immobilized in a cast.

Legg-Calvé-Perthes Disease (Perthes' Disease)
Clinical Manifestations

Legg-Calvé-Perthes disease (Perthes' disease) is a self-limiting condition in which there is avascular necrosis of the femoral head.

It usually occurs between the ages of 2 and 12 years, with an average age of 7 years at onset and about 4 times more commonly in males. Child may complain of hip pain and/or manifest a limp

The disease progresses in several stages over a time of approximately 2 years:

Prenecrosis	An insult or coagulation disorder causes loss of blood supply to the femoral head.
I Necrosis	Avascular stage (3–6 months); the child is asymptomatic, bone radiographs are normal, and the head of the femur is structurally intact but avascular.

II Revascularization	Period of 1–4 years characterized by pain and limitation of movement. Bone radiographs show new bone deposition and dead bone resorption. Fracture and deformity of the head of the femur can occur.
III Bone healing	Reossification takes place; pain decreases.
IV Remodeling	The disease process is over, pain is absent, and improvement in joint function occurs.

Diagnosis Tests

Diagnosis is made using standard anteroposterior and frog-leg radiographs.

Bone scans and MRI may show the disease process earlier than radiographs.

Laboratory studies of the blood, such as white blood cell count, help to rule out inflammatory synovitis of the hip.

Clinical Therapy

The femoral head must be contained within the hip socket by abduction until reossification is complete to promote healing and prevent deformity.

At the beginning of treatment, traction can be used to maintain the hips in an abducted and internally rotated position.

Once abduction is accomplished, treatment consists of Petrie (leg abduction) casting, or surgical soft tissue releases such as adductor tenotomy, followed by application of Toronto or Scottish Rite braces.

Nursing Management

Teach the parents and child about the course of the disease and expected treatment, emphasizing the importance of keeping the hip non–weight-bearing.

Offer suggestions for activities that redirect energy and promote normal development; these may include horseback riding, which promotes hip abduction; swimming to increase mobility; handcrafts to promote fine motor skills; and reading or computer activities to stimulate cognitive development.

Assist the family to work with the school to plan for the child's mobility to classes.

Teach cast or brace care as required by the child's treatment.

Slipped Capital Femoral Epiphysis

Slipped capital femoral epiphysis occurs when the femoral head is displaced from the femoral neck.

It is most common during the adolescent growth spurt, between the ages of 12–15 years in boys and 10–13 years in girls.

Boys are more often affected than girls; blacks are affected more often than other ethnic groups, as are children who are overweight, with sports injuries or other trauma, with a history of radiation therapy, or with endocrine disease (Acosta, Vade, Lomasney, et al. 2001).

Symptoms include limp, pain, and loss of hip motion.

Acute slipped capital femoral epiphysis has a sudden onset of less than 3 weeks' duration. The child with an acute slip has sudden, severe pain and cannot bear weight. This may be associated with traumatic injury.

Chronic slipped capital femoral epiphysis has a duration of longer than 3 weeks. It presents with persistent hip pain, which is generally aching or mild and can be referred to the thigh, knee, or both. A limp and decreased range of motion may also occur.

Acute-on-chronic is an additional slippage in a child with a chronic condition. The child with a chronic slip sustains a traumatic incident that causes further slippage of the femoral head, causing sudden, severe pain.

Radiographs are used to confirm the diagnosis. A bone scan, ultrasound, computed tomography, and MRI are sometimes performed to verify the extent of injury.

Surgical treatment is usually necessary; this involves fixation of the epiphysis with screws or pins.

Medical treatment, which is occasionally used, includes a regimen of no weight bearing, bed rest, a spica cast, and Buck or Russell traction.

Nursing care involves encouraging recommended weight among children and adolescents and recognizing and referring those with symptoms of the disorder.

Care during traction and after surgical correction are important nursing interventions (Tables 26–1 and 26–2).

Table 26–1   Types of Traction

Skin traction

Pull is applied to the skin surface, which puts traction directly on the bones and muscles. Traction is attached to the skin with adhesive materials or straps, or foam boots, belts, or halters.

  Dunlop traction (can be either skeletal or skin)

  Used for fracture of the humerus. The arm, which is flexed, is suspended horizontally with straps placed on both the upper and lower portions for pull from both sides.

  Bryant's traction

  Used specifically for the child 3 years of age or younger and weighing less than 17.5 kg (35 lb) who has developmental dysplasia of the hip or a fractured femur. This bilateral traction is applied to the child's legs and kept in place by wrapping the legs from foot to thigh with elastic bandages. The hips are flexed at a 90-degree angle, with knees extended. This position is maintained by attaching the traction appliance to weights and pulleys, which are suspended above the crib. The buttocks do not rest on the mattress, but are slightly elevated off the bed.

  Buck traction

  Used for knee immobilization; to correct contractures or deformities or for short-term immobilization of a fracture. It keeps the leg in an extended position, without hip flexion. Traction is applied to the extremity in one direction (straight line) with a single pulley system.

  Russell traction

  Used for fractures of the femur and lower leg. Traction is placed on the lower leg while the knee is suspended in a padded sling. The hips and knees, which are slightly flexed, are immobilized. One force is applied by a double pulley to the foot, and another force is applied upward using a sling under the knee and an overhead pulley.

Skeletal traction

Pull is directly applied to the bone by pins, wires, tongs, or other apparatus that have been surgically placed through the distal end of the bone.

  Skeletal cervical traction

  Used for cervical spine injuries to reduce fractures and dislocations. Crutchfield, Gardner-Wells, or Vinke tongs are placed in the skull with burr holes. Weights are attached to the apparatus with a rope and pulley system to the hyperextended head.

  Halo traction

  Used to immobilize the head and neck after cervical injury or dislocation. Also used for positioning and immobilization after cervical injury.

  90-90 traction

  Used for fractures of the femur or tibia. A skeletal pin or wire is surgically placed through the distal part of the femur; the lower part of the extremity is in a boot cast. Traction ropes and pulleys are applied at the pin site and on the boot cast to maintain the flexion of both the hip and knee at 90 degrees. This traction can also be used for treatment of an upper extremity fracture.

(*continued*)

Section III: Body Systems

Table 26–1   Types of Traction (Continued)

External fixators

These devices can be used in the treatment of simple fractures, both open and closed; complex fractures with extensive soft tissue involvement; correction of bony or soft tissue deformities; pseudoarthroses; and limb length discrepancy. They are attached to the extremity by percutaneous transfixing of pins or wires to the bone.

DISORDERS OF THE SPINE
Scoliosis
Clinical Manifestations

Scoliosis is a lateral S- or C-shaped curvature of the spine that is often associated with a rotational deformity of the spine and ribs; spinal curvatures of more than 10 degrees are abnormal.

Idiopathic scoliosis is the most common type and frequently occurs in girls, especially during the growth spurt between the ages of 10 and 13 years.

Scoliosis can also occur in congenital diseases involving the spinal structure and in the musculoskeletal changes seen in conditions such as myelomeningocele, cerebral palsy, or muscular dystrophy; it can also be acquired after injury to the spinal cord.

Truncal asymmetry, uneven shoulders and hips, a one-sided rib hump, and a prominent scapula occur; compensatory problems may develop

Table 26–2   Nursing Care of the Child with Traction

1. Assess the child in traction by first checking the equipment. Make sure that the equipment is in the proper position. Observe both the body appliance and the attached weights and pulleys. Make certain that the child's body is in proper alignment.
2. Assess the skin under the straps and pin insertion sites for any signs of redness, edema, or skin breakdown.
3. Assess the extremity by checking neurovascular status frequently (check warmth, color, distal pulses, capillary refill time, movement, sensation).
4. Provide pin care when ordered using sterile technique. Clean the area surrounding the pin with cotton-tipped applicators saturated with normal saline or half-strength hydrogen peroxide. Clean the area again with sterile water or more saline. Apply an antibacterial ointment, if ordered, using another cotton-tipped applicator.
5. When the traction equipment can be removed, skin care should be performed every 4 hr.
6. Place a sheepskin pad under the child's extremity if orders permit.

for curvatures of more than 40 degrees such as hip and back pain and lung compromise leading to fatigue or dyspnea with exertion.

Diagnostic Tests

Observation and radiographic examination are used to diagnose scoliosis.

MRI, computed tomography scan, and bone scan may be used to assess the degree of curvature.

Clinical Therapy

Treatment of children with mild scoliosis (curvatures of 10–20 degrees) consists of exercises to improve posture and muscle tone and to maintain, or possibly increase, flexibility of the spine.

Moderate scoliosis (curvatures of 20–40 degrees) includes bracing with either a Boston or Milwaukee brace, worn for 23 hours daily.

Electrical stimulation is used occasionally as an alternative treatment.

Children with severe scoliosis (curvatures of 40 degrees or more) require surgery, which involves spinal fusion and instrumentation.

Nursing Management

Nursing management focuses on screening and early detection, teaching about brace wear, caring for the adolescent having surgery for scoliosis, and partnering with the adolescent and family to provide support during all treatments.

Assessment

Assess all children for scoliosis, particularly those entering puberty:

- From the front
  - Is the head midline?
  - Are the shoulders at the same height?
  - Is there the same amount of space between arms and body on each side?
- From the back
  - Is the head midline?
  - Are the shoulders at the same height?
  - Are the scapula equally prominent and at the same height?
  - Is the spine straight?
  - Is there the same amount of space between arms and body on each side?
  - Are the hips at the same height?

- With the adolescent holding hands together and bent over slightly
  - Are the scapula humps even?
- With the adolescent holding hands together and bent over toward floor
  - Are the flank humps even?
  - Is the spine straight?
  - Is there a marked roundness when viewed from the side? (evidence of kyphosis)

Assess skin condition and hours of daily wear for the adolescent who wears a brace.

For the child who requires spinal fusion postoperative care requires intensive assessment of all systems, including respiratory, neurologic, musculoskeletal, integumentary, fluid and electrolytes, and pain control.

Intervention

Emphasize importance of continued care to monitor for continuation of curvature.

Provide information for families about the treatment that is prescribed for the child/adolescent.

Prepare the family and child when surgical intervention is planned.

Provide care for the child with spinal fusion, to include the following:
- Monitor respiratory status and use pulse oximeter; administer oxygen if needed; have the teen deep breathe and use incentive spirometer.
- Reposition at least every 2 hours.
- Perform neurovascular checks of each extremity, including color, circulation, capillary refill, warmth, sensation, motion every 2 hours for first 24 hours and then every 4 hours.
- Monitor presence of pedal and distal tibial pulses.
- Apply antiembolism stockings until the teen is ambulatory.
- Monitor for pain, swelling, or positive Homans' sign in legs.
- Evaluate for edema.
- Perform range of motion exercises when ordered.
- Assess level of pain, and initiate pain management strategies.
- Administer pain medication around the clock, especially in the first 48 hours.
- As the teen becomes ambulatory, instruct in brace or cast care as needed; provide instructions about activities that are allowed and those to avoid.

DISORDERS OF BONE
Osteoporosis and Osteopenia

Osteoporosis is a metabolic bone disease in which bone mineral density is more than 2.5 standard deviations below the norm; osteopenia is low bone mass between 1.0 and 2.5 standard deviations below norm (Bowman & Russell, 2001; Chan & Bishop, 2002).

Conditions associated with these disorders include osteopenia of prematurity, low mechanical loading due to inability to ambulate or treatment of a condition by immobilization, inadequate nutritional intake, Turner syndrome, growth hormone deficiency, osteogenesis imperfecta, juvenile rheumatoid arthritis, and diabetes.

The disorders are silent diseases and may go undetected for years until a fracture occurs.

Premature newborns at risk of osteopenia of prematurity need collaborative management by neonatologists, neonatal nutritionists, and neonatal nurses.

For children at risk of developing osteoporosis, calcium and vitamin D intake is encouraged, and oral supplements may be given.

Standing therapy for those who are nonambulatory can provide mechanical weight and enhance bone density (Caulton, Ward, Alsop, et al., 2004).

When a cast or other immobilizing device is removed from a child, a gradually increasing program of exercise in collaboration with physical rehabilitation professionals promotes bone strengthening and lowered risk for fractures or related sequelae.

Nurses perform dietary analysis of children at risk.

Refer children at risk to nutritionists and physicians for further education and diagnosis.

Administer nutritional supplements when prescribed, and teach families how to give these medications.

Partner with families to provide therapy for nonambulatory children that stimulates weight bearing.

Teach parents how to recognize fractures in children who may not have normal sensation and are unable to report them. Swelling, unusual shape of a limb, fussiness of the child, and falls should be reported promptly.

Osteomyelitis
Clinical Manifestations
Common causes of osteomyelitis include *Staphylococcus aureus*, *Escherichia coli*, group B streptococci, *Streptococcus aureus*, *Streptococcus pyogenes*, and *Haemophilus influenzae*.

Symptoms include constant bone pain, edema, decreased mobility of the infected joint, and fever.

Redness may be present over the area of infection.

The child may refuse to walk or may limp (Fernandez, Carrol, & Baker, 2000).

The onset of acute osteomyelitis is generally rapid and is therefore sometimes misdiagnosed as a sports injury.

Diagnostic Tests
A history suggestive of osteomyelitis includes an upper respiratory infection or blunt trauma followed by pain at the area of a growth plate.

Laboratory evaluation shows leukocytosis and an elevated erythrocyte sedimentation rate and C-reactive protein (Carek, Dickerson, & Sack, 2001); the degree of erythrocyte sedimentation rate elevation is directly related to the severity of the infection.

Radiographs and bone scans may identify the area of involvement.

A needle aspiration of the site or a blood culture can confirm the diagnosis and provide a culture of the causative organism.

Clinical Therapy
Medical management of infection begins with the intravenous administration of a broad-spectrum antibiotic, even before culture results are available.

When an adequate response to antibiotic is not obtained within 2–3 days, the area may be aspirated again, or surgical drainage may be performed.

Intravenous fluids may be administered to ensure adequate hydration.

Nursing Management
Assess the onset of symptoms and a history of recent infections or trauma; include questions about immunization status, especially tetanus.

Evaluate the affected area for signs of redness, swelling, pain, and decreased range of motion.

Measure vital signs; increased temperature and pulse may provide clues about worsening infection.

Blood cultures and other cultures of the body must be performed before the first dose of antibiotic when osteomyelitis is suspected.

Obtain continuing blood samples as needed to monitor erythrocyte sedimentation rate and C-reactive protein.

Administer intravenous fluids as ordered, and offer oral fluids frequently to maintain hydration status of the child.

Administer intravenous and oral antibiotics as ordered.

Monitor the intravenous site and provide care for the central or other lines.

Administer analgesics, and use other comfort measure to relieve bone pain and joint tenderness.

Strict aseptic technique and transmission-based precautions should be used during all nursing care; instruct the family in these techniques.

Osteogenesis Imperfecta
Clinical Manifestations

Osteogenesis imperfecta is a connective tissue disorder characterized by a biochemical defect in the production of collagen.

The disease is genetically transmitted, generally in an autosomal dominant inheritance pattern.

Clinical manifestations include multiple and frequent fractures; blue sclerae; thin, soft skin; increased joint flexibility; enlargement of the anterior fontanel; weak muscles; soft, pliable, brittle bones; and short stature; conductive hearing loss can occur by adolescence or young adulthood (Paterson, Monk, & McAllion, 2001); most children with osteogenesis imperfecta are short in height and may have decreased range of motion in several joints.

The disease is classified into four types:

- Type I: Most common form; children have fragile bones, blue sclerae, weakened tooth dentin, and hearing loss that manifests in adolescence.
- Type II: Ribs and skeleton are extensively involved; most children with this form of the disease die *in utero* or shortly after birth.
- Type III: The newborn or infant sustains numerous fractures and manifests blue sclerae; severe bone fragility and kyphoscoliosis

are observed; most children with type III disease die in childhood as a result of cardiorespiratory failure.

- Type IV: Characterized by fractures without other symptoms of the disease; bowing of the legs and other structural deformities can occur; however, the incidence of fractures decreases beginning in puberty.

Diagnostic Tests

Because the disease is genetic in origin, ultrasound or collagen analysis of chorionic villus cells can be used for diagnosis before birth in babies at known risk.

Diagnosis may be made only when the child has a delay in walking or sustains a fracture. Radiographic evaluation may detect both old and new fractures.

Tests such as dual energy x-ray absorptiometry can be used to measure bone density.

Serum alkaline phosphatase level may be elevated; other measures of bone metabolism such as serum osteocalcin, procollagen 1 C-terminal peptide, collagen 1 teleopeptide, and urine deoxypyridinoline may be performed occasionally to measure effects of experimental medication.

Clinical Therapy

There is no cure for osteogenesis imperfecta; clinical therapy consists primarily of fracture care and prevention of deformities.

Treatment includes physical therapy; casting, bracing, or splinting; surgical stabilization; nutritional management with high vitamin D and calcium intake; and bisphosphonate medication such as pamidronate.

Surgery to insert telescoping rods in long bones may be helpful to stabilize bones. Hematologic stem cell transplant has been used successfully in some children with severe osteogenesis imperfecta and is under further research (Horwitz, Prockop, & Gordon, et al., 2001).

Nursing Management

Assessment

Assess the child carefully and frequently for signs of fractures.

Ask about favorite activities of the child because they need to be integrated into plans for physical activity and developmental progression.

Perform careful growth measures and developmental screening.

Intervention

Handle the child gently: The trunk and extremities should be supported when the child is moved; perform tasks such as bathing and diapering carefully; use a blanket or pillow under the child for additional support when lifting and moving; do not pull the infant's legs upward when changing a diaper, as this can cause a fracture, but slip a hand under the hips to raise them, slide the diaper carefully in, and then bring it up as the legs are slightly abducted.

Partner with families to provide safe activities for the child. Discourage contact sports and other activities that are likely to lead to fractures.

Encourage a well-balanced diet with additional vitamin C, vitamin D, and calcium to encourage healing and bone growth; calories should be limited to maintain weight at recommended levels because immobility can lead to overweight and the child is generally short for age.

Provide preparatory teaching for the child who requires surgical intervention for management of fractures.

Parents may feel guilt, anger, and worry over the child; support them and refer to organizations such as the Osteogenesis Imperfecta Foundation.

Evaluate the child's developmental progress periodically, and make suggestions for interventions that parents can use to foster cognitive, social, and physical milestones.

DISORDERS OF MUSCLES
Muscular Dystrophy
Clinical Manifestations

The muscular dystrophies are a group of inherited diseases characterized by muscle fiber degeneration and muscle wasting; the disorders can begin early or late in life, and onset can be at birth or gradual during childhood.

With Duchenne muscular dystrophy, muscle weakness begins in the lower extremities in early childhood; parents may notice the child tripping, toe walking, and displaying enlargement of the calf muscles (in fact, the calf is not enlarged but muscle is replaced by fat). By the middle teen years, the child's condition has usually progressed so that walking is not possible. The disease continues to progress, potentially causing conditions such as scoliosis, other musculoskeletal conditions, cardiomyopathy, and respiratory difficulty. Fractures may occur when the child falls due to weakness. The child's life expectancy is the early 20s (Driscoll, 2001).

Becker's dystrophy is similar but emerges later and more slowly.

The dystrophies of infancy are manifested by generalized weakness and hypotonia. The baby may have difficulty with sucking and swallowing. Ocular problems may be present.

Diagnostic Tests

Diagnosis and classification are most often based on clinical signs and the pattern of muscle involvement.

Biochemical examinations such as serum enzyme assay, muscle biopsy, and electromyography confirm the diagnosis.

Serum creatine kinase level is elevated early in the disease.

Dystrophin, the muscle protein that is deficient in muscular dystrophy, can be measured by muscle biopsy.

Genetic testing establishes the specific abnormality and type of disease present.

Clinical Therapy

There is no effective treatment for childhood muscular dystrophy; research is being directed at several techniques to repair mutations by gene therapy and stem cell therapy (Papazian & Alfonso, 2002; Takeda & Miyagoe-Suzuki, 2001).

The steroids prednisone and deflazacort may preserve muscle function, preserving walking for a longer period (Biggar, Gingras, Feblings, et al., 2001).

Surgery may be used to correct scoliosis, a commonly accompanying disorder, to facilitate lung expansion.

Respiratory infections are vigorously treated with deep breathing, coughing, nebulizer treatments, and antibiotics when indicated.

Assessment

Monitor all vital signs as well as cardiac and respiratory functioning.

Assess urinary function and frequency of bowel movements.

Periodically measure strength and range of motion.

Assess mobility via ambulation or assisted device.

Perform periodic developmental assessments.

Evaluate the family's risk and protective factors for dealing with this chronic and fatal disorder.

Intervention

Nurses often provide home healthcare services to such children, work with them in school nursing positions, and partner with parents in clinics and other facilities to provide health promotion and maintenance as the child grows.

Administer oxygen or respiratory therapy as ordered.

Soft foods or enteral tube feedings may be needed to promote nutrition; the infant with a rare dystrophy in infancy may need gavage feedings.

Maintain bowel function with fluids, high-fiber foods, and medications as needed.

Monitor and ensure adequate fluid output.

Be alert for signs of infection.

Perform range of motion and provide for physical activity to level of ability.

Physical therapy helps the child ambulate and prevents joint contractures; provide good back support and posture by keeping the child's body in alignment when confined to a wheelchair; splints may be needed to maintain extremities in proper position.

Perform periodic developmental assessments, and provide parents with suggestions for encouraging the child's development.

Meet with teachers to evaluate the child's learning needs and functioning in the classroom; an individualized education plan should be established.

Partner with the school to provide tutors or home computers if needed.

Young children should be enrolled in early intervention programs before they are old enough for school.

Encourage the child to be independent for as long as possible, concentrating on what the child can accomplish.

Exercise as tolerated contributes to muscle strength and a general sense of well-being.

The family is challenged to manage the child's care, provide a nurturing environment for other children and family members, and obtain necessary financial resources over many years.

Refer the family to respite care, assist them in finding resources, and be certain that either a family member or health professional acts as case manager to coordinate various services needed; refer family members to resource and support groups such as the Muscular Dystrophy Association; refer for genetic counseling.

Parents need bereavement counseling and end-of-life care as the child becomes weaker and the disease progresses.

INJURIES TO THE MUSCULOSKELETAL SYSTEM
Fractures
Clinical Manifestations

Fractures, which may occur at any age, occur frequently in children because their bones are less dense and more porous than those of adults.

Due to their porous nature, the bones of children may bow leading to more common greenstick or spiral fractures in children (Eiff & Hatch, 2003).

Childhood fractures most often involve the clavicle, tibia, ulna, and femur, with distal forearm fractures the most common type. Fractures to the pelvis are often associated with motor vehicle crashes.

Epiphyseal (growth plate) injuries are dangerous in children, as they can interfere with future growth at the site. These constitute approximately 30% of childhood fractures (Eiff & Hatch, 2003).

Fractures are generally characterized by pain, abnormal positioning, edema, immobility or decreased range of motion, ecchymosis, guarding, and crepitus.

Types of fractures are described using the Salter-Harris classification system (Table 26–3).

Diagnostic Tests

Radiographs are used to diagnose fractures and to determine the exact location and type of fracture.

Clinical Therapy

Immobilization is essential for the bone healing process to take place.

A closed reduction aligns the bone by manual manipulation or traction.

An open reduction requires surgical alignment of the bone, often using pins, plates, wires, or screws.

For open fractures, surgery must also be performed for débridement to remove dead tissue and clean the wound.

Table 26–3 Salter-Harris Fracture Classification System

Type I
  Common
  Fracture between bone and growth plate
  Growth plate undisturbed
  Growth disturbances rare
Type II
  Most common
  Fracture through bone above growth plate
  Growth disturbances rare
Type III
  Less common
  Fracture through growth plate
  Serious threat to growth and joint
Type IV
  Fracture through growth plate and bone
  Serious threat to growth
Type V
  Rare
  Crush injury causes cell death in growth plate, resulting in arrested growth and limited bone length
  If growth plate is partially destroyed, angular deformities may result

Casting is the most common external method of immobilization.

Nursing Management

Assess the diets of all youth who might be at risk for fractures and insert dietary teaching in health promotion visits.

When dealing with an injured child, be alert to the signs and symptoms of fractures before moving the child; when in doubt about the nature of an injury, apply a splint.

Evaluate pain, swelling, and any abnormal positioning of the injured area.

When a child is admitted to the emergency department or hospital, nursing assessment includes the extent of the injury, the degree of pain, and the child's vital signs (respiratory status, pulse, blood pressure).

Nursing care focuses on care of the child before and after fracture reduction, encouraging mobility as ordered, maintaining skin integrity, preventing infection, and teaching the parents and child how to care for the fracture.

If conscious sedation or pain blocks are used, nursing care for these procedures is needed. When caring for a child who has undergone fracture reduction, it is important to be aware of the signs of complications; notify the physician immediately if these signs occur.

Document assessments and report changes and abnormal results immediately. The major serious complication is compartment syndrome, or a condition of increased pressure in a limited space such as the soft tissue of an extremity that is casted, which compromises circulation and nervous innervation (Harvey, 2001); manifestations of the syndrome begin approximately 30 minutes after tissue ischemia starts and include the following:

- Paresthesia (tingling, burning, loss of two-point discrimination)
- Pain (unrelieved by medication, characterized by crying in the young child)
- Pressure (skin is tense, cast appears tight)
- Pallor (pale, gray, or white skin tone)[1]
- Paralysis (weakness or inability to move extremity)[1]
- Pulselessness (weak or absent pulse)[1]

Check extremities every 15 minutes until stable and then every 1–2 hours for the following:

- Color
- Temperature
- Capillary refill
- Peripheral pulses
- Edema
- Sensation
- Motor ability
- Pain

Adapted from Kunkler, C. E. (1999). Neurovascular assessment. Orthopaedic Nursing, 18(3),63–71; and Harvey, C. (2001). Compartment syndrome: When it is least expected. Orthopaedic Nursing, 20(3),15–26.

See Box 26–1 for further details on cast care.

Teach the parents and child cast care, activity restrictions, and how to identify problems that should be reported.

Help parents to identify any modifications that may be needed at home and school; the child who has to manage steps at home or school may need special training with crutches or a temporary ramp.

---

[1]Indicates a late sign.

Refer parents to home health nurses or home teaching services if indicated.

Provide pertinent teaching to prevent future injuries.

Sports Injuries

Sports injuries are the most common type of injury in youth from 13 to 19 years.

Football, wrestling, soccer, and gymnastics are the sports most commonly associated with injury.

Fractures, described previously, are common sports injuries of young athletes.

See Table 26–4 for common sports injuries.

Children and adolescents should receive instruction in correct techniques from a person qualified to coach and supervise children.

Have parents inquire about the coach's experience and also verify that the coaching staff is prepared in emergency care.

Encourage youth to gradually increase time and intensity at a sport rather than immediately playing a new sport for long periods of time.

Ask about sports participation for all youth, but especially when there are complaints of sore muscles, edema of body parts, and bruises.

Table 26–4   Common Sports Injuries

Sport	Types of Injuries
Baseball	Hand and finger fractures and sprains
	Contusions and sprains of upper or lower extremities; wrists, elbows, knees, and ankles are common sites
	Injury to body parts when hit by a ball—i.e., broken teeth, face, head, eye, and chest injuries
Football	Head and neck injury such as skull or cervical vertebrae fracture
	Pulled muscles or dislocations in shoulders and legs
Gymnastics	Wrist and elbow fractures and strains
	Tendonitis in elbows and ankles/legs
Hockey (ice and inline)	Dental injuries
	Leg fractures
	Head and neck injuries
Soccer	Head and neck injuries
	Strains and fractures of legs
Wrestling	Fractures and dislocations of upper and lower extremities

Perform neurovascular assessment of extremities, including color, temperature, capillary refill time, edema, pulses, sensation, and pain.

Teach youth to warm up for 10–15 minutes before participation and to cool down for a corresponding period at the end of activity; they should not ignore pain.

Ensure that youth wear recommended gear for their sports, including equipment such as well-fitted protective helmet, face masks, eye protection, mouth guards, elbow and wrist guards, gloves, knee pads.

Injuries such as muscle strains should be treated promptly with the following:

- Resting the injury for 24–48 hours; applying ice for 20 minutes four times daily; compression with an elastic wrap to provide comfort and decrease edema; elevating the part affected above heart level
- Gradually increasing motion to the part
- Adding flexibility and resistance or strengthening exercises
- Returning gradually to the sport, usually in 2–3 weeks after injury (Harper, 2002)

27. ALTERATIONS IN INTEGUMENTARY FUNCTION

SKIN LESIONS

Skin lesions vary in size, shape, color, and texture characteristics. Primary lesions arise from previously healthy skin (Table 27–1). Secondary lesions result from changes in primary lesions (Table 27–2).

Acne

Acne is a chronic inflammatory disorder of the pilosebaceous hair follicles located on the face and trunk. The keratin and sebum that usually flow to the skin surface are obstructed in the follicular canal, causing *comedones* (whiteheads and blackheads). The sebum behind the comedone is an ideal environment for the anaerobic *Propionibacterium acnes,* and an inflammatory reaction results.

Clinical Manifestations

The three main types of acne are

1. Comedonal (characterized by open and closed comedones)
2. Papulopustular (characterized by red papules and pustules)
3. Cystic (characterized by nodules and cysts)

Lesions occur most often on the face, upper chest, shoulders, and back. Scars form when the surrounding dermis is damaged.

Inflammatory acne in adolescents with darker skin color is associated with a hyperpigmented macule that can last for 4 months or longer. Hyperpigmented areas may fade over time if inflammation is controlled (Rudy, 2003).

Clinical Therapy

Diagnosis is based on examination of the skin.

Treatment is customized to the predominant type of lesion present and severity of the lesions. Options include long-term use of keratolytics, retinoids, and oral antibiotics to suppress lesions and reduce scarring (Meds 27–1).

Isotretinoin (Accutane) is reserved for the most serious cases of acne that do not respond to other therapies.

- Parents and adolescents must sign informed consent about teratogenicity, monthly blood testing, and the potential for depression or suicide ideation (Woodard, 2002).

Table 27–1   Primary Skin Lesions

Lesion Name	Description	Example
Macule	Flat, nonpalpable, diameter <1 cm (0.5 in.)	Freckle, rubella, rubeola, petechiae
Papule	Elevated, firm, diameter <1 cm (0.5 in.)	Warts, pigmented nevi
Patch	Macule diameter >1 cm (0.5 in.)	Vitiligo, mongolian spot
Nodule	Elevated, firm, deeper in dermis than papule, diameter 1–2 cm (0.5 –1 in.)	Erythema nodosum
Tumor	Elevated, solid, diameter >2 cm (1 in.)	Neoplasm, hemangioma
Vesicle	Elevated, filled with fluid, diameter <1 cm (0.5 in.)	Early chickenpox, herpes simplex
Pustule	Vesicle filled with purulent fluid	Impetigo, acne
Bulla	Vesicle diameter >1 cm (0.5 in.)	Burn blister
Wheal	Irregular elevated solid area of edematous skin	Urticaria, insect bite

Table 27–2   Common Secondary Skin Lesions

Lesion Name	Description	Example
Crust	Dried residue of serum, pus, or blood	Impetigo
Scale	Thin flake of exfoliated epidermis	Dandruff, psoriasis
Lichenification	Thickening of skin with increased visibility of normal skin furrows	Eczema (atopic dermatitis)
Scar	Replacement of destroyed tissue with fibrous tissue	Healed surgical incision
Keloid	Overdevelopment or hypertrophy of scar, extends beyond wound edges and above skin line	Healed skin area after traumatic injury
Excoriation	Abrasion or scratch mark	Scratched insect bite
Fissure	Linear crack in skin	Tinea pedis (athlete's foot)
Erosion	Loss of superficial epidermis; moist but does not bleed	Ruptured chickenpox vesicle
Ulcer	Deeper loss of skin surface; bleeding or scarring may ensue	Chancre
Comedone	A plug of sebaceous and keratin material in a hair follicle opening	Acne
Burrow	A narrow, raised irregular channel caused by a parasite	Scabies
Telangiectasia	Dilated, superficial blood vessels	

Meds 27–1 Medications for Acne Based on Severity

Medication	Severity and Appearance
Tretinoin (Retin-A) 0.025% cream daily (to comedones only), in the evening Salicylic acid, adapalene, tazarotene	Grade I (mild) Comedonal acne
2.5% benzoyl peroxide gel Tretinoin in evening Topical antibiotics (clindamycin, erythromycin, tetracycline) twice a day Azelaic acid cream twice a day	Grade II (moderate) Papulopustular acne (red papules, pustules)
Tretinoin and benzoyl peroxide twice a day Oral antibiotics (tetracycline, minocycline, or doxycycline)	Grade III (severe) Cystic acne (red papules, many pustules, cysts)
Isotretinoin (Accutane) given twice a day for 15–20 weeks A second course of treatment for 8 weeks may be given to those who do not have a good response	Grade IV Pustulocystic nodular (severe, resistant to other treatment)

- Adolescent females need two negative pregnancy tests before starting treatment; a monthly pregnancy test during treatment; and two forms of contraception 1 month before, during, and 1 month after treatment (Buck, 2001).
- Monthly laboratory monitoring of liver function, cholesterol, and triglycerides is required. A 1-month supply of isotretinoin is provided to promote compliance.

Other medications prescribed include oral contraceptives and spironolactone.

Nursing Management
Assessment
Assess the distribution, predominant type, and severity of acne lesions.

Assess knowledge about the cause and treatment of acne and the home therapies used.

Explore the amount of emotional distress the acne is causing the adolescent.

Intervention
Encourage good nutrition to help the skin heal.

Teach correct procedures for taking prescribed drugs such as tetracycline and isotretinoin, and discuss possible side effects. Emphasize the importance of return visits to the adolescent's healthcare provider to monitor side effects of medications.

Provide psychological support to adolescents.

Patient and Family Education

Avoid picking and squeezing pimples. Wash your hands often, and avoid touching your face to reduce the transfer of oils and bacteria to the face.

Use gentle skin cleansers to wash the face twice a day. Do not use abrasive sponges or cloths. Wait 20 minutes until the skin is thoroughly dry before applying a topical retinoid.

For topical medications, use a pea-sized dose of topical medications to spread in a thin film over the skin. Avoid getting the topical medications near the eyes, lips, and mucous membranes.

Avoid the use of astringents and aftershaves that contain alcohol. They may further dry the skin and make it difficult to tolerate the prescribed treatments.

Avoid hats or gear that can cause friction and occlusion of the skin.

Greasy foods may leave a residual oil on the face and hands that can be occlusive. Wash your hands after handling greasy foods.

Limit the use of pomades or petrolatum-based hair products. Keep hair spray and mousse away from the face.

Use noncomedonic (for acne-prone skin) moisturizers to reduce irritation.

Use oil-free or water-based makeup. Avoid waterproof makeup.

Use noncomedonic sunscreen and protective clothing even on cloudy days, as the medications make the skin more sensitive to sun exposure.

Protect the face from cold, windy weather.

Sweating, heat and humidity, and emotional stress may exacerbate acne.

Do not get discouraged with daily treatments, as it will take 6–12 weeks before improvement is seen. Continue daily topical therapies when acne has improved significantly so that acne does not return.

Atopic Dermatitis (Eczema)

Atopic dermatitis is a chronic, superficial inflammatory skin disorder with intense pruritus. It affects 10–20% of children. The etiology is unknown. A family history of asthma or hay fever frequently predisposes a child to eczema.

The child's generally dry skin is more likely to crack and fissure.

Irritants have a greater chance to penetrate, and the child is more susceptible to infection.

Factors that exacerbate the condition include triggers (house mites, animal dander, and pollens), food allergies, irritants (soaps, detergents, chemicals, solvents, and abrasive clothing), hormonal changes, and emotional stress.

Clinical Manifestations

Acute atopic dermatitis is characterized by pruritus and erythematous patches with vesicles, exudate, and crusts. Subacute cases are characterized by scaling with erythema and excoriation. Erythema and warmth may indicate a secondary bacterial skin infection.

Infantile form—pruritic exudative, crusty, papulovesicular, and erythematous lesions on cheeks, scalp, forehead, neck, trunk, and extensor surfaces of extremities; diaper area spared; some patches weep; secondary infection; lichenification

Childhood form—pruritic, erythematous, dry scaly or weeping, well-circumscribed, papular lesions; buttocks become excoriated once toilet trained; thickened and lichenified lesions on antecubital, popliteal, and extensor surfaces of extremities, neck, and behind ears

Adolescent form—similar to childhood eczema in distribution and lesions; other affected areas may include the eyelids, where the earlobe touches the face, fingertips, toes, nipples, and the vulvar area

Diagnostic Tests

No laboratory tests are diagnostic. Cultures of the skin may be used when a secondary infection is suspected.

Clinical Therapy

The goals of treatment are to hydrate and lubricate the skin, reduce pruritus, minimize inflammatory changes, and identify flare-up triggers. Therapy includes the following:

- Apply occlusive topical ointment after bathing to trap moisture and prevent drying of the skin. Apply moisturizing ointments and creams three to four times a day and when skin feels dry (Meds 27–2).
- Apply topical corticosteroids twice daily before the skin moisturizer is used. Corticosteroids are discontinued when the rash disap-

Meds 27–2 Medication Used to Treat Atopic Dermatitis

Medications	Action	Adverse Effects
Emollients 　Eucerin cream 　Aquaphor ointment 　Vanicream 　Cetaphil cream 　SBR-lipocream 　White petrolatum	Lubricate the skin when applied immediately after bathing	Fragrances and preservatives in products may cause irritation. Fragrance-free or bland emollients should be used.
Oral antihistamines	Control of itching and sedating effect when given at night	Sleepiness and interference with school if given during the day.
Antibiotics 　Topical 　Oral	Treat cutaneous skin superinfections	Hypersensitivity reaction.
Corticosteroids 　Topical 　Oral	Anti-inflammatory	Skin atrophy; suppression of the hypothalamic-pituitary-adrenal axis; can induce glaucoma or cataract formation if used around eyes.
Immunomodulators 　Tacrolimus ointment 　Pimecrolimus (Elidel, SDZ ASM 981)	Inhibit T-lymphocyte activation; inhibit release of cytokines and inflammatory mediators from anti-immunoglobulin E–activated skin mast cells and basophils Often used on face rather than topical corticosteroids	Pruritus, burning or stinging sensation for up to 20 minutes in some children, but this response may be longer in the first week of therapy (Buck, 2001); sunscreens should be used because of potential increased risk for skin cancer. Approved for children older than 2 years.

SBR, skin barrier repair.

pears to reduce the risk of steroid side effects. Use lower-potency nonfluorinated ointments for infants and for thinner skin areas (face, diaper area, and skin folds). A higher-potency ointment is used for flare-ups.

- Oral corticosteroids may be used for a severe acute exacerbation, but a rebound effect occurs.
- Immunomodulator ointments may be the treatment of choice for some children not responsive to or intolerant of conventional therapy.
- Topical antibiotics are used to treat excoriated, open lesions that appear infected.

- Antihistamines do not help itching, but the sedative effect may help promote sleep. Humidification in the winter and air conditioning in the summer may help reduce pruritus.
- Avoidance of highly allergenic foods, such as eggs, wheat, milk, and peanuts, in the diets of infants and lactating mothers may improve the skin condition of some children.

Nursing Management

Assessment

Take a thorough history, including any family history of allergy, environmental or dietary factors, and past exacerbations.

Note the distribution and type of lesions; presence of weeping lesions or signs of infection.

Determine whether the sleep of the child or other family members is disturbed.

Identify whether the child's self-esteem is disturbed.

Intervention

If an oral antihistamine is ordered to promote sleep, make sure the parents understand the best time to give the medication for that purpose.

Help parents and children of all ages deal with the frustration of the acute flare-ups. Encourage good home care to improve the child's skin. Reassure parents that the condition usually improves with age and generally does not leave scars.

Identify activities that the child can participate in to improve self-esteem.

Help identify potential food allergens. Increased itching within hours of eating a certain food may be associated with the eczema flare-up. Provide alternative food options to fulfill daily nutritional requirements when allergens are identified. Refer the family to the Food Allergy and Anaphylaxis Network.

Patient and Family Education

Avoid wool clothing and clothing washed in harsh laundry detergents to decrease skin irritation and pruritus. Wear loose cotton clothing.

Bathe and let the child soak in tepid water for 5–15 minutes once or twice a day. Use mild soap, such as Dove or Tone, only on areas that are dirty. Rinse well. Pat the child dry with a towel or air dry rather than rubbing the skin.

Immediately apply the medication (corticosteroid, topical antibiotic, or immunomodulator) to the inflamed area and then the lubricant on top. Apply the lubricant to the entire body. Use an ointment or cream, as lotions have less oil.

Consider the cost of ointments and creams, as large quantities are needed to cover the body at least twice a day. Petrolatum or Vaseline is inexpensive, safe, and easily applied.

In areas where the humidity is low, more frequent application of lubricants to the skin is needed. Corticosteroids should be applied no more than twice a day.

Help assure that parents use enough corticosteroids for effective treatment. It takes 5–8 g to cover the entire body of a child who weighs 10 kg, so a 15 g tube of corticosteroid ointment is enough for only *1* day. It takes 45 g to cover the entire body of an adolescent once (Hansen, 2003). The steroid is only used where there is inflammation.

For immunomodulators, a pea size amount should cover a 2-in. circle.

When a skin flare-up occurs, wet occlusive dressings increase penetration of corticosteroid ointments and help decrease itching. Apply the topical ointment, then wrap the child in a wet towel for 10 minutes, and then reapply the topical ointment followed by an emollient (Raimer, 2000).

Cellulitis

Cellulitis is an acute inflammation of the dermis and underlying connective tissue that usually occurs on the face and extremities after injury to the skin barrier, an abscess, or sinusitis. Common causative organisms are *Staphylococcus aureus, Streptococcus pneumoniae, Haemophilus influenzae*, group A beta-hemolytic *Streptococcus*, and group B *Streptococcus*.

Clinical Manifestations

Rapid onset of erythema, edema of the face or infected limb, warmth, and tenderness

Fever, chills, malaise, and enlargement and tenderness of regional lymph nodes; the child appears ill

Diagnostic Tests

A complete blood count with differential may show an increase in white blood cells.

Cultures of the site; blood cultures if the child has a toxic appearance.

Clinical Therapy

Intravenous antibiotics if the face is involved; intravenous or oral antibiotics when other sites are involved. The child may be hospitalized. Analgesics are given for pain.

Nursing Management

Administer prescribed oral or intravenous antibiotics and analgesics as scheduled.

Apply warm compresses to the affected area four times daily.

Elevate head or affected limb, and keep child on bed rest.

Monitor for complications such as abscess formation, spread of the infected area in the 24- to 48-hour period after the start of treatment, increased lethargy, and fever.

Contact Dermatitis

Contact dermatitis is an inflammation of the skin that occurs in response to direct contact with an allergen or irritant. Sweating and friction enhance the absorption of the allergen or irritant.

An external irritant causes an inflammatory reaction, but no memory T-cell function or antigen-specific immunoglobulins are activated. Common irritants include soaps, detergents, fabric softeners, bleaches, lotions, urine, and stool.

An allergy antigen is absorbed from the skin surface during the initial sensitization phase and an immune memory is created. Common allergens include nickel, poison ivy, poison oak, lanolin, neomycin, rubber, potassium dichromate (a leather tanning agent), thimerosal, fragrances, and latex.

Clinical Manifestations

Irritant Contact Dermatitis

A discrete area of redness matching the exposure location is followed by edema, vesiculation, dryness of the skin, scaling, fissuring, and necrosis.

A rash develops within a few hours of contact, peaks within 24 hours, and quickly resolves with removal of the irritant.

Allergic Contact Dermatitis

Erythema, edema, pruritus, and vesicles or bullae that rupture, ooze, and crust characterize the rash of allergic contact dermatitis that develops within 12–24 hours after exposure.

The rash is usually limited to the area of contact. Symptoms can last up to 3–4 weeks without treatment.

Clinical Therapy

The distribution of the lesions provides clues about the source and identity of the allergen or irritant.

Remove the offending agent (e.g., clothes, plant, soap).

Skin care may involve calamine lotion, cool compresses with aluminum acetate (Burow's solution) to promote drying, and wet dressings or colloidal oatmeal soaks to relieve itching.

Antihistamines may be given to reduce itching or for a sedative effect when the child is too irritable to sleep.

Corticosteroids—medium-potency topical corticosteroids may be used for 2–3 weeks for allergic contact dermatitis when less than 10% of the body surface area (BSA) is affected; oral corticosteroids are used for 7–10 days when more than 10% of the BSA is affected, followed by tapering doses over the next 7–10 days.

Nursing Management

Assessment

Assess the skin, and identify the potential source of inflammation. Identify the family's knowledge of potential allergens and irritants.

Intervention

Teach parents proper application of topical corticosteroids and to continue use of the ointments, even when the skin shows signs of healing, to prevent rebound dermatitis.

Inform parents to use Burow's solution or aluminum acetate (Domeboro solution) for blistered or oozing lesions for 20 minutes daily to help dry lesions.

Familiarize parents with the symptoms of infection and need for follow-up care.

Teaching the child and family how to avoid exposure to the allergen or irritant is an important nursing role.

- Wash all clothes before the first wearing. Rinse clothes an extra time to remove all soap. Use mild soap to clean the skin.
- Place a barrier between the allergen and the skin (e.g., cover all metal snaps on clothing with cloth, wear socks to avoid exposure to shoe leather), or seek clothing or shoes made without allergens.
- Avoid use of nickel jewelry and belt buckles if a nickel allergy exists.
- Remove clothing worn after outside activities and shower, and then put on clean clothes.

Dermatophytoses (Ringworm)

Dermatophytoses are fungal infections that affect the skin, hair, or nails.

Tinea capitis involves the hair of the scalp and is usually seen in children between 1 and 10 years old.

Tinea corporis involves the skin of the body but not the scalp, beard, groin, hands, or feet. It is seen in children and adolescents.

Clinical Manifestations

Tinea Capitis

Circumscribed hair loss, erythema; broken hairs, dotted stubbed appearance where weakened hair has broken off; diffuse fine scaling, may appear as seborrhea, with yellow, greasy scales; mild itching

May have large, purulent, tender boggy mass on scalp with drainage (kerion); papules, pustules, and crusting on scalp; enlarged suboccipital or posterior cervical nodes

Tinea Corporis

Pink, scaly circular patch with an expanding border, may be scaly or erythematous throughout; slightly raised borders with a clearing center.

Multiple lesions on the face, neck, and arms may be associated with cuddling an infected kitten.

Diagnostic Tests

Microscopic examination of the hair and scale scrapings using a potassium hydroxide wet mount or a fungal culture

Clinical Therapy

Tinea Capitis

Griseofulvin orally for 6–8 weeks or 2 weeks after symptoms disappear (alternate antifungal agents include fluconazole, itraconazole, and terbinafine); selenium sulfide shampoo two to three times weekly, leave on for 10 minutes before rinsing to help eliminate scalp spores.

Children being treated may develop a hypersensitivity reaction to the fungal antigen, an extensive, itchy rash similar to atopic dermatitis. This *id* reaction is not a medication reaction. Mild topical corticosteroids and an antihistamine are used to treat it. Continuing the antifungal agent is critical to resolving the fungal infection (Williams, Godfrey, & Friedlander, 2003).

Tinea Corporis

Topical antifungal cream (e.g., clotrimazole, miconazole, ketocona-zole, naftifine, terbinafine) twice a day for 4 weeks; wash with sele-nium sulfide shampoo.

An oral antifungal agent may be needed when lesions are extensive, involve hair follicles, or there is no response to topical therapy.

Nursing Management

Emphasize the need to take the oral antifungal medication for at least 6 weeks. Medication absorption is enhanced if given with a high-fat food such as whole milk or peanut butter.

Assess all family members and household pets for fungal lesions.

Educate the child and family to avoid personal contact with hair and sharing of hair accessories, brushes, and hats.

Inform parents and children with tinea capitis that hair regrowth is slow and may take 6–12 months.

Diaper Dermatitis

An irritant contact dermatitis in infants from 4 to 12 months of age. Caused when urine and feces interact with the skin. *Candida albi-cans* is a secondary infection that may occur after antibiotic therapy for another condition.

Clinical Manifestations

Primary irritant rash—glazed red plaques over the skin in direct con-tact with the diaper area; the skin folds are spared; in severe cases, a fiery-red, raised, and confluent rash may be seen

Candida albicans secondary infection—bright-red scaly plaques with sharp margins; small papules and pustules may be seen, along with satellite lesions; skin folds are involved

Clinical Therapy

Diagnosis is usually based on appearance.

Irritant rash—with each diaper change for 5–7 days, apply barrier or protective sealant, such as zinc-oxide paste, Desitin, or Balmex; ap-plication of low- to moderate-potency (0.25–1.0%) hydrocortisone cream before application of protective sealant.

Candida albicans—alternate applications of 1% hydrocortisone cream and antifungal creams (clotrimazole or nystatin) to the af-fected areas at each diaper change, so that each medication is applied several times a day; an oral antifungal agent may be given to clear the candidiasis from the intestines.

Nursing Management

Change the diaper as soon as it is wet, or at least every 2 hours during the day and once during the night. Use superabsorbent disposable diapers. Expose the diaper area to air.

Wash the perianal area with warm water and a mild soap (e.g., unscented Dove or Tone) or a nonwater cleanser (Aquanil HC lotion or Cetaphil) only after a bowel movement. Use soft paper towels with warm tap water or baby wipes without alcohol.

Avoid use of powders until the skin has healed.

Apply A&D ointment, zinc oxide, Desitin, and Balmex to protect the skin from urine and stool.

Observe for signs of infection. Encourage parents to return if significant improvement is not seen within a week.

Impetigo

Impetigo is a highly contagious, superficial infection of minor skin abrasions, lacerations, insect bites, burns, or dermatitis caused by streptococci, staphylococci, or both.

Clinical Manifestations

The lesion begins as a vesicle or pustule surrounded by edema and redness at an injured site. The serous vesicular fluid becomes cloudy, and the vesicle ruptures, leaving a honey-colored crust covering an ulcerated base. Pruritus and regional lymphadenopathy may be present.

Diagnostic Tests

Impetigo is diagnosed by appearance. A Gram stain and bacterial culture may be used.

Clinical Therapy

Soak crusts in warm water and gently scrub them off with an antiseptic soap.

Apply topical bactericidal ointment (e.g., bacitracin or mupirocin) for 5–7 days. If there is no response to topical antibiotics; a skin culture and a systemic oral antibiotic may be needed.

Nursing Management

Educate parents to cleanse the lesions and apply topical medications. Emphasize the need to use the topical or oral antibiotic for the full number of days prescribed.

The infection is communicable for 48 hours after antibiotic ointment treatment is begun. Inform parents of ways to reduce spread of infection to others. Inform the childcare center about the child's infection, so that toys and surfaces can be sanitized.

Pediculosis Capitis (Lice)

Pediculosis capitis is an infestation of the hair and scalp with lice. Head lice live and reproduce only on humans and are transmitted by direct hair-to-hair contact or indirect contact by sharing hair accessories, brushes, hats, towels, and bedding.

Clinical Manifestations

Intense pruritus, sesame-sized bugs or nits in the hair, open sores from scratching.

Nits look like silvery white, yellow, or darker 1-mm teardrops adhering to one side of the hair shaft, commonly behind the ears and at base of head.

Posterior cervical nodes may be palpable.

Clinical Therapy

Lice are diagnosed by their presence in the hair.

Use pediculicide shampoo, such as pyrethrin with an enzymatic lice egg remover, or an ovicidal rinse, such as permethrin (Nix). A second-line therapy is malathion (Ovide); however, toxicity, flammability, odor, and higher cost are a concern. Products without pesticides include Lice B Gone, Lice Away Enzyme Shampoo, and Hair Clean 1-2-3.

The hair is towel dried, and the nits are removed with a fine-toothed comb. A second treatment is needed in 7 days because the neurotoxin is ineffective on nits.

Nursing Management

Assessment

Use a bright light and magnifying glass to see the lice and nits along the hair shaft, close to the scalp. Distinguish lice and nits from dandruff flakes. Examine all family members and contacts for lice.

Intervention

Educate parents to use the pediculicide for the time specified on the directions. If the child has extra long hair, use a second bottle of pediculicide.

Remove the nits with a fine-toothed comb, tweezers, and a basin filled with water or isopropyl alcohol to dip and clean the comb and tweezers. Nits adhere to the hair shaft and must be manually pulled down it. If the nit cannot be removed, cut the hair shaft below the level of the nit.

Check the hair every 2–3 days, and remove any lice or nits seen. Repeat treatment 1 week later, as lice may hatch in 6–8 days. The child may return to childcare or school after the first pediculicide treatment.

Teach the child not to share clothing, headwear, or combs. Bedding and clothing used by the child should be changed daily, laundered in hot water with detergent, and dried in a hot dryer for 20 minutes. Seal toys and other personal items that cannot be washed or dry cleaned in a plastic bag for 2 weeks.

Scabies

A highly contagious infestation caused by the mite *Sarcoptes scabei* and spread by skin-to-skin contact, often within a household. The female mite burrows into the outer layer of the epidermis to lay her eggs, leaving a trail of debris and feces. The larvae hatch in approximately 2–4 days and proceed toward the surface of the skin. The cycle is repeated 14–17 days later.

Clinical Manifestations

Papules on hands, lesions in webs of fingers and skin folds, lesions on palms and wrists of hands, irritation and intense pruritus

Linear, threadlike, grayish burrows 1–10 cm in length

Secondary infection from scratching

Diagnostic Tests

Microscopic view of burrow scrapings often reveals actively moving mites, fecal pellets, and eggs or nits.

Clinical Therapy

A scabicide, such as 5% permethrin lotion, is applied over the entire body, including the scalp and forehead after a bath when the skin is cool and dry. Do not apply to an infant's face. The lotion can be applied to an older child's face if lesions are present. The lotion is left in place for 8–12 hours (overnight) before washing it off. A second treatment is used 1 week later. Treat all family members and childcare givers at the same time, even if not symptomatic. An oral antihistamine may be prescribed to help relieve itching.

Nursing Management

Advise parents that scabies is highly contagious and transmitted by close contact. All clothing, bedding, and pillowcases used by the child should be changed daily, washed with hot water, and ironed before reuse. Nonwashable toys and other items should be sealed in plastic bags for 5–7 days.

VASCULAR TUMORS (HEMANGIOMAS)

Vascular tumors, or *hemangiomas*, are neoplasms of endothelial cells and increased numbers of small blood vessels that undergo rapid growth and proliferation during the first 6–10 months during infancy. This phase is followed by a slow decrease in size over several years.

Clinical Manifestations

Superficial hemangiomas—bright-red vascular cutaneous plaques that resemble strawberries.

Deep hemangiomas—bluish tumors covered with normal-appearing epidermis.

Mixed hemangiomas have features of both superficial and deep tumors.

The lesions are minimally compressible and have no bruit or thrill. Ulceration of the vascular tumor may occur during the period of rapid growth.

Diagnostic Tests

Initial diagnosis is by physical examination and monitoring the growth of the vascular tumor. Ultrasound, computed tomography scanning, or magnetic resonance imaging may also be used.

Clinical Therapy

Systemic corticosteroids are used during the proliferation phase for infants with extensive facial hemangiomas. A daily dose of oral prednisone is given for 7–10 days, and the dose is then tapered to the lowest effective dose for a 4–6 week course of treatment. Two- to four-week rest periods between courses of corticosteroid treatment may be prescribed (Dinehart, Kincannon, Geronemus, 2001). Injections of corticosteroids into small localized hemangiomas are sometimes performed.

Pulsed dye laser treatment is used for superficial hemangiomas during the proliferative phase.

Nursing Management
Assessment

Assess the distribution of the hemangioma, and consider the potential for pressure on vital structures as it goes through a rapid growth stage.

Monitor for ulceration of the hemangioma or compression on the airway.

Monitor the infant's growth, because corticosteroid treatment may slow growth.

Assess the parents' response to the infant's appearance.

Intervention
Educate parents about the type of vascular lesion, administration of corticosteroids, and potential medication side effects (gastrointestinal upset, sleep disturbance, temporary growth retardation, decreased appetite, and transient facial edema).

Inform parents about possible ulceration as the hemangioma grows rapidly and signs to expect. Tell them to cover and protect the skin from infection until seen by the physician.

Help parents see positive characteristics in the infant (e.g., responsiveness to interaction and smiling). Show parents photographs of other children who have completed therapy to show that gradual improvements are possible.

Prepare parents for changes to the child's appearance with pulsed dye laser therapy (initial appearance will be darkening of the hemangioma for 1–2 weeks, followed by fading to red and eventual lightening of the treated skin surface). Protect treated skin from sun exposure, and use sunscreen in the future.

INJURIES TO THE INTEGUMENTARY SYSTEM
Animal Bites
Children are at a higher risk for animal bites, and most cases involve dogs. Bites are commonly associated with inappropriate behavior by the child, such as teasing, playing, or interfering with feeding.

Clinical Manifestations
Dog bites tend to be crushing, rather than clean, sharp lacerations. Dog bites are more commonly on the upper torso, face, and scalp in children, rather than on the arms and legs. Cat bites tend to be puncture wounds.

Diagnostic Tests
Damage to nerves, muscles, tendons, and vascular structures is identified by physical examination. Head and neck bites require radiographic examination to rule out any associated injury, such as airway trauma or a depressed skull fracture.

Clinical Therapy
Initial treatment includes irrigation of the wound, removal of devitalized tissue, and a clean dressing. Conscious sedation and pain man-

agement may be needed. Some wounds require surgical closure or reconstruction. Antibiotics may be prescribed.

Arrange to have the animal observed for 10 days for signs of rabies.

Human rabies immune globulin or human diploid cell rabies vaccine should be given to all children bitten by any animal proven to be rabid, or in which rabies cannot be excluded.

Nursing Management
Assessment
Observe and document the extent of the injury, circumstances surrounding the attack, present location of the animal, and attempts to assess the animal's health.

Intervention
Irrigate the wound with large quantities of sterile saline or lactated Ringer's solution. Apply a clean pressure dressing, and elevate the affected part to reduce bleeding.

Determine whether a tetanus booster is needed.

Teach parents how to care for the wound and how to identify signs of infection.

Patient and Family Education to Prevent Animal Bites
General guidelines for pets in the home:
- Never leave a young child alone with an animal.
- Do not buy a pet unless you are confident of your child's ability to respect it.
- Spay or neuter the pet to reduce aggression.

If an animal (wild or unknown) is sick or acting strangely, notify the health department.

Teach children the following rules:
- Avoid unfamiliar animals, and report them to a parent.
- Avoid contact with all wild animals.
- Do not touch an animal when it is eating, sleeping, or nursing.
- Never overexcite an animal. Do not roughhouse or play games that stimulate aggressive behavior.
- Never tease or throw objects at an animal.
- Never put your face close to an animal. Seek permission before hugging or petting an animal.
- If approached by a dog, stay calm, stand still, talk softly, and back away slowly until the dog loses interest; do not run.

- If attacked, pretend to be a tree or a log, and protect the face.

Burns

Burns result from different mechanisms.

- Thermal burns, the most common burns in children, may occur through exposure to flames, scalds, or contact with a hot object.
- Chemical burns occur when children touch or ingest caustic agents.
- Electrical burns occur from exposure to direct or alternating current in electrical wires, appliances, or high-voltage wires, as well as lightning strikes.
- Radiation burns result from exposure to radioactive substances or sunlight.

A full-thickness burn can occur in adults after a 2-second immersion in water with a temperature of 65°C (149°F). Infants and children have more sensitive skin and burn more quickly (Stewart, 2000).

After the burn, intense vasoconstriction results in ischemia that may increase the depth of the burn injury. Vasoactive hormone release increases capillary permeability resulting in edema and decreased circulating blood volume. Water and heat is lost through the injured skin. The child's metabolic rate and need for calories increase as the child tries to maintain body temperature.

Clinical Manifestations

Burns are classified by depth.

Partial-thickness burns, in which the injured tissue can regenerate and heal, encompass first- and second-degree burns. Severe pain is associated with partial-thickness burns.

Full-thickness burns, in which the injured tissue cannot regenerate, are known as third-degree burns.

Diagnostic Tests

Burn severity is determined by the depth of the burn injury, percentage of BSA affected, and involvement of specific body parts. BSA is calculated using a Lund-Browder chart.

Major burns involve a partial thickness burn on >20% BSA, full thickness ≥10% BSA, and all burns that involve the face, eyes, ears, hands, feet, and perineum. Circumferential burns (injury completely surrounding the thorax or an extremity), anterior chest burns, and smoke inhalation are also classified as major burns.

Moderate burns involve partial thickness burns over 10–20% BSA or full thickness burns over 3–10% BSA.

Minor burns involve partial thickness burns over <10% BSA or full thickness burns over <2% BSA.

Clinical Therapy

Initial care involves ensuring that the child has an airway, is breathing, and has a pulse. Use moist soaks or ice over small areas to stop the burning process and to relieve pain. Treatment focuses on decreasing burn fluid losses, preventing infection, controlling pain, promoting nutrition, and salvaging all viable burned tissue. Intravenous fluid replacement with lactated Ringer's or normal saline is given to prevent hypovolemic shock in cases of major burn injury using the Parkland or Galveston formula for calculation. The child's temperature is maintained.

Continuous enteral feedings are often initiated within 6 hours of the burn injury to support the child's increased nutritional requirements. These children often need nearly twice the basal metabolic caloric requirements and nearly 2-g/kg body weight of protein (Smith, 2000).

Débridement (removal of dead tissue to speed the healing process) is performed using sedation and anesthesiology support for pain management. Hydrotherapy may be used to help clean the wound before débridement. Antibacterial topical creams [sulfadiazine, mafenide acetate (Sulfamylon), or bacitracin] may be applied and covered with a dressing. Dressing changes occur once or twice daily. Superficial second-degree burns re-epithelialize within 3 weeks.

Skin grafting is necessary with any deep second- or third-degree burn. The graft or a skin-replacement product, such as TransCyte, is placed after the wound is débrided in the operating room. This protective barrier decreases infection risk and protects against fluid loss.

Physical therapy and occupational therapy are important in promoting joint and muscle function, as well as self-care skills. Splints may help prevent contractures and reduce scarring. Jobst or pressure garments are used to reduce development of hypertrophic scarring and contractures.

Nursing Management

Assessment

Perform an initial emergency assessment of airway, breathing, and circulation. Assess for signs of smoke inhalation, burns to the face and neck, or other potential injuries when the mechanism of injury also includes a fall or explosion.

Inspect the location, extent, and shape of the burn injury. Consider the potential for child abuse with burns having the following characteristics: glove and stocking burns, burns that spare flexor surfaces, contact burns from cigarettes or irons, or zebra burn lines from contact with a hot grate.

Frequently monitor vital signs, circulatory and respiratory status, pain control, intake and output, and daily weight measurement. Be alert to signs of infection.

Assess the child's and family's concerns over appearance and the stress of hospitalization. Identify how well the family is coping with the child's injury and other family stressors.

Intervention
Provide nursing care that includes dressing changes, hydrotherapy, antibiotic therapy, fluid and nutrition management, analgesic support, and play therapy.

Prevent complications, such as infections, pneumonia, renal failure, and irreversible loss of function. Perform range-of-motion exercises.

Provide wound care according to guidelines and physician orders.

Increase the child's fluid intake to compensate for fluid loss through damaged skin. Encourage a high-calorie, high-protein diet to meet the increased nutritional requirements of healing.

Encourage the child and parents to voice concerns, and show understanding and support.

Children with minor burns are cared for at home after an initial visit to the emergency department to débride any open blisters and apply topical antibiotic and dressing. Provide pain medication before dressing changes. Educate the parents to observe for signs of infection.

Patient and Family Education: Care of Minor Burns
Place burn under cool, running water to stop the burning process and to help pain. Do not use ice.

Remove all clothing and jewelry from the burned area.

Apply a topical antibiotic, such as Neosporin.

Insect Bites and Stings
Insect and spider bites, as well as stings in some cases, are venomous or produce an allergic reaction.

Clinical Manifestations

Bee or Wasp Sting

Venoms contain enzymes that affect vascular tone and permeability. Local reaction includes mild, local pain; erythema; and edema. Systemic reaction includes generalized urticaria, flushing, angioedema, pruritus, and wheezing. Anaphylaxis is rare.

Fire Ants

Venom is hemolytic and neurotoxic, causing a histaminelike response. Local reaction includes a black center at the point of the bite or a trail of lesions across the skin; initial wheal turns into a vesicle within a few hours, and, in 24 hours, the fluid is cloudy, and the vesicle is surrounded by a red halo; pruritus; and erythema, edema, and induration. Systemic and anaphylactic reactions can occur.

Black Widow Spider

Venom is neurotoxic. Local reaction includes stinging sensation at time of bite, localized edema and erythema, two fang marks, and petechiae branching from site. A systemic reaction occurs in 1–3 hours with muscle rigidity of torso and abdomen, priapism, muscle cramps near the bite; malaise, sweating, nausea, vomiting, dizziness, hypertension and arrhythmias; oliguria; and restlessness and insomnia. Symptoms peak in 3–12 hours and diminish within 72 hours.

Brown Recluse Spider

Venom contains proteolytic enzymes and a cytotoxic factor. Reaction includes erythema and edema evolving to a purple bull's-eye lesion with an outer white zone of induration, progression to severe necrosis with scab that hardens and falls off in 7–14 days, and an ulcerated depression that heals in 6–8 weeks with scarring. Necrosis is more extensive on adipose tissue. Severe systemic reactions may occur in 12–72 hours, including fever, chills, restlessness, malaise, joint pain, and nausea and vomiting.

Clinical Therapy

Ice, cool compresses; elevate the extremity; antihistamine medication; remove bee stinger.

Children with a severe allergic reaction to insects should wear a medical alert identification and carry an emergency kit with epinephrine. Teach the child, parents, and school personnel how to administer epinephrine.

Desensitization injections may be given to children with an anaphylactic reaction or severe systemic reaction to bees, wasps, and fire ants.

Antivenom, diazepam, and opioids may be given for black widow spider bites.

Excision and skin grafting may be performed in cases of severe necrosis due to brown recluse spider bites.

Nursing Management

Encourage parents and children to become familiar with insects and spiders in the geographic area. Teach children to avoid spiders and other biting or stinging insects.

Use an insect repellent. Avoid the use of perfumed shampoos, powders, soaps, lotions, or bright-colored or floral-print clothing when outdoors. Avoid eating sweet foods and beverages outdoors, as these attract bees and wasps.

Teach children to stay calm when a bee or wasp approaches and to slowly walk away without swatting.

Pressure Ulcers

Tissue ischemia due to pressure deprives cells of oxygen and nutrients and can result in a soft tissue injury. Without intervention, the injury rapidly progresses and a pressure ulcer forms. Children at greatest risk are those with paralysis, limited mobility or low activity, sensory deficits, or the inability to change positions and chronic fecal or urinary soiling.

Sites and potential causes of pressure ulcers include

- Occipital region of scalp—inability to lift head
- Sacrum and buttocks—confinement to bed or wheelchair
- Legs and feet—orthotics, leg braces, casts
- Spine and neck—scoliosis brace
- Knees and elbows—rubbing against bed sheet

Clinical Manifestations

Stage 1—an area of redness that does not dissipate within 30 minutes of removing the pressure or skin irritant

Stage 2—the skin looks rubbed or raw (superficial or partial-thickness injury), similar to an abrasion or blister

Stage 3—an ulcer forms as skin damage extends through the epidermis and dermis

Stage 4—the injury deepens to underlying tissue, muscles, bone, or connective tissue

Clinical Therapy

Diagnosis is based on appearance of the skin.

Remove pressure from the affected site until the skin has healed. Frequent repositioning is needed.

A transparent film may be applied to affected red skin to minimize friction.

Pressure ulcers are treated with various dressings, such as hydrocolloids, gels or hydrogels, and calcium alginates.

Nursing Management

Assessment

Inspect the dependent skin surfaces of all infants and children confined to bed at least three times in each 24-hour period. Identify the size (diameter and depth) and character of the skin lesion.

Note any signs of infection, the appearance of wound edges, and the type of tissue at the wound base. Describe drainage amount, color, and type.

Intervention

Develop protocols for pressure ulcer prevention for children at high risk.

- Increase ambulation, post a turning schedule or encourage frequent position changes, and encourage use of pressure-reducing surfaces and use of moisture barriers.
- Ensure adequate intake of fluids, proteins, and vitamins.
- Provide wound care and dressing changes according to agency guidelines.
- Avoid the use of tape to hold dressings in place unless a protective skin barrier is used.

Teach children with impaired mobility and diminished pain sensation and the parents to inspect the braces and skin under the braces daily for signs of irritation (redness or blisters). Check all edges of the braces for roughness that can pinch or scrape the skin. Brace should not be worn if any redness does not diminish within 30 minutes. Have the child wear cotton socks under the braces to prevent rubbing of bare skin.

Sunburn

Sunburn is a burn injury to the outer layer of skin caused by excess ultraviolet light exposure, or sun exposure after taking phototoxic drugs. Sunburn occurs more often in children with red or blond hair and fair skin that freckles easily. The risk for melanoma and basal cell carcinoma is strongly related to a history of one or more severe blistering sunburns during childhood or adolescence.

Clinical Manifestations

Erythema and skin tenderness usually develop between 30 minutes and 4 hours after exposure to sunlight. Prolonged exposure can result in edema, vesiculation, bullae, or ulceration.

Clinical Therapy

Increase oral fluids. Relieve pain with cool compresses followed by the application of a low-potency topical corticosteroid (on unblistered skin) to relieve discomfort. Nonsteroidal anti-inflammatory drugs may be used for pain relief and to reduce inflammation.

Nursing Management

Teach adolescents how to monitor for changes in moles that could signal the development of skin cancer and to seek care immediately. Characteristics of moles that indicate a need for evaluation include those that are asymmetric, have an irregular border, have color variations, and have a diameter larger than 0.6 cm.

Patient and Family Education: Preventing Sunburn

Keep children out of direct sunlight as much as possible. Avoid scheduling outdoor activities during the hours of maximum exposure (10 AM to 2 PM).

When outdoors, minimize exposure by wearing hats and long-sleeve, closely woven cotton clothing and pants; wear T-shirts while swimming. Special sun-protection clothing is now available from some manufacturers.

Water, concrete, and sand reflect sunlight and increase exposure reflecting up to 85% of the ultraviolet rays.

Use sunscreen (of at least 15 skin protection factor). For optimal protection, apply as thickly as directed to all exposed areas 30–45 minutes before sun exposure. Reapply every 2 hours as needed, or sooner if swimming, toweling off, or perspiring heavily.

Use a waterproof sunscreen when swimming; this provides protection in water for approximately 60–80 minutes. Then reapply. Call the poison control center immediately if sunscreen gets in the eyes as it causes a chemical burn.

Avoid using sunscreens in infants younger than 6 months because of the possibility of absorption of the chemicals through their skin.

A child can be burned even on a cloudy day, as 80% of ultraviolet rays can penetrate the cloud cover.

Some medications cause hypersensitivity to sunlight. Check with your healthcare practitioner for guidance.

REFERENCES

Acosta, K., Vade, A., Lomasney, L. M., Demos, T. C., & Bielski, R. (2001). Radiologic case study. Orthopedics, 24,737–745.

Adekoya, N., Thurman, D. J., White, D. D., & Webb, K. W. (2002). Surveillance for traumatic brain injury deaths—United States, 1989–1998. Morbidity and Mortality Weekly Report, 51(SS-10),1–14.

Adesman, A. (2003). A diagnosis of ADHD? Don't overlook the probability of comorbidity! Contemporary Pediatrics, 20(12),91–106.

Advisory Committee on Childhood Lead Poisoning Prevention. (2000). Recommendation for blood lead screening of young children enrolled in Medicare: Targeting a group at high risk. Morbidity and Mortality Weekly Report, 49(RR14),1–13.

Alcorn, D. M. (2001). Red eye: When to treat and when to refer. Infectious Diseases in Children, 3–8.

Alemzadeh, R., & Wyatt, D. T. (2004). Diabetes mellitus in children. In R. E. Behrman, R. M. Kliegman, & H. B. Jenson. (Eds.), Nelson Textbook of Pediatrics (17th ed.) (pp. 1947–1972). Philadelphia: Saunders.

Alexander, M. (2003). Ocular allergy: Treatment options for children. Contemporary Pediatrics, Suppl,3–6.

American Academy of Pediatric Dentistry. (2000). Policy on early childhood caries (ECC): Unique challenges and treatment options. http://www.aapd.org, accessed 8/31/2003.

American Academy of Pediatrics. (2000). Types of learning disabilities. http://www.aap.org/pubed/ZZZ0QSFNQ7C.htm?&sub_cat=1, accessed 9/24/2005.

American Academy of Pediatrics. (2001). Diagnosis and management of autistic spectrum disorder. Pediatrics, 107,1221–1226.

American Academy of Pediatrics. (2003). Red book: 2003 Report of the Committee on Infectious Diseases (26th ed.). Elk Grove Village, IL.

American Academy of Pediatrics. (2004). Car safety seats: A guide for families. Elk Grove Village, IL.

American Academy of Pediatrics. (2004a). Pediatric nutrition handbook (5th ed.). Elk Grove Village, IL.

American Academy of Pediatrics. (2004b). Management of hyperbilirubinemia in the newborn infant 35 or more weeks of gestation. Pediatrics, 114 (1),297–316. http://aappolicy.aappublications.org/cgi/content/full/pediatrics;114/1/297, accessed 1/20/05.

American Academy of Pediatrics Committee on Practice and Ambulatory Medicine and Section on Ophthalmology. (2003). Eye examination in infants, children, and young adults by pediatricians. Pediatrics, 111,902–907.

American Academy of Pediatrics Committee on Infectious Diseases and Committee on Fetus and Newborn. (2003). Revised indications for the use of palivizumab and respiratory syncytial virus immune globulin intravenous for the prevention of respiratory syncytial virus. Pediatrics, 112,1442–1446.

American Academy of Pediatrics Committee on Quality Improvement, Subcommittee on Attention-Deficit/Hyperactivity Disorder. (2001). Clinical practice guideline: Treatment of the school-aged child with attention-deficit/hyperactivity disorder. Pediatrics, 108,1033–1044.

American Association of Mental Retardation. (2004). Definition of mental retardation. http://www.aamr.org/Policies/faq_mental_retardation.shtml, accessed 7/15/2004.

American Heart Association. (2002). Pediatric advanced life support provider manual. Dallas, TX.

American Psychiatric Association. (2000). Diagnostic and statistical manual of mental disorders (4th ed., text revision). Washington, D.C.

American Psychiatric Association Working Group on Eating Disorders. (2000). Practice guidelines for the treatment of patients with eating disorders. American Journal of Psychiatry, 157,1–39.

Anderson, P. M. (2004). Neoplasms of the kidney. In R. E. Behrman, R. M. Kliegman, & H. B. Jenson (Eds.), Nelson textbook of pediatrics (17th ed.) (pp. 1554–1556). Philadelphia: Saunders.

Arceci, R. J., & Cripe, T. P. (2002). Emerging cancer-targeted therapies. Pediatric Clinics of North America, 49,1339–1368.

Arguin, A. L., & Swartz, M. K. (2004). Gastroesophageal reflux in infants: A primary care perspective. Pediatric Nursing, 30,45–52.

Arvin, A. M. (2002). Antiviral therapy for varicella and herpes zoster. Seminars in Pediatric Infectious Diseases, 13,12–21.

Ashfield, J. E., Nickel, K. R., Siemens, D. R., MacNeily, A. E., & Nickel, J. C. (2003). Treatment of phimosis with topical steroids in 194 children. Journal of Urology, 169,1106–1108.

Baggott, C. R., Kelly, K. P., Fochtman, D., & Foley, G. V. (2002). Nursing care of children and adolescents with cancer (3rd ed.). Philadelphia: Saunders.

Baird, G., Charman, T., Cox, A., Baron-Cohen, S., Swettenham, J., Wheelwright, S., & Drew, A. (2001). Screening and surveillance for autism and pervasive developmental disorders. Archives of Disease in Childhood, 84,468–475.

Baron, M. L. (2002). Crohn disease in children. American Journal of Nursing, 102(10),26–34.

Barst, R. J. (1999). Recent advances in the treatment of pediatric pulmonary artery hypertension. Pediatric Clinics of North America, 46,331–345.

Behrman, R. E., Kliegman, R. M., & Jenson, H. B. (2004). Nelson textbook of pediatrics (17th ed.). Philadelphia: Saunders.

Bell, F. (2000). Post-renal transplant compliance. Journal of Child Health Care, 4,5–9.

Berul, C. I. (2000). Cardiac evaluation in the young athlete. Pediatric Annals, 29,162–165.

Betcher, D. L., Simon, P. J., & McHard, K. M. (2002). In C. R. Baggott, K. P. Kelly, & D. Fochtman (Eds.), Nursing care of children and adolescents with cancer (3rd ed.) (pp. 575–588). Philadelphia: Saunders.

Biggar, W. D., Gingras, M., Feblings, D. L., Harris, V. A., & Steele, C. A. (2001). Deflazacort treatment of Duchenne muscular dystrophy. Journal of Pediatrics, 138,45–50.

Bindler, R. C., & Ball, J. W. (2003). Clinical skills manual for pediatric nursing: Caring for children (3rd ed.). Upper Saddle River, NJ: Prentice Hall.

Blackburn, S. T. (2003). Maternal, fetal, and neonatal physiology: A clinical perspective (pp. 656–669). St. Louis: Saunders.

Blair, J., & Selekman, J. (2004). Epilepsy. In P. J. Allen, & J. A. Vessey (Eds.), Primary care of the child with a chronic condition (4th ed.) (pp. 469–497). St. Louis: Mosby.

Blevins, J. Y. (2003). Primary herpetic gingivostomatitis in young children. Pediatric Nursing, 29, 199–202.

Bleyer, A. (2004). Principles of diagnosis: Principles of treatment. In R. E. Behrman, R. M. Kliegman, & H. B. Jenson (Eds.), Nelson textbook of pediatrics (17th ed.) (pp. 1684–1693). Philadelphia: Saunders.

Boland, E. A., & Grey, M. (2004). Diabetes mellitus (types 1 and 2). In P. J. Allen & J. A. Vessey. Primary care of the child with a chronic condition. (4th ed.) (pp. 426–444). St. Louis: Mosby.

Bolton-Maggs, P. H. B. (2000). Idiopathic thrombocytopenic purpura. Archives of Disease in Childhood, 83,220–223.

Bowman, B. A., & Russell, R. M. (2001). Present knowledge of nutrition (8th ed.). Washington, D.C.: International Life Sciences Institute.

Brambilla, F. (2001). Social stress in anorexia nervosa: A review of immuno-endocrine relationships. Physiology and Behavior, 73,365–369.

Brook, M. M. (1999). Pediatric bacterial endocarditis: Treatment and pro-phylaxis. Pediatric Clinics of North America, 46,275–287.

Buck, M. L. (2001). Isotretinoin: Improving patient education and reducing risk. Pediatric Pharmacology, 7(7),1–6.

Buck, M. L. (2003). Clinical applications for botulinum toxin type A in pedi-atric patients. Pediatric Pharmacology, 9(3). http://www.medscape.com/viewarticle/451626, accessed 4/18/2003.

Burd, A. J., & Burd, R. S. (2002). Inguinal hernia in the premature infant: Management of a common problem. Neonatal Network, 21(7),39–47.

Busen, N.H., Modeland, U. & Kouzekananni, K. (2001). Adolescent ciga-rette smoking and health risk behavior. Journal of Pediatric Nursing, 16,187–193.

Cade, M., & Tidwell, S. (2001). Autism and the school nurse. Journal of School Health, 71,96–100.

Campbell, S. (2003). Prenatal cocaine exposure and neonatal/infant out-comes. Neonatal Network, 22,19–21.

Capper-Michel, B. (2004). Bronchopulmonary dysplasia. In P. J. Allen & J. A. Vessey (Eds.), Primary care of the child with a chronic condition, (4th ed.) (pp. 282–298). St. Louis: Mosby.

Carek, P. J., Dickerson, L. M., & Sack, J. L. (2001). Diagnosis and management of osteomyelitis. American Family Physician, 63,2413–2420.

Carley, A. (2003). Anemia: When is it iron deficiency? Pediatric Nursing, 29,128–133.

Cash, S. (2004). Guideline offers direction for prompt diagnosis, treatment of hyperbilirubinemia. American Academy of Pediatrics News. Reprinted from American Academy of Pediatrics (July 2004). AAP news. Elk Grove Village, IL: American Academy of Pediatrics.

Castiglia, P. T. (2000a). Depression in children. Journal of Pediatric Health Care, 14,73–75.

Castiglia, P. T. (2000b). Depression in adolescents. Journal of Pediatric Health Care, 14,180–182.

Caulton, J. M., Ward, K. A., Alsop, C. W., Dunn, G., Adams, J. E., & Mughal, M. Z. (2004). A randomized controlled trial of standing programme on bone mineral density in non-ambulant children with cerebral palsy. Archives of Disease in Childhood, 89,131–135.

Centers for Disease Control and Prevention (2002). Sexually transmitted diseases treatment guidelines 2002. Morbidity and Mortality Weekly Recommendations and Reports, 51(RR-6),1–82.

Centers for Disease Control and Prevention (2004). Diabetes projects. http://www.cdc.gov/diabetes/projects/cda2.htm, accessed 12/12/2004.

Centers for Disease Control and Prevention (2005). Recommended childhood and adolescent immunization schedule—United States, 2005. http://www.cdc.gov, accessed 2/3/2005.

Champi, C. (2002). Primary immunodeficiency disorders in children: Prompt diagnosis can lead to lifesaving treatment. Journal of Pediatric Health, 16(1),16–21.

Chan, Y. Y., & Bishop, N. J. (2002). Clinical management of childhood osteoporosis. International Journal of Clinical Practice, 56,280–286.

Cheng, K. K., Molassiotis, A., Chang, A. M., Wai, W. C., & Cheung, S. S. (2001). Evaluation of an oral care protocol in the prevention of chemotherapy-induced oral mucositis in paediatric cancer patients. European Journal of Cancer, 37,2056–2063.

Clayden, G., & Keshtgar, A. S. (2003). Management of childhood constipation. Postgraduate Medical Journal, 79,616.

Cohen, H., Chen, X. C., Sunkle, S., Davis, L., Geromanos, K., Xanthos, G., et al. (2000). Ability of caregivers to read delayed hypersensitivity skin tests in children exposed to and infected by HIV. Journal of Pediatric Health Care, 14,50–55.

Committee on Pediatric AIDS and Committee on Adolescence. (2001). Adolescents and human immunodeficiency virus infections: The role of the pediatrician in prevention and intervention. Pediatrics, 107,188–190.

Conway, E. E., Asuncion, A., & DaRosso, R. (1999). Diagnosing and managing brain tumors: The pediatrician's role. Contemporary Pediatrics, 16,84–97.

Cook, E. H., & Higgins, S. S. (2004). Congenital heart disease. In P. J. Allen & J. A. Vessey (Eds.), Primary care of the child with a chronic condition (4th ed.) (pp. 382–403). St. Louis: Mosby.

Cook, L. S. (2000). A simple case of anemia: Pathophysiology of a common symptom. Journal of Intravenous Nursing, 23,271–281.

Cooper, C. S., Andrews, J. I., Hansen, W. F., & Yankowitz, J. (2002). Antenatal hydronephrosis: Evaluation and outcome. Current Urology Reports, 3,131–138.

Cooper, M. A., Pommering, T. L., & Koranyi, K. (2003). Primary immunodeficiencies. American Family Physician, 68,2001.

Corrales, K. M., & Utter, S. L. (1999). Failure to thrive. In P. Q. Samour, K. K. Helm, & C. E. Lang (Eds.), Handbook of pediatric nutrition (2nd ed.) (pp. 395–412). Gaithersburg, MD: Aspen.

Curry, H. (2004). Bleeding disorder basics. Pediatric Nursing, 30,402–429.

Cystic Fibrosis Foundation. (2004). Genetic carrier testing for CF. http://www.cff.org, accessed 3/10/2004.

Derivan, M., & Ferrante, C. (2000). Aplastic anemia. Clinical Journal of Oncology Nursing, 5,228–229.

Dinehart, S. M., Kincannon, J., & Geronemus, R. (2001). Hemangiomas: Evaluation and treatment. Dermatologic Surgery, 27,475–485.

Ditmyer, S. (2004). Hydrocephalus. In P. J. Allen, & J. A. Vessey (Eds.), Primary care of the child with a chronic condition (4th ed.) (pp. 543–560). St. Louis: Mosby.

Driscoll, D. A. (2001). Duchenne and Becker muscular dystrophies. Contemporary OB/GYN, October,97–102.

Duchene, T. M. (2000). Managing sinusitis in children. Nurse Practitioner, 25(9),42–55.

Duitsman, D. M., Suddaby, E. C., & Masterson, G. (1999). Unique considerations for the pediatric heart transplant recipient: The role of the school nurse. Journal of School Nursing, 15(3),10–13.

Dulczak, S., & Frothingham, B. (2002). Retinoblastoma. In C. R. Baggott, K. P. Kelly, D. Fochtman, & G. V. Foley, Nursing care of children and adolescents with cancer (3rd ed.) (pp. 589–597). Philadelphia: Saunders.

Edmunds, M. W., & Mayhew, M. S. (2004). Pharmacology for the primary care provider (2nd ed.). Philadelphia: Elsevier Mosby.

Eiff, M. P., & Hatch, R. L. (2003). Boning up on common pediatric fractures. Contemporary Pediatrics, 20(11),30–59.

Elder, M. E. (2000). T-cell immunodeficiencies. Pediatric Clinics of North America, 47,1253–1274.

Ellsworth, P. I., Cendron, M., & McCullough, M. F. (2000). Surgical management of vesicoureteral reflux. Association of Operating Room Nurses Journal, 71,498–513.

English, M. (2002). Challenges in managing profound hypokalemia. British Medical Journal, 324,269–270.

Erickson, C. C., & Jones, C. S. (2000). Pediatric sudden cardiac death: What the pediatrician needs to know. Pediatric Annals, 29,509–518.

Fernandez, J, Carrol, C. L., & Baker, C. J. (2000). Discitis and vertebral osteomyelitis in children: An 18-year review. Pediatrics, 105,1299–1304.

Ferrer, F. A., & McKenna, P. H. (2000). Current approaches to the undescended testicle. Contemporary Pediatrics, 17(1),106–111.

Ferrieri, P., Gewitz, M. H., Gerber, M. A., Newburger, J. W., Dajani, A. S., Shulman, S. T., et al. (2002). Unique features of infective endocarditis in children. Pediatrics, 109,931–943.

Fish, K. B. (2000). Suicide awareness at the elementary school level. Journal of Psychosocial Nursing, 38,20–23.

Flynn, J. T. (2003). Recognizing and managing the hypertensive child. Contemporary Pediatrics, 20(8),38–60.

Foster, G. T., Vaziri, N. D., & Sassoon, C. S. H. (2001). Respiratory alkalosis. Respiratory Care, 46,384–391.

Freeman, J. M. (2003). What every pediatrician should know about the ketogenic diet. Contemporary Pediatrics, 20(5),113–127.

Froh, D. L. (2002). Alterations in pulmonary function in children. In K. L. McCance, & S. E. Huether (Eds.), Pathophysiology: The biologic basis for disease in adults and children (4th ed.) (pp. 1145–1169). St. Louis: Mosby.

Gadomski, A. (2002). Bronchiolitis dilemma: A happy wheezer and his unhappy parent. Contemporary Pediatrics, 19(11),40–59.

Gance-Cleveland, B. (2003). Adaptation to Addison's disease in a child: A case study. Journal of Pediatric Health Care, 17,301–310.

Gibson, F., & Nelson, N. (2000). Mount care for children with cancer. Pediatric Nursing 12,18–22.

Gilmore, A., & Thompson, G. H. (2003). Common childhood foot deformities. Consultant for Pediatricians, 2,63–71.

Gilstrap, L. C., & Oh, W. (Eds.). (2002). Guidelines for perinatal care (5th ed.). Elk Grove Village, IL: American Academy of Pediatrics and The American College of Obstetricians and Gynecologists.

Glaser, N. S., Shirali, A. C., Styne, D. M., & Jones, K. L. (1998). Acid–base homeostasis in children with growth hormone deficiency. Pediatrics, 102,1407–1414.

Gokhale, R. (2001). Chronic abdominal pain: Inflammatory bowel disease and eosinophilic gastroenteropathy. Pediatric Annals, 30,49–55.

Goldrick, B. A. (2003). Endocarditis associated with body piercing. American Journal of Nursing, 103,26–27.

Green, M., & Palfrey, J. S. (Eds.). (2002). Bright futures: Guidelines for health supervision of infants, children, and adolescents (2nd ed.). Arlington, VA: National Center for Education in Maternal and Child Health.

Gross, R. D. (2002). Understanding ocular infections and strategies for management. Contemporary Pediatrics, Suppl, 4–7,10–12.

Gungor, N., & Arslanian, S. (2004). Progressive beta cell failure in type 2 diabetes mellitus of youth. Journal of Pediatrics, 144,656–659.

Guskiewicz, K. M., Weaver, N. L., Padua, D. A., & Garrett, W. E. (2000). Epidemiology of concussion in collegiate and high school football players. American Journal of Sports Medicine, 28,643–650.

Halec, I., & Zimmerman, D. (2004). Coordinating care for children with Turner syndrome. Pediatric Annals, 33,189–196.

Harper, R. S. (2002). Back in the game: Preventing and treating athletic injuries in adolescents. Advance for Nurse Practitioners, 10,55–66.

Harvey, C. (2001). Compartment syndrome: When it is least expected. Orthopaedic Nursing, 20(3),15–26.

Hayes, R. O. (2001). State programs for universal newborn hearing screening. Pediatric Clinics of North America, 46,89–94.

Hazinski, M. F. (1999). Manual of pediatric critical care. St. Louis: Mosby.

Hedrick, H. L., Crombleholme, T. M., Flake, A. W., Nance, M. L., von Allmen, D., Howell, L. J., et al. (2004). Right congenital diaphragmatic hernia: Prenatal assessment and outcome. Journal of Pediatric Surgery, 39,319–323.

Hendricks-Ferguson, V. L. (2000). Crisis intervention strategies when caring for families of children with cancer. Journal of Pediatric Oncology Nursing, 17,3–11.

Herman-Giddens, M. E., Slora, E. J., Wasserman, R. C., Bourdony, C. J., Bhapkar, M. V., Koch, G. G., et al. (1997). Secondary sexual characteristics and menses in young girls seen in office practice: A study from the Pediatric Research in Office Settings network. Pediatrics, 99,505–512.

Herpertz-Dahlmann, B., Muller, B., Herpertz, S., Heussen, N., Hedebrand, J., & Remschmidt, H. (2001). Prospective 10-year follow-up in adolescent anorexia nervosa—course, outcome, psychiatric comorbidity, and psychosocial adaptation. Journal of Child Psychology and Psychiatry, 42,603–612.

Hillerman, W. L., Russell, C. L., Barry, D., Brewer, B., Bianchi. L., Cundiff, W., et al. (2002). Evaluation guidelines for adult and pediatric kidney transplant programs: The Missouri experience. Progress in Transplantation, 12,30–35.

Hogg, R. J., Furth, S., Lemley, K. V., Portman, R., Schwartz, G J, Coresh, J., et al. (2003). National Kidney Foundation's kidney disease outcomes quality initiative clinical practice guidelines for chronic kidney disease in children and adolescents: Evaluation, classification, and stratification. Pediatrics, 111,1416–1421.

Home Safety Council. (2004). Resource center. http://www.homesafety council.org/resource_center/resourcecenter.aspx, accessed 7/4/2004.

Horwitz, E. M., Prockop, D. J., Gordon, P. L., Koo, W. W., Fitzpatrick, L. A., Neel, M. D., et al. (2001). Clinical responses to bone marrow transplantation in children with severe osteogenesis imperfecta. Blood, 97,1227–1231.

Howard, E. R. (2001). Hirschsprung's disease and allied disorders. Gut, 49,741–742.

Hudson, G. T., & Dixon, D. (2003). Autism: Challenges in diagnosis and treatment. Clinician Reviews, 13,45–52.

Hussong, M. R. (2002). Non-Hodgkin's lymphoma. In C. R. Baggott, K. P. Kelly, D. Fochtman, & G. V. Foley, Nursing care of children and adolescents with cancer (3rd ed.) (pp. 536–544). Philadelphia: Saunders.

Hyman, P. E., & Danda, C. E. (2004). Understanding and treating childhood bellyaches. Pediatric Annals, 33,97–104.

Ilowite, N. T. (2002). Current treatment of juvenile rheumatoid arthritis. Pediatrics, 109,109–115.

Ishibashi, A. (2001). The needs of children and adolescents with cancer for information and social support. Cancer Nursing, 24,61–67.

Jakubik, L. D., Colfer, A., & Grossman, M. B. (2000). Pediatric short bowel syndrome: Pathophysiology, nursing care, and management issues. Journal of the Society of Pediatric Nurses, 5,111–121.

Jellinek, M., Patel, B. P., & Froehle, M. C. (Eds.) (2002). Bright futures in practice: Mental health (Vols. I & II). Arlington, VA: National Center for Education in Maternal and Child Health.

Jung, A. D. (2001). Gastroesophageal reflux in infants and children. American Family Physician, 64,1853–1860.

Kaplowitz, P. B., Oberfield, S. E., & the Drug and Therapeutics and Executive Committees of the Lawson Wilkins Pediatric Endocrine Society (1999). Reexamination of the age limit for defining when puberty is precocious in girls in the United States: Implications for evaluation and treatment. Pediatrics, 104,936–941.

Katz, D. A. (2001). Evaluation and management of inguinal and umbilical hernias. Pediatric Annals, 30,729–735.

Kaufman, M. W., Clark, J. Y., & Castro, C. L. (2001). Neonatal circumcision. Maternal Child Nursing, 26,197–201.

Kavey, R. E. W., Daniels, S. R., Lauer, R. M., Atkins, D. L., Hayman, L. L., Taubert, K., et al. (2003). American Heart Association guidelines for primary prevention of atherosclerotic cardiovascular disease beginning in childhood. Journal of Pediatrics, 142,368–372.

Kelly, D. A. (2002). Managing liver failure. Postgraduate Medical Journal, 78,660–667.

Kieckhefer, G., & Ratcliffe, M. (2004). Asthma. In P. J. Allen, & J. A. Vessey (Eds.), Primary care of the child with a chronic condition (4th ed.) (pp. 174–197). St. Louis: Mosby.

Kingsbury, K. J. (2003). Understanding the essentials of blood lipid metabolism. Progressive Cardiovascular Nursing, 18,13–18.

Kinsella, J. P., Parker, T. A., Ivy, D., & Abman, S. H. (2003). Noninvasive delivery of inhaled nitric oxide therapy for late pulmonary hypertension in newborn infants with congenital diaphragmatic hernia. Journal of Pediatrics, 142,397–401.

Kirschner, B. S. (2001). Management of abdominal pain. Pediatric Annals, 30,12–14.

Klein, E. J., Kapoor, D., & Shugerman, R. P. (2004). The diagnosis of intussusception. Clinical Pediatrics, 43,343–347.

Kliegman, R. M., & Willoughby, R. E. (2005). Prevention of necrotizing enterocolitis with probiotics. Pediatrics, 115,171–172.

Kline, M. W., Calles, N. R., Simon, C., & Schwarzwald, H. (2000). Pilot study of hydroxyurea in human immunodeficiency virus–infected children receiving didanosine and/or stavudine. Pediatric Infectious Disease Journal, 19,1083–1086.

Knight, J. R. (1997). Adolescent substance use: Screening, assessment, and intervention. Contemporary Pediatrics, 14,45, 51–56, 61–72.

Koleilat, M. A., Williams, L. W., & Ryan, M. E. (2003). Read the warning signs of primary immunodeficiency. Contemporary Pediatrics, 20(6),65–81.

Koo, H. P. (2001). Is it really cryptorchidism? Contemporary Urology, 13, 12–16, 31.

Kotb, M. A., Kotb, A., Sheba, M. F., & El Koofy, N. M. (2001). Evaluation of the triangular cord sign in the diagnosis of biliary atresia. Pediatrics, 108,416–420.

Kraus, S. J. (2001). Genitourinary imaging in children. Pediatric Clinics of North America, 48,1381–1423.

Kuehne, E. A., & Reilly, M. W. (2004). Prenatal cocaine exposure. In P. J. Allen, & J. A. Vessey (Eds.), Primary care of the child with a chronic condition (4th ed.) (pp. 708–721). Mosby: St. Louis.

Lam, J. P. H., Eunson, G. J., Munro, F. D., & Orr, J. D. (2001). Delayed presentation of handlebar injuries in children. British Medical Journal, 322,1288–1289.

Lang, M. M., & Towers, C. (2001). Identifying poststreptococcal glomerulonephritis. The Nurse Practitioner, 26(8),34–49.

Larsson, A., & Therrell, B. L. (2002). Newborn screening: The role of the obstetrician. Clinical Obstetrics and Gynecology, 45,697–732.

Lashley, F. R. (2002). Newborn screening: New opportunities and new challenges. Newborn and Infant Nursing Reviews, 2,228–242.

Leonard, M. (2002). Diagnostic evaluations and staging procedures. In C. R. Baggott, K. P. Kelly, D. Fochtman, & G. V. Foley, Nursing care of children and adolescents with cancer (3rd ed.) (pp. 66–89). Philadelphia: Saunders.

Leone, A. (2003). Relationship between cigarette smoking and other coronary risk factors in atherosclerosis: Risk of cardiovascular disease and preventive measures. Current Pharmacological Design, 9,2417–2423.

Lesperance, L., Wu, A. C., & Bernstein, H. (2002). Putting a dent in iron deficiency. Current Pediatrics, 19(7),77+.

Letton, R. W. (2001). Pyloric stenosis. Pediatric Annals, 30,745–750.

Leung, A. K. C., & Kellner, J. D. (2004). Acute sinusitis in children: Diagnosis and management. Journal of Pediatric Health Care, 18,72–76.

Lewin, M. B. (2000). The genetic basis of congenital heart disease. Pediatric Annals, 29,469–480.

Lewis, D. W., Scott, D., & Rendin, V. (2002). Treatment of pediatric headache. Expert Opinion in Pharmacotherapeutics, 3,1433–1441.

Lieberman, L. J., & McHugh, E. (2001). Health-related fitness of children who are visually impaired. Journal of Visual Impairment & Blindness, 5,272–287.

Lipshultz, S. E., Sleeper, L. A., Towbin, J. A., Lowe, A. M., Orav, E. J., Cox, G. F., et al. (2003). The incidence of pediatric cardiomyopathy in two regions of the United States. New England Journal of Medicine, 348,1647–1655.

Litovitz, T. L., Klein-Schwartz, W., White, S., Cobaugh, D. J., Youniss, J., Drab, A., et al. (2000). 1999 annual report of the American Association of Poison Control Centers Toxic Exposure Surveillance System. American Journal of Emergency Medicine, 18,517–574.

Lupus Foundation of America. (2001). Education. http://www.lupus.org/education/types.html, accessed 12/4/2004.

Maltezou, H. C., Spyridis, P., & Kafetzis, D. A. (2000). Extra-pulmonary tuberculosis in children. Archives of Disease in Childhood, 83,342–346.

March of Dimes (2004). Newborn screening: March of Dimes Newborn screening recommendations: Professionals and researchers. http://www.marchofdimes.com/professionals/681_1200.asp, accessed 2/25/2005.

McManus, J., & Gilchrist, G. S. (2000). Neuroblastoma. In R. E. Behrman, R. M. Kliegman, & H. B. Jenson (Eds.), Nelson textbook of pediatrics (16th ed.) (pp. 1552–1554). Philadelphia: Saunders.

McMullen, A. H., & Bryson, E. A. (2004). Cystic fibrosis. In P. J. Allen, & J. A. Vessey (Eds.), Primary care of the child with a chronic condition (4th ed.) (pp. 404–425). St. Louis, Mosby.

Meltzer-Brody, S., Hidalgo, R., Connor, K. M., & Davidson, J. R. T. (2000). Posttraumatic stress disorder: Prevalence, health care use and costs, and pharmacologic considerations. Psychiatric Annals, 30,722–730.

Merkel, S. (2002). Pain assessment in infants and young children: The finger span scale. American Journal of Nursing, 102(11),55–56.

Merkel, S. I., Voepel-Lewis, T., Shayevitz, J. R., & Malviya, S. (1997). The FLACC: A behavioral scale for scoring post-operative pain in young children. Pediatric Nursing, 23,293–297.

Metayer, C., Lynch, C. F., Clarke, E. A., Glimelius, B., Storm, H., Pukkala, E., et al. (2000). Second cancers among long-term survivors of Hodgkin's disease diagnosed in childhood and adolescence. Journal of Clinical Oncology, 18,2435–2443.

Michaud, L. J., Semes-Concepcion, J., Duhaime, A. C., & Lazar, M. F. (2002). Traumatic brain injury. In M. L. Batshaw (Ed.), Children with disabilities (5th ed.) (pp. 525–545). Baltimore: Paul H. Brooks Publishing Co.

Miller, B. S., & Zimmerman, D. (2004). Idiopathic short stature in children. Pediatric Annals, 33,177–181.

Mindell, J. (2003). Sleep, infants, and parents. National Sleep Foundation. http://www.sleepfoundation.org/ask/infantsandparents.html, accessed 8/28/2003.

Mitchell, J. C., & Wood, R. J. (2000). Management of cleft lip and palate in primary care. Journal of Pediatric Health Care, 14,13–19.

Morbidity and Mortality Weekly Report. (2005). Blood lead levels—United States, 1999–2002. Morbidity and Mortality Weekly Report 54,513–516.

Morcuende, J. A., Dolan, L. A., Dietz, F. R., & Ponseti, I. V. (2004). Radical reduction in the rate of extensive corrective surgery for clubfoot using the Ponseti method. Pediatrics, 113,376–380.

Mulvihill, K. (2003). Systemic lupus erythematosus: Early identification, co-management are key KP contributions. Advances for Nurse Practitioners, 11(1),32–36.

Mundy, A. R. (1999). Metabolic complications of urinary diversion. Lancet, 353,1813–1814.

Murdock, A. M., & Johnston, S. D. (2005). Diagnostic criteria for celiac disease: Time for change? European Journal of Gastroenterology & Hepatology, 17,41–43.

Murray, K. F., & Christie, D. L. (2000). Vomiting in infancy: When should you worry? Contemporary Pediatrics, 17,81–115.

Murray, R. B., & Zentner, J. P. (2001). Health promotion strategies through the life span (7th ed.). Upper Saddle River, NJ: Prentice Hall.

National Association of Pediatric Nurse Practitioners. (2002). NAPNAP position statement on the pediatric health care home. http://www.napnap.org/practice/positions/healthcarehome.html, accessed 8/25/2003.

National Asthma Education and Prevention Program. (2002). NAEPP Expert Panel Report: Guidelines for the diagnosis and management of asthma—Update on selected topics 2002 (NIH Publication No. 02-5075). Bethesda, MD: National Institutes of Health, NHLBI.

National Center for Learning Disabilities. (2004). Learning disabilities basics. http://www.ldanatl.org/aboutld/parents/ld_basics/index.asp, accessed 9/24/2005.

National Initiative for Children's Healthcare Quality. (2003). Improving care for children with ADHD. Boston: Author.

National Safety Council. (2003). Injury facts. Itasca, IL: National Safety Council.

National Strategy for Suicide Prevention. (2001). http://www.mentalhealth.org/suicideprevention, accessed 11/5/2001.

Nechyba, C., & Gunn, V. (Eds.). (2002). Harriet Lane handbook. Baltimore: Johns Hopkins University Press.

Neidlinger, N. A., Madan, A. K., & Wright, M. J. (2001). Meckel's diverticulum causing cecal volvulus. The American Surgeon, 67,41–43.

Odim, J., Laks, H., Burch, C., Komanapalli, C., & Alejos, J. C. (2000). Transplantation for congenital heart disease. Advances in Cardiac Surgery, 12,59–76.

Otitis Media with Effusion, Clinical Practice Guideline (2004). Pediatrics, 113,1412–1429.

Owens, P. L., Thompson, J., Elixhauser, A., & Ryan, K. (2003). Care of children and adolescents in U.S. hospitals. In HCUP Fact Book No. 4. Rockville MD: Agency for Healthcare Research and Quality.

Pakakasama, S., & Tomlinson, G. E. (2002). Genetic predisposition and screening in pediatric cancer. Pediatric Clinics of North America, 49,1393–1413.

Palma Sisto, P. A. (2004). Endocrine disorders in the neonate. Pediatric Clinics of North America, 51,1141–1168.

Papazian, O., & Alfonso, I. (2002). Adolescents with muscular dystrophies. Adolescent Medicine, 13,511–532.

Park, M. K. (2002). Pediatric cardiology for practitioners (4th ed.). St. Louis: Mosby.

Paterson, C. R., Monk, E. A., & McAllion, S. J. (2001). How common is hearing impairment in osteogenesis imperfecta? Journal of Laryngology and Otolaryngology, 115,280–282.

Patrick, K., Spear, B., Holt, K., & Sofka, D. (Eds.) (2001). Bright futures in practice: Physical activity. Arlington, VA: National Center for Education in Maternal and Child Health.

Paulson, E. K., Kalady, M. F., & Pappas, T. N. (2003). Suspected appendicitis. New England Journal of Medicine, 348,236–242.

Pearson, D. A., McGrath, N. M., Nozyce, M., Nichols, S. L., Raskino, C., Brouwers, et al. (2000). Predicting HIV progression in children using measures of neuropsychologic and neurologic functioning. Pediatrics, 106(6), e76. http://www.pediatrics.org/cgi/content/full/106/6/e76, accessed 1/15/ 2002.

Pender, N. J., Murdaugh, C. L., & Parsons, M.A. (2002). Health promotion in nursing practice (4th ed.). Upper Saddle River, NJ: Prentice Hall.

Perkin, R. M., & Swift, J. D. (2002). Infectious causes of upper airway obstruction in children. Pediatric Emergency Medicine Reports, 7(11),117–128.

Persing, J., Hector, J., Swanson, J., & Kattwinkel, J. (2003). Prevention and management of positional skull deformities in infants. Pediatrics, 112,199–202.

Prakash, J., Sen, D., Kumar, N. S., Kumar, H. Tripathi, L. K., & Saxena R. K. (2003). Acute renal failure due to intrinsic renal diseases: Review of 1122 cases. Renal Failure, 25,225–233.

Prober, C. G. (2004). Central nervous system infections. In R. E. Behrman, R. M. Kliegman, & H. B. Jenson (Eds.), Nelson textbook of pediatrics (17th ed.) (pp. 2038–2047). Philadelphia: Saunders.

Quality Standards Subcommittee, American Academy of Neurology. (1997). Practice parameters: The management of concussion in sports. Neurology, 48,581–585.

Raimer, S. S. (2000). Managing pediatric atopic dermatitis. Clinical Pediatrics, 39(1),1–14.

Reimschisel, T. (2003). Breaking the cycle of medication overuse headache. Contemporary Pediatrics, 20(10),101–114.

Rezvani, I. (2004). Defects in metabolism of amino acids. In R. E. Behrman, R. M. Kliegman, & H. B. Jenson. (Eds.), Nelson textbook of pediatrics (17th ed.) (pp. 398–402). Philadelphia: Saunders.

Robinson, D., & Drumm, L. (2001). Maple syrup urine disease: A standard of nursing care. Pediatric Nursing, 27,515–522.

Robinson, R. F., Nahata, M. C., Mahan, J. D., & Batisky, D. L. (2003). Management of nephrotic syndrome in children. Pharmacotherapy 23,1021–1036.

Rogers, A. S. (2000). Serologic examination of hepatitis B infection and immunization in HIV-positive youth and associated risks. AIDS Patient Care and STDs, 14,651–657.

Roizen, N. J. (2002). Down syndrome. In M. Batshaw (Ed.), Children with disabilities (5th ed). Baltimore: Paul H. Brookes Publishing Co.

Rowley, A. H., & Shulman, S. T. (1999). Kawasaki syndrome. Pediatric Clinics of North America, 46,313–329.

Rudy, C. A. (2001). Dental trauma. School Nurse News, 18(1),33–35.

Rudy, S. J. (2003). Overview of the evaluation and management of acne vulgaris. Pediatric Nursing, 29,287–293.

Ryan-Murray, J., & Petriccione, M. M. (2002). Central nervous system tumors. In C. R. Baggott, K. P. Kelly, D. Fochtman, & G. V. Foley, Nursing care of children and adolescents with cancer (3rd ed.) (pp. 503–523). Philadelphia: Saunders.

Sadovsky, R. (2001). Meckel's diverticulum: Review and management. American Family Physician, 64,2000–2001.

Salihu, H. M., Boos, R., & Schmidt, W. (2002). Omphalocele and gastrochisis. Journal of Obstetrics and Gynecology, 22,489–492.

Santen, S. A., & Altieri, M. F. (2001). Pediatric urinary tract infection. Emergency Medicine Clinics of North America, 19,675–690.

Schulman, C. S. (2003). Emergency care focus: A FASTer method of detecting abdominal trauma. Nursing Management, 34(9),47.

Scolapio, J. S. (2002). Short bowel syndrome. Journal of Parenteral and Enteral Nutrition, 26,S11–S16.

Sectish, T. C., & Prober, C. G. (2004). Pneumonia. In R. E. Behrman, R. M., Kliegman, & H. B. Jenson, (Eds.), Nelson textbook of pediatrics (17th ed.) (pp. 1432–1435). Philadelphia: Saunders.

Seidenfeld, M. E., & Rickert, V. I. (2001). Impact of anorexia, bulimia and obesity on the gynecologic health of adolescents. American Family Physician, 64,445–450.

Shaw, N. M. (2003). Assessment and management of the hematologic system. In C. Kenner & J. W. Lott (Eds.), Comprehensive neonatal nursing: A physiologic perspective (3rd ed.) (pp. 586–602). St. Louis: Saunders.

Shelov, S. P. (Ed.). (2002). Caring for your baby and young child: Birth to age 5. Elk Grove, IL: American Academy of Pediatrics.

Shugart, M. A., & Lopez, E. M. (2002). Depression in children and adolescents. Postgraduate Medicine, 112(3),53–61.

Smillova, A., & Walker, E. (2000). Meningococcemia: A critical care emergency. Critical Care Nurse, 20(5),28–38.

Smith, M. L. (2000). Pediatric burns: Management of thermal, electrical, and chemical burns and burnlike dermatologic conditions. Pediatric Annals, 29,367–378.

Smith, P. C. K. (2003). The role of the primary care advanced practice nurse in evaluating and monitoring childhood cancer survivors for a second malignant neoplasm. Journal of Pediatric Oncology Nursing, 19,84–96.

Sondheimer, J. (2003). Gastroesophageal reflux. In W. Hay, A. Hayward, M. Levin, & J. Sondheimer (Eds.), Current pediatric diagnosis & treatment (16th ed.) (pp. 614–615). New York: Lange Medical Books/McGraw-Hill.

Spiro, D. M., Arnold, D. H., & Barbone, F. (2003). Association between antibiotic use and primary idiopathic intussusception. Archives of Pediatric and Adolescent Medicine, 157,54–59.

Starr, N. B., & Freitas-Nichols, J. (2000). Cardiac arrhythmias in children. Journal of Pediatric Health Care, 14,127–129.

Steeg, C. N., Walsh, C. A., & Glickstein, J. S. (2000). Rheumatic fever: No cause for complaisance. Contemporary Pediatrics, 17(1),128–141.

Stewart, C. (2000). Emergency care of pediatric burns. Pediatric Emergency Medicine Reports, 5(10),101–112.

Subcommittee on Management of Acute Otitis Media, American Academy of Pediatrics. (2004). Diagnosis and management of acute otitis media. Pediatrics, 113,1451–1465.

Suddaby, E. C. (2001). Contemporary thinking for congenital heart disease. Pediatric Nursing, 27,233–238, 270.

Surer, I., Ferrer, F. A., Baker, L. A., & Gearhart, J. P. (2003). Continent urinary diversion and the exstrophy-epispadias complex. The Journal of Urology, 169,1102–1105.

Swenson, O. (2002). Hirschsprung's disease. Pediatrics, 109,914–918.

Takeda, S., & Miyagoe-Suzuki, Y. (2001). Gene therapy for muscular dystrophies: Current status and future prospects. Biodrugs, 15,635–644.

Tang, A. W. (2003). Practical guide to anaphylaxis. American Family Physician, 68,1325.

Tanyi, R.A. (2003). Sickle cell disease: Health promotion and maintenance and the role of primary care nurse practitioners. Journal of the American Academy of Nursing Practitioners, 15,389–397.

Thompson, J. (2001). Intussusception, pyloric stenosis and Hirschsprung's disease. Community Practitioner, 74,312–313.

Towbin, K. E., Mauk, J. E., & Batshaw, M. L. (2002). Pervasive developmental disorders. In M. Batshaw (Ed.), Children with disabilities (5th ed). Baltimore: Paul H. Brookes Publishing Co.

Trachtman, H., Cnaan, A., Christen, E., et. al. (2003). Effect of an oral Shiga toxin-binding agent on diarrhea-associated hemolytic uremic syndrome in children. Journal of the American Medical Association, 290,1337–1344.

Traggiai, C., & Stanhope, R. (2003). Disorders of pubertal development. Best Practice & Research Clinical Obstetrics & Gynaecology, 17(1),41–56.

Trigg, M. E. (2004). Hematopoietic stem cells. Pediatrics, 13,1051–1057.

Trimarchi, T. (2001). Endocrine critical care problems. In M. A. Q. Curley & P. A. Moloney-Harmon. (Eds.), Critical care nursing (2nd ed.) (pp. 805–819). Philadelphia: Saunders.

Umpaichitra, V., Bastian, W., & Castells, S. (2001). Hypocalcemia in children: Pathogenesis and management. Clinical Pediatrics, 40,305–312.

U.S. Department of Health and Human Services (2000). Healthy people 2010. Washington, D.C.: U.S. Department of Health and Human Services. http://www.health.gov/healthypeople/document/html, accessed 4/13/2001.

U.S. Department of Labor. (2003). OSHA Technical Manual. http://www. osha.gov, accessed 2/19/2004.

Van Eerden, P., & Bernstein, P. S. (2003). Summary of the publications, "Neonatal encephalopathy and cerebral palsy: Defining the pathogenesis and pathophysiology" by the ACOG Task Force on Neonatal Encephalopathy and Cerebral Palsy, Medscape OB/GYN & Women's Health 8(2). http://www.medscape.com/viewarticle/457882, accessed 7/10/2003.

Varade, W. S. (2000). Hemolytic uremic syndrome: Reducing the risks. Contemporary Pediatrics, 17(9),54–64.

Vegunta, R. K., Ali, A., Wallace, L. J., Switzer, D. M., & Pearl, R. H. (2004). Laparoscopic appendectomy in children: Technically feasible and safe in all stages of acute appendicitis. American Surgeon, 70,198–202.

Virdis, R., Street, M. E., Bandello, M. A., Tripodi, C., Donadio, A., Villani, A. R., et al. (2003). Growth and pubertal disorders in neurofibromatosis type 1. Journal of Pediatric Endocrinology Metabolism, 16(Suppl 2), 289–292.

Vogt, B. A. (2002). A newborn with a urinary tract anomaly: What role for the general pediatrician? Contemporary Pediatrics, 19(10),131–153.

Weir, E. (2003). Congenital abdominal wall defects. Canadian Medical Association Journal, 169,809.

Weller, E. B., Calvert, S. M., & Weller, R. A. (2003). Bipolar disorder in children and adolescents: Diagnosis and treatment. Current Opinions in Psychiatry, 16,383–388.

Westlake, S. K., & Bertolone, K. L. (2002). Acute lymphoblastic leukemia. In C. R. Baggott, K. P. Kelly, D. Fochtman, & G. V. Foley, Nursing care of children and adolescents with cancer (3rd ed.) (pp. 466–490). Philadelphia: Saunders.

White, J. H. (2000). The prevention of eating disorder: A review of the research on risk factors with implications for practice. Journal of Child and Adolescent Psychiatric Nursing, 123,76–88.

Williams, J. V., Godfrey, J. C., & Friedlander, S. F. (2003). Superficial fungal infections: Confronting the fungus among us. Contemporary Pediatrics, 20(1),58–80.

Williams, P. G., Dalrymple, N., & Neal, J. (2000). Eating habits of children with autism. Pediatric Nursing, 26,259–264.

Wilson, T. A., Rose, S. R., Cohen, P., Rogol, A. D., Backeljauw, P., Brown, R., et al. (2003). Update of guidelines for the use growth hormone in children: The Lawson Wilkins Pediatric Endocrinology Society Drug and Therapeutics Committee. Journal of Pediatrics, 143,415–421.

Woodard, I. (2002). Adolescent acne: A stepwise approach to management. Topics in Advanced Practice Nursing eJournal, 2(2). http://www.medscape.com/viewarticle/430534, accessed 9/24/2003.

Woolf, A. S., & Thiruchelvam, N. (2001). Congenital obstructive uropathy: Its origin and contribution to end-stage renal disease in children. Advances in Renal Replacement Therapy, 8,157–163.

World Health Organization. (1996). Basic document, ed. 36. Geneva, Switzerland: World Health Organization.

Wright, R. B, Pomerantz, W. J., & Luria, J. W. (2002). New approaches to respiratory infections in children. Emergency Medicine Clinics of North America, 20(1),93–114.

Zelnik, N., Pacht, A., Obeid, R., & Lerner, A. (2004). Range of neurological disorders in patients with celiac disease. Pediatrics, 113,1672–1677.

Zuckerman, G. B., & Conway, E. E. (2000). Drowning and near-drowning: A pediatric epidemic. Pediatric Annals, 29,360–366.

INDEX

Page numbers followed by italic *f* indicate figures and those followed by italic *t* indicate tables or boxes.

Endocrine system, *continued*
    precocious puberty. *See* Precocious puberty
    syndrome of inappropriate diuretic hormone. *See* Syndrome of inappropriate diuretic hormone (SIADH)
    Turner syndrome, 478–79
Enterobiasis, 392*t*
Enterobius vermicularis, 392*t*
Enuresis:
    clinical manifestations, 433
    clinical therapy, 434, 435*t*
    description and etiology, 433
    diagnostic tests, 433–34
    nursing management
        assessment, 434
        implementation, 434
Eosinophils:
    in immunodeficiency conditions, 291*t*
    normal values, 318*t*
Ependymomas, 354. *See also* Brain tumors
Epinephrine, for anaphylaxis, 312, 314
Epispadias:
    clinical manifestations, 435–36
    clinical therapy, 436
    description and etiology, 434–35
    diagnostic tests, 436
    nursing management
        assessment, 436
        implementation, 436–37
        patient and family education, 437
Epistaxis:
    clinical manifestations, 220
    clinical therapy, 220–22
    nursing management, 222
Epoetin alfa:
    in cancer treatment, 346*t*
    for chronic renal failure, 450*t*
Epogen. *See* Epoetin alfa
Epstein-Barr virus, 169
Ergot, for migraine, 512
Erikson, Erik, nursing applications of theories, 2–4*t*
Erosion, skin, 596*t*
Erythema infectiosum (fifth disease):
    clinical manifestations, 164–65
    clinical therapy, 165
    complications, 165
    epidemiology, 164
    nursing management, 165

Erythema marginatum, 282
Escherichia coli:
    in hemolytic uremic syndrome, 452
    in osteomyelitis, 584
Esophageal fistula, 374. *See also* Tracheo-esophageal atresia and fistula
ESRD (end-stage renal disease), 447, 449. *See also* Chronic renal failure
Ethambutol, for tuberculosis, 252*t*
Ethosuximide, for seizure disorders, 525*t*
Etoposide, for cancer chemotherapy, 343*t*
Ewing's sarcoma, 360. *See also* Cancer
Exanthem subitum. *See* Roseola (exanthem subitum, sixth disease)
Excoriation, 596*t*
Exposure assessment, 162
External fixators, 580*t*
Extracellular fluid volume:
    deficit. *See* Dehydration
    excess, 180–82
Eyes. *See also* Visual disorders; Visual impairment
    assessment, 21–22
    foreign bodies in, 214*t*
    injuries, 213, 214–15*t*
    in review of systems, 17*t*

F
Face, assessment, 20
Failure to thrive (FTT), 558. *See also* Feeding disorder of infancy and early childhood
Falls, teaching topics, 91*t*
Farsightedness (hyperopia), 203
Fat, recommended dietary allowance by age group, 70*t*
Fatty acid oxidation defects:
    clinical manifestations, 480
    clinical therapy, 480
    description and etiology, 479–80
    diagnostic tests, 480
    nursing management, 480
Febrile seizures, 524. *See also* Seizure disorders
Feeding disorder of infancy and early childhood:
    clinical manifestations, 558–59
    clinical therapy, 559
    description and etiology, 558
    nursing management, 559–60
    risk factors, 558
Felbamate, for seizure disorders, 525*t*

Kidneys. *See also* Renal replacement
therapy
alterations in function
acute postinfectious glomerulonephritis. *See* Acute postinfectious glomerulonephritis
acute renal failure. *See* Acute renal
failure
chronic renal failure. *See* Chronic
renal failure
hemolytic uremic syndrome, 452–
53
nephrotic syndrome. *See* Nephrotic
syndrome
polycystic kidney disease, 458–59
palpation, 39
Klinefelter syndrome:
clinical manifestations, 478
clinical therapy, 478
description and etiology, 477–78
diagnostic tests, 478
nursing management, 478
Knock-knees. *See* Genu valgum
Koplik's spots, 168
Korotkoff's sound, 36
Kussmaul respirations, 484

L

L-asparaginase, for cancer chemotherapy,
342t
Labia minor, assessment, 41–42
Laboratory values, blood, 76–80
Lactulose, for cystic fibrosis, 244t
Lamotrigine, for seizure disorders, 526t
Lantus, 487t
Laryngotracheobronchitis (croup):
clinical manifestations, 246
clinical therapy, 247, 247t
description and etiology, 246
diagnostic tests, 246
nursing management
assessment, 247
implementation, 247–48
Lasix (furosemide). *See* Diuretics
Latency stage (Freud), 3t
Latex allergy:
description and etiology, 314–15
nursing management, 315–16
protective measures, 315t
Lazy eye. *See* Amblyopia
Lead:
normal values, blood, 79

poisoning
clinical manifestations, 157t, 428t
clinical therapy, 429–30
diagnostic tests, 429
etiology, 428–29
incidence, 427
nursing management, 430
sources, 428, 428t
Learning disabilities:
clinical manifestations, 563t
clinical therapy, 563
description and etiology, 562–63
nursing management, 563
Legal blindness, 210. *See also* Visual
impairment
Legg-Calvé-Perthes disease:
clinical manifestations, 576–77
clinical therapy, 577
diagnostic tests, 577
nursing management, 577
Lente, action time, 487t
Lesions, skin, 595, 595t
Leukemia. *See also* Cancer
clinical manifestations, 360–61
clinical therapy, 362
diagnostic tests, 361–62, 361t
nursing management
assessment, 362–63
intervention, 363–64
patient and family education, 364
Leukokoria, 367
Level of conscious (LOC):
altered. *See* Altered level of consciousness
Lice. *See* Pediculosis capitis
Lichenification, 596t
Light palpation, 38
Lipoproteins, normal values, 77
Lisinopril. *See* Angiotensin-converting
enzyme inhibitors
Lispro, action time, 487t
Liver:
alterations in function
biliary atresia, 412–13
hepatitis. *See* Hepatitis
hyperbilirubinemia. *See* Hyperbilirubinemia
palpation, 39
LOC (level of consciousness):
altered. *See* Altered level of consciousness
Long QT syndrome, 283–84

Musculoskeletal system, *continued*
  developmental dysplasia of the hip.
    See Developmental dysplasia
    of the hip
  genu valgum, 48, 574
  genu varum, 48, 574
  Legg-Calvé-Perthes disease. *See*
    Legg-Calvé-Perthes disease
  metatarsus adductus, 569
  muscular dystrophy. *See* Muscular
    dystrophy
  osteogenesis imperfecta. *See* Osteo-
    genesis imperfecta
  osteomyelitis, 584–85
  osteoporosis and osteopenia, 583
  scoliosis. *See* Scoliosis
  slipped capital femoral epiphysis.
    See Slipped capital femoral
    epiphysis
  injuries
    fractures. *See* Fractures
    in sports, 593–94, 593*t*
    in review of systems, 18*t*
Mycobacterium tuberculosis, 249
Mycoplasma pneumoniae, 248
Myelodysplasia:
  clinical manifestations, 517
  clinical therapy, 518
  description and etiology, 516–17
  diagnostic tests, 518
  nursing management
    assessment
      child, 519
      newborn, 518–19
    implementation
      newborn before surgery, 519
      postsurgical care, 519–20
    patient and family education, 520
Myopia (nearsightedness), 203
Myringotomy, 216

N
Nasopharyngitis, 222–23
National Childhood Vaccine Injury Act,
  Vaccine Injury Table 2005,
  139–40*t*
Near drowning, 528. *See also* Hypoxic-
  ischemic brain injury
Nearsightedness (myopia), 203
Necator americanus, 394*t*
Neck, assessment, 26–27
Necrotizing enterocolitis:
  clinical manifestations, 401
  clinical therapy, 401–2
  description and etiology, 400
  diagnostic tests, 401
  nursing management
    assessment, 402
    intervention, 402–3
Neisseria gonorrhoeae, in conjunctivitis,
  201
Neisseria meningitidis:
  in bacterial meningitis, 505
  in meningococcemia, 334
Neonatal abstinence syndrome:
  clinical manifestations, 520–21
  clinical therapy, 521
  description and etiology, 520
  diagnostic tests, 521
  nursing management
    assessment, 521–22
    implementation, 522
Neonatal infant pain scale, 147, 148*t*
Neonatal lupus, 301. *See also* Systemic
  lupus erythematosus
Nephroblastoma, 358–59
Nephrocaps, for chronic renal failure,
  450*t*
Nephrotic syndrome:
  clinical manifestations, 454
  clinical therapy, 454, 455–57*t*
  description and etiology, 453–54
  diagnostic tests, 454
  nursing management
    assessment, 454, 457
    implementation, 457–58
    patient and family education, 458
Nervous system. *See* Neurologic system
Neural tube defects. *See* Myelodysplasia
Neuroblastoma. *See also* Cancer
  clinical manifestations, 356
  clinical therapy, 357
  diagnostic tests, 356–57
  nursing management, 357–58
Neurofibromatosis 1:
  clinical manifestations, 522–23
  clinical therapy, 523
  description and etiology, 522
  diagnostic tests, 523
  nursing management, 523
Neurologic system:
  assessment, 51–57, 54*t*
  injuries
    concussion, 527–28

traumatic brain injury. *See* Traumatic brain injury (TBI)
in review of systems, 18*t*
significant medical conditions
  altered levels of consciousness.
    See Altered level of consciousness
  bacterial meningitis. *See* Bacterial meningitis
  cerebral palsy. *See* Cerebral palsy
  encephalitis, 510–11
  headaches. *See* Headaches
  hydrocephalus. *See* Hydrocephalus
  myelodysplasia. *See* Myelodysplasia
  neonatal abstinence syndrome. *See* Neonatal abstinence syndrome
  neurofibromatosis 1. *See* Neurofibromatosis 1
  seizure disorders. *See* Seizure disorders
Neutrophils:
  in immunodeficiency conditions, 291*t*
  normal values, 318*t*
Newborns:
  health promotion and health maintenance
    general observations, 85
    growth and developmental surveillance, 85–86, 86*t*
    injury and disease prevention, 91–93*t*, 91–94
    mental health, 88–89
    nutrition, 87
    oral health, 88
    physical activity, 87–88
    relationships, 89–91, 90*t*
    timing of visits, 85
90-90 traction, 579*t*
Nissen fundoplication, 386
Nitrosoureas, for cancer chemotherapy, 344*t*
Nix. *See* Permethrin
Nodule, 596*t*
Non-Hodgkin lymphoma, 365–66. *See also* Cancer
Noncarbonic acid excess. *See* Metabolic acidosis
Nonsteroidal anti-inflammatory drugs (NSAIDs), for nephrotic syndrome, 457*t*

Normal values:
  blood, 76–80, 194*t,* 318*t,* 330*t*
  cerebrospinal fluid, 81
  electrolytes, 179*t*
  sweat, 81
  thyroid hormones, 500*t*
  urine, 80–81, 432*t*
Normocytic anemia, 321
Nose and sinuses:
  assessment, 24
  disorders
    epistaxis. *See* Epistaxis
    nasopharyngitis, 222–23
    sinusitis, 223
  in review of systems, 17*t*
NPH, action time, 487*t*
Nuchal rigidity, 505
Nutrition:
  in kidney disease, 448*t*
  screening
    adolescents, 123
    infants, 96, 99
    newborns, 87
    school-age children, 116–17
    toddlers and preschoolers, 105–6
  teaching
    infants, 98–99*t*
    toddlers and preschoolers, 108*t*

O

Obsessive-compulsive disorder, 547
Obstructive uropathy:
  clinical manifestations, 438
  clinical therapy, 438
  description and etiology, 437–38
  diagnostic tests, 438
  nursing management
    assessment, 438
    implementation, 439
Omphalocele, 379–80
Ophthalmia neonatorium, 201
Opiates, clinical manifestations of abuse, 554*t*
Opium, clinical manifestations of abuse, 554*t*
Oprelvekin, in cancer treatment, 346*t*
Oral health, screening:
  infants, 100
  newborns, 88
  school-age children, 118
  toddlers and preschoolers, 106–7, 109–10